Foundations of

ADULT NURSING

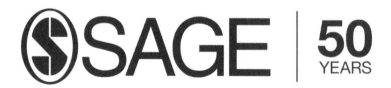

SAGE was founded in 1965 by Sara Miller McCune to support the dissemination of usable knowledge by publishing innovative and high-quality research and teaching content. Today, we publish more than 750 journals, including those of more than 300 learned societies, more than 800 new books per year, and a growing range of library products including archives, data, case studies, reports, conference highlights, and video. SAGE remains majority-owned by our founder, and after Sara's lifetime will become owned by a charitable trust that secures our continued independence.

Los Angeles | London | Washington DC | New Delhi | Singapore

Foundations of

ADULT NURSING

Edited by
DIANNE BURNS

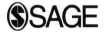

Los Angeles | London | New Delhi
Singapore | Washington DC

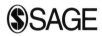

Los Angeles | London | New Delhi
Singapore | Washington DC

SAGE Publications Ltd
1 Oliver's Yard
55 City Road
London EC1Y 1SP

SAGE Publications Inc.
2455 Teller Road
Thousand Oaks, California 91320

SAGE Publications India Pvt Ltd
B 1/I 1 Mohan Cooperative Industrial Area
Mathura Road
New Delhi 110 044

SAGE Publications Asia-Pacific Pte Ltd
3 Church Street
#10-04 Samsung Hub
Singapore 049483

Editor: Alex Clabburn
Associate editor: Emma Milman
Production editor: Katie Forsythe
Copyeditor: Audrey Scriven
Proofreader: Clare Weaver
Indexer: Elske Janssen
Marketing manager: Tamara Navaratnam
Cover design: Wendy Scott
Typeset by: C&M Digitals (P) Ltd, Chennai, India
Printed and bound by CPI Group (UK) Ltd,
Croydon, CR0 4YY

Editorial arrangement, Introduction, Introduction to Part 2 and
Chapter 8 © Dianne Burns 2015
Chapter 1 © Elizabeth Lee-Woolf, Julia Jones, Jane Brooks and
Joanne Timpson 2015
Chapter 2 © Caroline Jagger, Heather Iles-Smith and Julia
Jones 2015
Chapter 3 © Jean Rogers 2015
Chapter 4 © Julie Gregory 2015
Chapter 5 © Deborah Ward 2015
Chapter 6 © Georgina Taylor 2015
Chapter 7 © Mary Cooke 2015
Chapter 9 © Helen Davidson 2015
Chapter 10 © Judith Ormrod and Dianne Burns 2015
Chapter 11 © Paul Tierney, Samantha Freeman and Julie
Gregory 2015
Chapter 12 © Emma Stanmore and Christine Brown Wilson 2015
Chapter 13 © John Costello 2015

First published 2015

Library of Congress Control Number: 2014954829

British Library Cataloguing in Publication data

A catalogue record for this book is available from
the British Library

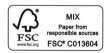

MIX
Paper from
responsible sources
FSC® C013604
www.fsc.org

ISBN 978-1-4462-6790-5
ISBN 978-1-4462-6791-2 (pbk)

Dedicated to Jack, Aimee, Rebecca and Jacob

Contents

About the Editor and Contributors

Dianne Burns (RGN, RNT, MSc, BSc Hons, PGCE, SFHEA) is a Lecturer and Unit Lead for the B Nurse Leadership and Management Units in the School of Nursing, Midwifery and Social Work at the University of Manchester. A Registered General Nurse since 1984, Dianne worked in a variety of clinical settings as a staff nurse (Acute Medical/ Surgical, Orthopaedics) and latterly as a nursing sister (Accident/Emergency) before moving into a community setting; working as a practice nurse then Nurse Practitioner/ Nursing Team Co-ordinator within a large semi–rural GP Practice. She joined the University of Manchester as a Lecturer in Nursing in 2003.

Dianne currently teaches across a variety of programmes within school and co-leads the Faculty HEA Senior Fellowship Programme alongside Dr Judith Williams. She is a University Link Lecturer with Central Manchester NHS Foundation Trust.

Over the last 10 years, Dianne, a current member and former steering committee member of the RCN Education Forum, has held a number of key programme management roles including Examinations Officer, Adult Branch Co-ordinator and Deputy Programme Director (DPSN/BSc Programme) and Adult Field Lead (B Nurs programme). She currently has three strategic leadership roles within the school: Academic Lead for Portfolio Development (B Nurs programme), Peer Educator Programme Lead (B Nurs programme) and Academic Lead for Employability (SNMSW). Each of these roles provides a perfect opportunity for her to draw upon her enthusiasm and passion for engaging with students, colleagues and healthcare practitioners in order to enhance learning within the school, the University and the wider community.

Jane Brooks is a Lecturer in the School of Nursing, Midwifery and Social Work at the University of Manchester, Deputy Director for the UK Centre for the History of Nursing and Midwifery and Editor of the UK Association for the History of Nursing Bulletin. Her most recent publications include articles on the feeding work of nurses after the liberation of Bergen-Belsen and nursing during the 1943/4 typhus epidemic in Naples. Dr Brooks is co-editor of *One Hundred Years of Wartime Nursing Practices, 1854–1953* (MUP, 2015). She has previously published on the history of nursing work with older adults in the UK. In 2014 she received the Monica Baly Bursary from the Royal College of Nursing for her work on nursing in the Second World War.

Christine Brown Wilson was formerly a Senior Lecturer in the School of Nursing, Midwifery and Social Work, University of Manchester, United Kingdom. She is currently Associate Professor/Director of Teaching and Learning in the School of Nursing and Midwifery, University of Queensland. Christine has extensive experience of working with older people in the statutory and private sectors in intermediate and long-term care. At the University of Manchester, Christine designed and led the Caring for Older People Unit for pre-registration nurses until 2012 when she became Programme Director for the

UoM post-registration undergraduate degree programme. Her research involves older people, including those with dementia, focusing on the development of relationships and implementation of relationship-based approaches to care. Christine is committed to improving care for older people, including those with dementia, through education, research and practice development. She is particularly interested in how technology supports decision making by healthcare professionals and is part of an interdisciplinary research team considering these issues. She has published widely and regularly peer reviews for academic journals and the National Institute of Health Research Programme.

Mary Cooke is a Lecturer in Emergency and Urgent Care Nursing at the School of Nursing, Midwifery and Social Work, the University of Manchester. Her most recent publications report research into carer's needs for looking after people with cancer at end of life in the home, and comparing professional and patient expected outcomes from interventions in treatment for COPD using qualitative and quantitative method among others. This interest in outcomes from involving patients, service users and carers in changing health services, policy, and relationships with professionals has developed over 15 years. Her clinical specialism in emergency and trauma nursing is the basis for the decision making chapter, where theory in decision making is explored, and clinical examples offered to demonstrate the critical assessment and decisions made around nursing interventions.

John Costello is Associate Professor and Programme Director for the BSc (Hons) Nursing Practice degree course being provided in Singapore as a project of the University of Manchester School of Nursing, Midwifery and Social Work. Before this he was a Senior Lecturer in Palliative Care in the School. John has been a teacher of Palliative Care at undergraduate and postgraduate levels for over 25 years. His research interest is focused on the social management of death, dying and bereavement. He has published extensively on these topics nationally and internationally and is the author of four books.

Helen Davidson BNurs (Hons), MSc, PGCE, HV Cert is based at the School of Nursing, Midwifery and Social Work at the University of Manchester and works as a Lecturer and Academic Lead for Practice Learning. After graduating from the School in 1998, Helen worked for a number of years as a Health Visitor in South Manchester, whilst also developing an interest in practice education and mentorship. Helen recognises the increased emphasis on Health Promotion and Public Health across the field of adult nursing, within a range of settings. Helen's chapter on Health Promotion explores a number of key concepts in relation to this area, including the various models of practice.

Sam Freeman's career so far has been largely clinical and educationally focused. She is currently a Lecturer in nursing supporting educational delivery within both undergraduate and postgraduate programmes. Within undergraduate education, she teaches critical and acute care nursing. Sam is the Unit Lead for Communication and Interpersonal skills for Nursing unit and Lecturer for the Complex Care unit and Systematic Approaches to Nursing Care unit. In post-registration Sam supports the Intensive Care Continuing Professional Development (CPD) module. Prior to this role she enjoyed 12 years within critical care nursing.

Julie Gregory PhD, MSc Pain Management. BA (Hons), RN is a Nurse Lecturer at the University of Manchester. She strongly believes that it is essential that nurses are educated and have the knowledge and skills to provide high quality compassionate care for the increasingly complex individual patient requirements. Julie has extensive clinical experience, initially in orthopaedics and trauma, caring for a wide range of age groups and conditions. She was a nurse specialist for acute pain until 2011 and has been an Independent Nurse Prescriber since 2005. An important aspect of her specialist nurse role was teaching and developing pain management practice at the hospital. She was also a member of the team delivering the Acute Illness Management (AIM) course for all the members of the healthcare team highlighting the importance of pain management and its impact on an acutely ill patient.

Heather Iles-Smith is Head of Nursing Research and Innovation, Leeds Teaching Hospitals Trust (LTHT) and Visiting Associate Professor, Faculty of Health, University of Leeds. Her role encompasses the development of clinical academic careers for nurses, midwives and Allied Healthcare Professionals (AHP) and leadership of the Clinical Research Nurses. Additionally she is responsible for the strategic direction for nursing and AHP research and innovation at LTHT. Heather is also an active researcher and having completed her PhD in 2012 she continues to investigate the psychological health of heart attack patients. Her other research interests relate to renal medicine and the care of dementia patients. In October 2014 Heather led the Lancashire Care NHS Foundation Trust, Dementia Research Nursing Team to successfully win the Inaugural Nursing Times Clinical Research Nurse award, a very proud moment!

Caroline Jagger Msc, Bsc (Hons) RN, NMP, Dip HE, qualified in 2001 and worked initially in the speciality of orthopaedics, looking after the holistic needs of both elective and trauma patients and undertaking key trainer roles in manual handling and practice development at Calderdale and Huddersfield NHS Foundation Trust. Caroline transferred to Manchester working as a specialist nurse in osteoporosis in 2007. Since 2011, she has been working as a seconded teaching fellow at the University of Manchester, lecturing on the undergraduate programme for nurses. She has recently been appointed as Deputy Programme Director for the Independent Prescribing Programme for pharmacists and nurses at the University of Manchester.

Julia Jones graduated from the University of Manchester's School of Nursing and Midwifery in 2009 following which she worked in the Intensive Care Unit of the Royal Bolton Hospital. Prior to embarking on a nursing career, Julia held a number of senior positions, predominantly in safety and regulated industries where safety and quality are paramount. Julia initially spent 12 years in human resources before moving into more buisness-focused roles and she has extensive experience in commercial and project management and the management of multidisciplinary teams. Julia is now based in France and is currently working for one of the world's largest international research projects. She is also a volunteer and the secretary of a registered 'Association' providing bereavement support. Julia has a keen interest in mentoring and, whilst studying for her nursing degree was a mentor as part of the University's Widening Participation Scheme and has maintained her links with the University including acting as a mentor within the wider mentoring programme.

Elizabeth Lee-Woolf is a Lecturer in the School of Nursing, Midwifery and Social Work at the University of Manchester and is the current Adult Field Lead for the BNurs programme. Her experience in nurse education spans across the last 30 years and she has been involved in the development and delivery of several curricula with particular emphasis on the biosciences applied to nursing and recently the development of e-learning strategies. Understanding the changing needs of students as they make their transition from new student to registrant has been a major influence in facilitating a caring yet thorough student experience to ensure that students are ready for the challenge of their first post. Liz has significant experience in the development of processes through which challenges to a student's fitness to practise are managed, including how a student is supported before during and after a fitness to practice hearing.

Judith Ormrod spent the majority of her clinical nursing experience working as a staff nurse and Senior Ward Sister in Intensive Care Units and acute admission wards in Central London Hospitals. Since moving to Manchester she has taught undergraduate and postgraduate nursing students at the University of Manchester. Her clinical and research interests include psychosocial factors affecting women across the lifespan, interpersonal violence and FGM/C, family estrangement, clinical supervision and the ethics of research. Her PhD considered the psychosocial factors affecting pregnant women who were living with Type 1 Diabetes Mellitus. She is also a Chartered Psychologist and works part time in a local NHS Trust.

Jean Rogers qualified as a registered nurse (RGN) in 1988 from Salford NHS Foundation Trust. She has worked in a number of areas including elective orthopaedics, acute trauma and ENT, rheumatology and endocrinology, acute medicine and acute rehabilitation. She undertook the orthopaedic course at the Robert Jones and Agnes Hunt Orthopaedic Hospital in 1991 where she was in the last group to follow the 12-month course and in her spare time completed a certificate in higher education. Following this Jean held post as senior staff nurse, junior sister and lecturer/practitioner and completed a BSc (hons) in nursing practice. She has undertaken the practice educators' Master's module and passed an MSc with merit in practice development (nursing practice) and is a co-author of Oxford University Press's *Handbook of Orthopaedic and Trauma Nursing* as well as numerous articles.

She is chair of the Northwest Orthopaedic and Trauma Forum, chair of RCN Cheshire East, sits on the North West regional board and is a staff governor. Her main interests lie in orthopaedics, nurse education and the politics of nursing, and she takes an active role in both areas being a member of the orthopaedic forum, the practice educator's special interest group and the RCN Education forum. Jean is currently undertaking a professional doctorate in Health and Social Care at the University of Salford.

Her current post is as practice education facilitator for Stockport NHS Foundation Trust where she believes that she has the best of both worlds educating nurses of the future in a practice setting.

Emma Stanmore is a registered nurse, a specialist community practitioner and has worked as a nurse academic at the School of Nursing, Midwifery and Social Work in the University of Manchester since 2005. Emma has both a clinical and research background in using new innovations to improve healthcare for older people and those with musculoskeletal problems. Emma is Chief Investigator in a number of research projects that include the development of new remote monitoring technologies in rehabilitation and the development of Kinect exergames to improve function and prevent falls in older people and those with arthritis. Emma is committed to improving the care of older people in practice, research and through the education of undergraduate and postgraduate nursing education. Her research is informed by experience as a District Nursing Sister, a Rehabilitation Project Manager, and a Clinical Manager of an interdisciplinary team.

Georgina Taylor is an Honorary Researcher in the School of Health and Education at Middlesex University. Research interests include health inequalities, the health of refugees and asylum seekers, living and working in multicultural environments and compassion in healthcare. She has previously taught interprofessional working to undergraduate nursing students.

Paul Tierney is a Lecturer in the School of Nursing and Midwifery, Queen's University Belfast. He teaches into the undergraduate nursing programme and is Pathway Coordinator for the Specialist Practice Cardiology programme. Paul began his nursing career in the Coronary Care Unit in the Royal Victoria Hospital, Belfast. He subsequently worked in a variety of cardiology posts progressing to Deputy Ward Manager in a medical cardiology ward. Later, Paul worked as a research nurse with cardiac clinical trials before moving into nurse education in 2008. He has a keen interest in resuscitation and is an Advanced Life Support (ALS) instructor with the Resuscitation Council UK.

Joanne Timpson is a Senior Lecturer and currently enacts the dual roles of Academic Lead for the Student Experience and Senior Academic Advisor in the School of Nursing, Midwifery and Social Work at the University of Manchester. These roles complement perfectly her interests in nursing theory, the therapeutic frame, the impulse to nurse and the necessity to secure supportive student strategies, privileging and enhancing empathic and empowering learning environments. Her clinical expertise lies in supportive and palliative care and she endeavours to bring her experience of humanistic nursing philosophy, family-centred care and collegiality to all her professional pursuits.

Deborah Ward has been a Lecturer at the University of Manchester since 2007 and teaches across a range of pre- and post-registration programmes, particularly in those relating to infection prevention and control. Her publications have focused on this area of practice, in particular the clinical education of pre-registration nursing students.

Acknowledgements

I am particularly grateful to all of the practitioners, educators, students and others I have met over the years who have helped and guided me in my own nursing and teaching practice. I would like to thank all reviewers, families, friends and colleagues for their support. In particular, special thanks to:

Margaret Lynch

Dr Tommy Dickenson

Dr Sarah Kendal

Sarah Booth

Professor Christine Hallett

John Vernon

Dr Shaun Speed

Publisher's Acknowledgements

Figure 1.1 The Gibbs Reflective Cycle is republished with permission of Oxford Brookes University.

Table 7.2 Types of clinical decisions made by nurses in acute and primary care settings is republished with permission BMJ Publishing Group Ltd.

Figure 8.3 NHS Change Model is republished with permission of NHS Improving Quality.

Table 8.8 Six-stage Framework for Service Improvement is republished with permission of NHS Improving Quality.

Figure 10.4 The overlap between long-term conditions and mental health problems is republished with permission of The King's Fund.

Figure 10.7 The House of Care Model is republished with permission of The King's Fund.

Figure 11.1 The enhanced recovery pathway © Crown copyright.

Table 11.3 NEWS score and Table 11.4 Outline clinical response to NEWS triggers are copyright of the Royal College of Physicians, 2012. Republished with permission of the Royal College of Physicians.

Table 11.5 Standards for critical care outreach teams © Crown copyright.

About the Companion Website

Visit the website for this book at https://study.sagepub.com/burns for access to resources which will support you in your learning or teaching if you are a lecturer.

The website includes:

For students

Multiple choice questions to test your knowledge of each chapter when you are revising

Test yourself on key terms in adult nursing

Free SAGE journal articles to use as examples in assignments and support evidence-based practice

Links to **websites in the activities**

For lecturers

Seminar plans with discussion questions to use with your class

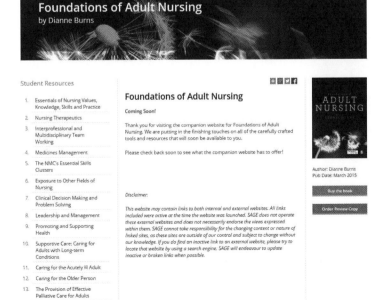

Introduction

This book aims to provide a concise, easy to read introductory text for those individuals who are undertaking their studies within the *adult field* of nursing at undergraduate level (i.e. students on Nursing and Midwifery Council (NMC) approved undergraduate programmes). However, we recognise that it will also be of interest to mentors as well as those involved in supporting adult nursing students (e.g. lecturers and nurse teachers), those on 'associate' level courses (e.g. Foundation Degree students in health and social care) and students from other fields of nursing.

As a core text for 'beginners', the book is written in an easy to access, user-friendly style and examines in detail the essential knowledge and skills needed to provide therapeutic care to adults with a range of health needs. Taking a broad rather than a deep approach, we will be encouraging you as the reader to explore the core principles and key aspects of an adult nurse's role, reflecting upon current nursing theory and the factors that underpin high quality, evidence-based care delivery in practice. By incorporating a variety of activities and case scenarios we intend to bring to life many of the contemporary issues faced by adult nurses today. By also guiding you to other resources as appropriate, our primary aim is to assist you in the development of an understanding of the importance of *person-centred care* and an *evidence-based approach* to adult nursing. In doing so we hope that this will not only help you demonstrate your knowledge in written assignments and examinations but also more importantly that you will use each of these fundamental aspects to underpin the care you provide for patients in practice.

The *Modernising Nursing Careers Framework* (DHSSPS, 2006) identifies the changing context for healthcare and a need for the current nursing workforce to reflect those changes and become more adaptable. This approach will be illustrated throughout this book in terms of its relevance to current UK healthcare provision and policy, namely with regard to:

- an expanding older population;
- increasing incidence of long-term conditions;
- the growing impact of preventable conditions due to lifestyle choices (i.e. smoking, obesity, alcohol intake, etc..);
- and the need for nurses to demonstrate skills in caring for people in a variety of settings.

The content of this book will be underpinned throughout by the Nursing and Midwifery Council's *UK Competency Frameworks for Adult Nursing* (NMC, 2010a, 2010b) which clearly define both what adult nursing students must achieve before entering the professional register and what qualified adult nurses must continue to meet throughout their professional career. It will also reflect current UK policy and practice, taking into account the fact that contemporary adult field nursing is delivered to a diverse client group in a number of settings. Focusing primarily on the top morbidity and mortality indicators across the UK (i.e. Circulatory Disease, Cardiovascular Disease, Respiratory Disease, Diabetes, Cancers, Infectious Disease, and Dementia), it also includes specific content to support the development of knowledge and skills related to the EU Directive 2005/36EC (European Commission, 2011) which demands that adult nurses gain exposure to the following:

- General and Specialist Medicine.
- General and Specialist Surgery.
- Child Care and Paediatrics.
- Maternity Care.
- Mental Health and Psychiatry.
- Care of the Older Person (Geriatrics).
- Home Nursing (Community Nursing).

The Nursing and Midwifery Council demand that *all* nurses are able to demonstrate (and maintain) competencies relating to *professional values, communication* and *interpersonal skills, clinical decision making* and *leadership, management and team working* (NMC, 2010a). In addition adult nurses are required to demonstrate a set of competencies comprised of field-specific elements.

Making reference throughout to the NMC Code (2015), the current evidence base and relevant legislation policies from across the UK, it is upon these frameworks and competencies that the book is based. The book is composed of two parts.

Part One: Theory and context in relation to adult nursing

Made up of Chapters 1 to 8, this part of the book provides an introduction to the overarching theoretical and contemporary practice issues faced by adult nurses today.

Chapter 1: Essentials of nursing values, knowledge, skills and practice

This chapter introduces you to the key principles, core values, legal and professional issues that influence contemporary nursing practice, recognising the importance of self-awareness and professional regulation in developing professional practice. The significance of core values is explored (e.g. empathy, compassion, dignity, respect, cultural competence, communication) to help you develop an appreciation of how such values must underpin your nursing practice. The chapter also focuses on the legal, ethical and professional aspects of adult care provision and the importance of evidence-based care and nursing research.

Chapter 2: Nursing therapeutics

In this chapter we encourage you to consider appropriate philosophies, models and frameworks for the delivery of safe and competent care. We identify the factors which contribute to the development of therapeutic partnerships, exploring the concept of safe and effective person-centred care and introducing you to systematic approaches to nursing care, the nature of nursing interventions and the mechanisms by which interventions can be selected and evaluated. The overall focus of the chapter is on challenging routine and tradition in nursing practice.

Chapter 3: Interprofessional and multidisciplinary team working

This chapter explores how multi-agency working has the potential to positively impact on health highlighting the importance of accurate record keeping, effective communication, accountability and delegation. You will begin to understand the significance and the benefits of team working in the provision of effective healthcare. We also identify useful strategies for overcoming common barriers to interprofessional and multidisciplinary working in practice settings.

Chapter 4: Medicines management

This chapter outlines the theoretical underpinning knowledge related to the management and review of medicines, exploring the role and responsibilities of adult nurses to promote patient safety in the context of medicines management. We review the policies, legal requirements and the practical application of medicines and go on to evaluate various procedures for the safe management and administration of medicines, including an awareness of Patient Group Directives (PGD). Concentrating on the mechanisms and actions of medicines administered for commonly encountered adult medical and mental health conditions, we help you identify and evaluate the likely side effects and interactions of commonly used medications.

Chapter 5: The NMC essential skills clusters

This chapter summarises the importance of key themes discussed in Part One of the book which will help you make links with the relevant NMC skills clusters. Setting the scene for Part Two, the chapter outlines NMC skills cluster (NMC, 2010c) requirements, suggesting how you can demonstrate your achievement of these in practice.

Chapter 6: Exposure to other fields of nursing

Reflecting the principles set out by the NMC (2010a) which emphasise the need for adult nurses to have shared core competencies in the other fields of nursing (i.e. child, learning disability, mental health and maternity) this chapter looks specifically on the competencies which require adult nurses to be able to recognise and respond appropriately to the various needs of individuals: those of babies, children and young people; pregnant and postnatal women; people with mental health problems; people with physical disabilities; people with learning disabilities; older people; and people with long-term problems such as cognitive impairment. You are encouraged to consider and explore the ethical, legal and professional dilemmas around common situations to which an adult nurse may be exposed amid suggestions that should help you identify opportunities that will demonstrate your achievement of these competencies in practice.

Chapter 7: Clinical decision making

This chapter explores the underpinning theories related to clinical judgement and decision-making processes within a healthcare setting, examining the key issues in managing complexity and critically reviewing determinants that can impact on clinical decision-making processes. It also includes a critical consideration of the higher order intellectual skills associated with clinical (diagnostic) reasoning, empirical (diagnostic) judgements and discerning clinical decision making.

Chapter 8: Leadership and management

This chapter reviews current leadership approaches within contemporary healthcare settings and encourages you to critically evaluate the importance of effective leadership and management within the modern healthcare arena. Exploring contemporary leadership research and management theory, concepts related to the management of change, service improvement, resource management, risk management, quality assurance and professional accountability associated with the effective management of nursing care, the aim of this chapter is to help you develop your knowledge and understanding in order to enhance your own leadership and management skills.

Part Two: Caring for adults in a variety of settings

This section of the book highlights specific areas of care which are commonly encountered within adult nursing practice.

Chapter 9: Promoting health

This chapter begins by introducing you to the principles and practice of epidemiology, public health, health promotion/health education and preventative healthcare, thereby enabling you to gain a basic understanding of how demographic health information and epidemiological data inform national and global priorities for health and health promotion/public health initiatives. We explore the role of the adult nurse in contemporary public health practice and the relationship between the health of the public, the social determinants influencing health and the tools and structures that underpin the assessment of health and healthcare needs. In particular we look at the impact of 'risky behaviours' (unhealthy eating, physical inactivity, alcohol and substance misuse and sexual health), focusing on national health promotion initiatives and services to provide a clear overview of both the government agenda and legislative practice.

Chapter 10: Supportive care: caring for adults with long-term conditions

This chapter helps you to develop knowledge and understanding of the role of the adult nurse in the provision of supportive care to individuals living with long-term conditions (LTC). It examines the bio-psychosocial impact of living with and caring for individuals experiencing long-term ill health, exploring ways in which an adult nurse can work effectively to support individuals and their families/carers by promoting self-care and empowerment within a variety of settings.

Chapter 11: Caring for the acutely ill adult

This chapter considers the impact of acute and severe illness on normal daily functioning and explores the principles of working towards recovery from acute illness utilising contemporary surgical and medical approaches with a particular focus on acute assessment and technological advances. Highlighting the significance of risk assessment, prioritising care and the prevention of deterioration, the importance of the application of critical thinking and evaluation to competently provide safe, knowledgeable and competent individualised client care is explored. The chapter also discusses the use of technology in the management of individuals with severe and/or complex illness and considers the limitations as well as the importance of professional competence and its incorporation within patient care. We go on to explore evidence-based rationales for the management of severe illness in order to promote recovery and independence.

Chapter 12: Caring for the older person

The aim of this chapter is to help you develop an understanding of the principles of health promotion, quality of life, dignity in care, independence, empowerment and choice in relation to older people. We explore the needs of older people and their carers in a variety of care settings, taking into account the nature of care that older people may require. A key focus here is promoting an understanding of the principles of anti-discriminatory practice with reference to age and then considering how this is applied in practice with a particular emphasis on the 'frail' older person. In particular, we look at the challenges faced by those with dementia.

Chapter 13: The provision of effective palliative care for adults

This chapter focuses on the role of the adult nurse in supporting patients with a life-limiting illness within a palliative care context. It centres around the provision of care within a multidisciplinary framework that involves the holistic assessment of physical and bio-psychological needs in relation to patients with malignant and non-malignant conditions. An exploration of contemporary palliative care services, including hospice care and care at home, highlights the provision of care to family members and significant others who are associated with grief and bereavement after care.

References

Department of Health, Social Services and Public Safety (2006) *Modernising Nursing Careers: Setting the Direction*. Belfast: DHSSPS.

European Commission (2011) *European Union Directive 2005/36/EC* (consolidated version). Available at: http://eur-lex.europa.eu/LexUriServ/LexUriServ.do?uri=CONSLEG:2005L0036:2 0110324:EN:PDF (last accessed 28 September 2014).

Nursing and Midwifery Council (2010a) *Standards of Proficiency for Pre-Registration Nursing Education*. London: NMC.

Nursing and Midwifery Council (2010b) *Standards of Competence for Registered Nurses*. London: NMC.

Nursing and Midwifery Council (2010c) *The Essential Skills Clusters*. London: NMC.

Nursing and Midwifery Council (2015) *The Code: Professional Standards of Practice and Behaviour for Nurses and Midwives*. London: NMC.

Theory and Context in Relation to Adult Nursing

PART ONE

Theory and Context in
Relation to Adult Nursing

1   Essentials of Nursing: Values, Knowledge, Skills and Practice

ELIZABETH LEE-WOOLF, JULIA JONES, JANE BROOKS AND JOANNE TIMPSON

As you begin your studies in nursing we hope that you will be as full of questions as you are enthusiasm for your chosen profession and we trust that you are ready for the challenge. Our aim is to engage you with our passion for nursing and instil an ethos of nursing as a privilege. We will review the essentials of nursing knowledge and values, exploring together how these will underpin your practice in a way that we hope will excite your professional imagination and intelligence.

After reading this chapter you should be able to:

- Outline the landmarks of nursing history and highlight how these have influenced modern nursing practice across the UK.
- Explain how legal and ethical principles provide a core framework for our professional practice.
- Define the core values that underpin nursing and recognise their application to practice.
- Understand the principles of The Code (NMC, 2015) by which we practise and how these define our *fitness to practise*.
- Highlight the challenges to modern nursing and relate these to recognised core values.

Related NMC competencies

The overarching NMC requirement is that all nurses

> ... must act first and foremost to care for and safeguard the public. They must practise autonomously and be responsible and accountable for safe, compassionate, person-centred, evidence-based nursing that respects and maintains dignity and human rights. They must show professionalism and integrity and work within recognised professional, ethical and legal frameworks. They must work in partnership with other health and social care professionals and agencies, service users, their carers and families in all settings, including the community, ensuring that decisions about care are shared. (NMC, 2010a: 13, 2010b: 6)

--------------------- To achieve entry to the register as an adult ---------------------
nurse you should be able to:

- Practise with confidence according to *The Code: Professional Standards of Practice and Behaviour for Nurses and Midwives* (NMC, 2015) and within other recognised ethical and legal frameworks.
- Practise in a holistic, non-judgemental, caring and sensitive manner that avoids assumptions, supports social inclusion, recognises and respects individual choice and acknowledges diversity.
- Appreciate the value of evidence in practice.
- Understand and apply current legislation to all service users.
- Be responsible and accountable for keeping your knowledge and skills up to date through continuing professional development, learning from experience, supervision, feedback, reflection and evaluation. Recognise your own limitations and seek to address these.
- Be self-aware and recognise how your own values, principles and assumptions may impact upon your practice and communication with others.

(Adapted from the NMC Standards of Competence for Adult Nursing, 2010a, 2010b.)

Background

To understand the role of the contemporary adult nurse in the UK it is useful to know a little of nursing's history and to recognise key landmarks over the last 150 years that signal the development towards the professional nursing practice we have today. However it is not our intention to provide a detailed history of nursing here and you are advised to explore the Further Reading which illustrates in more detail the historical threads that bring us to this point (see the suggested Further Reading at the end of this chapter).

Although caring and the role of carer have existed throughout history, nursing in its modern sense is a relatively recent concept. It is recognised that the words 'nurse' and 'nursing' are derived from the Old French *nourice* and the Late Latin *nutrire*, meaning to nourish and care (*Oxford English Dictionary*, 2014a), but their use in today's sense has only occurred from the seventeenth century onwards. It is often suggested that nursing can be traced back through history to its earliest times. If you accept that this reflects the act of carer and caring then this is undoubtedly true. The themes that run through the earliest annals of history involve those who provided succour (i.e. assistance and support in times of hardship or distress) for families, communities or for those injured in battle for example. What is perhaps more important here for modern notions of nursing are those involved with what Susan Reverby, Patricia D'Antonio, and Barbra Mann Wall have called 'professed-nursing', namely the care of sick strangers (Reverby, 1987; O'Brien D'Antonio, 1993; Mann Wall, 1998). This distinction is crucial because if we understand modern professional nursing as caring for those people who are not our friends or family this means it is a very different undertaking from caring for those who are. Nevertheless, often the carers who nursed 'sick strangers' were influenced by religious values and altruism believing that it would be wrong to gain monetarily from their work. There was, however, a more insidious ideology at work: once a lady worked for money, she was no longer considered a lady. To cite historian Sue Hawkins, ' … they forfeited their respectability' (Hawkins, 2010: 29). Given that nursing reformers in the nineteenth century wished to increase the number of educated middle-class women in the occupation this was clearly a problem. Hence the vocation or *calling* to nurse has been the province of those who had a desire to care with little thought of reward, or perhaps more pertinently, were felt not to want such financial reward because they were respectable. Either way, whilst philanthropy may indeed be admirable, such notions influenced the status of the nurse, and perhaps, some might argue, limited the evolution of nursing as a highly skilled profession (Helmstadter, 1993, 1996).

Throughout the eighteenth century we can see the appearance of what might be termed the 'modern hospital' in Britain. This was also the Age of Enlightenment – a movement made up of intellectuals who wished to see development in many areas of life through reasoned argument and science rather than adhering to traditions without thought. This influence can be seen in the funding of modern 'voluntary hospitals' by wealthy benefactors such as Thomas Guy who funded Guy's Hospital in London (1719) followed by the Edinburgh Royal Infirmary (founded in 1729), St Bartholomew's Hospital (opened in 1730, funded by public subscription), the Middlesex Hospital (opened in 1745, funded by public subscription) and the Manchester Royal Infirmary (in 1752). These hospitals had a charitable remit to provide treatment for the poor which was recognised by an Act of Parliament in 1836. However, they only needed to provide care for the 'deserving poor' and all voluntary hospitals also tended to focus on acute illnesses that could be treated and would therefore provide excellent advertisements for future possible benefactors. This system excluded the chronically sick, the elderly and infirm, the mentally ill and those with learning disabilities. The latter two types of patients were cared for in separate 'asylums for the insane' while the elderly and chronically sick were cared for in Poor Law Hospitals. The Poor Law Hospitals were described as 'murderous pesthouses' into which 'the dense mass of living creatures were crammed' (cited in White, 1978: 18).

STOP AND THINK

- How do people today consider the work carried out by nurses in intensive care units in acute hospitals?
- How do people view the nursing of older people with dementia?
- What sort of facilities do we offer to each of these groups of patients?

The thing about history is that there are often reasons in our past which go some way to explain the ways in which services develop over time.

- Are you able to identify any links with history for the care of older people that exist today?

Modern nursing has its roots in the nineteenth century. (We do not wish to ignore the notion that there were significant examples of nursing-type activities in earlier times but it would be difficult to present their importance here without sounding superficial.) As the Industrial Revolution changed the face of our national landscape the need to care and manage the sick faced equal challenges. The choices surrounding who did what were primarily influenced by industry and the developing urban communities employed therein, but also by gender role. As a result those individuals who nursed tended to be women. Living conditions were often crowded, unsanitary and polluted. Disease flourished and work-based accidents were common.

SOME EARLY NURSING PIONEERS IN BRITAIN

Florence Nightingale was born in 1820 to a wealthy family. She was encouraged and taught to think and question in a way that was unusual for a girl of those times. Her parents did not approve of her wish to nurse which they deemed unconventional. However, in 1851 she travelled to Kaiserswerth for three months to learn to be a nurse and two years later Nightingale became superintendent of a hospital for gentlewomen in Harley Street. The outbreak of the Crimean War, and the plight of wounded soldiers in terrible conditions, saw her initiate a campaign to take a team of nurses to military hospitals in Turkey where, despite relentless opposition, she improved the care and conditions for patients. Even before her return to Britain in 1856 the Nightingale Fund – which the grateful public of Britain had established in her name following her work in the Crimea – had accrued significant monies. Although initially not enthused by the project, in 1860 the Nightingale Training School for nurses at St Thomas's Hospital in London was established in her name (Baly, 1997; Bostridge, 2008). The purpose of the school was to train nurses who would then establish similar schools based on her principles. By 1867 probationer nurses were able to pay to attend and this facilitated a two-tier system of nurses where, by the turn of the twentieth century, only those who had paid for their training would be offered a post as Sister.

    Mary Seacole was another Crimean pioneer (Alexander and Dewjee, 1984: Griffon, 1998). Born in Jamaica in 1805 (her father was a Scot and her mother Jamaican), Seacole was well travelled and had gained perspectives on medicines and care wherever she went. Like Florence Nightingale, in 1854 Seacole asked the British government to send her to Crimea to assist in the army hospital. In her autobiography, Seacole recalled being turned down. However she did then fund her own travel to the Crimea, where she cared for soldiers. On returning to the UK her health was poor and she had little money and no family to support her. She achieved a great deal but died in 1910 and thus did not live to see the achievement of nurse registration.

    Ethel Gordon Manson (who later became known as Mrs Bedford Fenwick) was passionate about the improvements to nursing and nurse training. She trained as a nurse at the Nottingham Children's Hospital and then at Manchester's Royal Infirmary between 1878 and 1879. She became the matron of St Bartholomew's Hospital in London at the age of only 24 years old. In 1888 she married Dr Bedford Fenwick, retired from nursing and devoted her life to national and international nursing matters. As the founder of the Royal British Nurses' Association (1887), the International Council of Nurses (1899) and editor of the first professional nursing journal *The Nursing Record/The British Journal of Nursing* from 1893–1946, she was a staunch advocate that nursing should be regulated and that every nurse should be registered. She is nevertheless considered to have contributed to phenomenal achievements in nursing's development (Griffon, 1995). She died on 13 March 1947.

ACTIVITY 1.1

Find out more about the pioneers of nursing practice and identify their contribution to the development of nursing and nurse education.
    You can start by accessing the UK Centre for the History of Nursing and Midwifery at www.nursing.manchester.ac.uk/ukchnm
    (See also the suggested Further Reading at the end of the chapter.)

We should not deny the fact that whilst nursing was struggling for recognition, this aspect also reflects an earlier period in medicine where doctors had little recognisably organised training as such. *The Medical Act* of 1858 responded to a need for the public to be able to determine whether or not a doctor was qualified to practise and resulted in the inauguration of the General Medical Council. This professional body was (and remains to this day) charged with registering practitioners and ensuring the public have access to that information (although this is now governed under *The Medical Act* of 1983). Following on from this, many recognised the logic for nurses to be registered in a similar fashion. The debate and will for this became more organised, especially after the beginnings of nurse training in 1860.

By 1880 the Hospitals' Association (HA) was in agreement that some form of nurse registration was a necessity and therefore voluntary registration was introduced. Ethel Bedford Fenwick (a member of the Matrons' Committee) passionately believed in professionalism and that nurses should be registered in a similar fashion to doctors. She set up the British Nurses' Association which provided an alternative voluntary register that noted completion of a programme of study, but also more importantly aligned itself with a remit to protect the public.

The First World War provided the pivotal impetus for registration. Many women had answered a call to go and nurse which had, incidentally, raised its profile with the public. Womens' role in society was changing and their contribution to working life whilst soldiers were away was generally noted and applauded. Meanwhile the College of Nursing was founded in 1916 (later to become the Royal College of Nursing). This organisation led and supported initiatives to further develop and raise the profile of nursing and the need for a nursing register. In 1919 one MP (Major Barnet) was persuaded to propose a Private Members Bill which resulted in the *Nurse Registration Act*. This called upon the General Nursing Council to maintain and monitor a nursing register as well as provide central guidance to inform nurse training programmes. It was replaced by the United Kingdom Central Council in 1983 and subsequently by the Nursing and Midwifery Council in 2002. All had similar duties in their role to maintain the register, provide educational guidance and ensure protection of the public. It is interesting to note that women still had no right to vote and nursing would not be officially recognised as a profession for almost another one hundred years but at least they had registration and regulation.

The NHS was born in 1948 which again reflected the changes that war had brought to society. However, and despite the work of many groups, nurse education and the role of the nurse were slow to evolve. Graduate education for nurses was embryonic although several university medical schools began offering some form of nurse education at degree level. The University of Edinburgh offered the first degree in nursing in 1960 and the University of Manchester's Bachelor of Nursing degree soon followed. It was at the University of

Manchester that the first Professor of Nursing was appointed – Jean Kennedy McFarlane later to become Baroness McFarlane of Llandaff. Other 'experimental' courses were tried throughout the 1960s and 1970s, with some at degree and some at diploma level.

The birth of modern nursing

Several reports during the twentieth century culminated in the Briggs Committee's remit to consider various concerns surrounding the methods, content and quality of nurse education and its interface with the NHS. Scott Wright was an influential member of this committee and the report which followed in 1972 recommended a step change: a move away from *training* towards *professional education* and the development of research into all aspects of education and nursing practice. After much wrangling the Nurses, Midwives and *Health Visitors Act* (passed in 1979) saw the beginnings of a modern-day nurse education. Project 2000 was introduced in 1988 and diploma education for nurses was piloted in a number of schools prior to it being rolled out across Britain. Student nurses now had student status and were no longer employees of the hospital in which the School of Nursing was based. This created some challenges for nursing practice but these were not insurmountable and many nurses at all levels engaged with this new approach to education with enthusiasm. Between 1990 and 2010 diploma and degree courses in nursing ran side by side but in 2010 legislation was enacted to ensure that every nurse in England would be educated to degree level, reflecting previous changes already effected in Scotland, Northern Ireland and Wales for both nursing and other allied health professions such as physiotherapy, radiography, and occupational therapy.

———————— TWENTIETH-CENTURY PIONEERS ————————
IN NURSING

Lisbeth Hockey was born Lisbeth Hochsinger on the 17 October 1918 in Graz, Steiermark, Austria. In 1936, at the age of eighteen, she commenced her medical studies at the Karl-Franzens University of Graz. However, following the Nazi occupation of Austria in 1938 she left for England. Hockey was not able to recommence her medical studies in England for three reasons: she was a woman (and few British women went to university at that time); she did not speak English; and she had no money. British friends recommended nursing as an alternative and so Hockey began her training at the London Hospital in Whitechapel in 1939 (Mason, 2005: 2–5). Her importance to the nursing profession came from her natural desire to ask questions. However, during her training this was to cause her problems with those in authority:

> What intrigued me or alarmed me was the number of pressure sores and bed sores of course in those days. But what interested me more, was why some people did not get bed sores ... And I went to the sister one day and said, 'please explain to me why some patients have got bed sores and others didn't' seeing as I was interested in the ones that didn't, and she said, 'it's not your place to ask questions, go back and do your work'. (Hockey, 2001)

She was not put off, and after qualifying as a nurse she trained as both a district nurse and then a health visitor before becoming a tutor at the Royal College of Nursing. In 1971,

Hockey became the Director of the first Nursing Research Unit at the University of Edinburgh (Weir, 2004). She was awarded her PhD on 3 December 1979 and on 4 December the same year was invested Order of the British Empire in recognition of her contribution to nursing research (Mason, 2005: 2). She died on 15 June 2004.

Baroness Jean McFarlane of Llandaff (Jean Kennedy McFarlane) was born on 1 April 1926. The youngest child of a large family, she did well at school and went to study sciences at London University. However, her voluntary work with people experiencing difficult life situations led her to undertake a nursing course at Manchester Royal Infirmary, and then later qualified as both a midwife and health visitor. Her career in nursing saw her lead a project, sponsored by the then Department of Health and Social Security and RCN (1967) to research nursing care in depth and provide evidence for quality care. McFarlane's role was to summarise the project and produce a literature review on 'The proper study of the nurse' (McFarlane, 1970). McFarlane returned to Manchester in the early 1970s to work with the Department of Community Medicine, pursuing her vision that nurses' education should be of graduate standing and prepare them to work equally in a hospital or community setting. This resulted ultimately in the development of a Bachelor's degree in Nursing with additional health visiting and district nursing qualifications. Her work was renowned both on the national and international stage. McFarlane was awarded a chair in nursing at Manchester in 1974 – the first in England – and her subsequent work for the Royal Commission on the NHS led to her parliamentary seat in the House of Lords and further influence on a number of select committees. Although Baroness McFarlane died in 2012, her influence on people and undergraduate nurse education continues to evolve and respond to the dynamic world of healthcare provision.

Margaret Scott Wright (a contemporary of both Jean McFarlane and Lisbeth Hockey) enjoyed significant nursing and nurse management roles at St George's and The Middlesex Hospitals in London before embarking on a challenging career as a nursing researcher both in Edinburgh and several Canadian universities. Her clinical work spanned a period of immense development of the nursing role in care, the advance of technology in diagnostics and treatment and a stronger dialogue between medical practitioners and nurses which would evolve into clinical specialist nursing opportunities. Scott Wright was passionate about the development of nursing research as she believed it would enhance the quality of care provision by adding academic rigour to the clinical nurse's expertise. She was also one of the first UK nurses to study for a Doctorate of Philosophy (1961) and in 1971 was awarded the first chair of nursing studies in Europe whilst at Edinburgh University. Her desire to see nursing research as a central theme in nurse education was helped by her role in the influential Briggs Committee which reported to government in 1972 and strongly supported the development of nursing research units across the UK. Her career finally took her to Canada where she continued to have international influence on the development of nursing research.

So what can we learn from our nursing history?

Nursing has at its roots *nurture, caring, comfort* and *compassion*, ministered by those committed to humanitarian values and often enduring significant hardship in the process. Several conflicts have given rise to ground-breaking innovations and discoveries in medical technology and treatment and the evolution of nursing has taken place alongside. As a result advances in nursing practice, and more recently, nursing research, have often followed the development of medical practice. One thing of which we can be absolutely sure is that as a nursing student you will study, learn, practise and develop your knowledge and skills in the light of new discoveries and treatments. Indeed nursing in the future will surely be different from what it is today. However, in this regard we must advise some caution: we must be careful not to live in our history as this can distract us from the importance of our present and the potential for nursing's future. A healthy interest in events that have shaped the profession will often provide the impetus and courage to ensure that our nursing practice continues to evolve and can meet the needs of service users in a dynamic world.

STOP AND THINK

- Are you able to identify your reasons for becoming a nurse?
- What is it that you wish to achieve?
- What skills and attributes do you feel you can offer the profession?

Keep a note of your answers to these questions as we shall re-visit this topic later in the chapter.

Where are we now?

Professional nurses of today can access the benefits of established educational programmes which are both validated and monitored by a professional body – the Nursing and Midwifery Council (NMC) – and the Higher Education Institution (HEI) in which courses take place. As new registrants launch their careers, the Modernising Nursing Careers (DHSSPS, 2006), NHS Knowledge and Skills (NHS Employers, 2014) and Preceptorship Frameworks (DH, 2010a; NHS Education for Scotland, 2006; NHS Wales, 2012; Northern Ireland Practice and Education Council, 2013) help nurses to grow and develop their skills whilst continuing effective patient contact in practice and/ or following management, education or research pathways.

The role of the nurse has also been extended and nurses are now significant partners with other health professionals and service users in care provision. Increasingly, specialist nurses are the leaders of care and take additional responsibilities in areas such as prescribing, implementing complex care interventions and performing minor surgery or other invasive treatments. It is clear that as a profession we are facing an unprecedented rate of change. This is partly in response to the changing face of healthcare itself as we move towards a more community-based focus of care, but is also as a result of improvements in treatments and technologies. We face targets and the competitive aspects of a free market economy which has been introduced to the NHS where it is almost impossible to put a price on the time you spend with a frightened patient waiting for uncertain news in an A&E for example. We also face increased scrutiny from our service users and those who provide support to carers. Increased media coverage has led to an atmosphere of alarm, ambiguity and a perception of neglect, especially in the context of ongoing chronic disease and end of life care. This lack of compassion and kindness was highlighted in its starkest form in the Francis Reports (DH, 2010b, 2013) which provoked a necessary period of professional introspection and an avowed reclaiming of our core values (DH, 2012a, 2012b; Moore, 2012; NHS Wales, 2013) and the seven principles of the NHS Constitution (2013) which will be explored and discussed in more detail later in the chapter.

It is our hope that as an adult nurse you will develop the knowledge, skills and confidence that will enable you to provide high quality, evidence-based nursing in a variety of settings. Further, we hope that you will always be sensitive to the needs of those in your care, their families or carers and to the multidisciplinary colleagues with whom you work and communicate in the provision of holistic care.

The parameters for your programme of study are laid down by the NMC's Standards for Pre-registration Nurse Education (NMC, 2010a). These standards provide a framework to which your university or Higher Educational Institution (HEI) will add the appropriate knowledge and experience that will help you meet these essential requirements. During your studies you will undoubtedly learn about nursing theory and practice, anatomy and physiology in health and illness, psychology and communication, sociology, pharmacology, microbiology, health promotion and education, law and ethics. These topics when applied to nursing will form the building blocks that will then inform your practice. As you move through a number of practice placements you will begin to appreciate the diverse nature of the adult field of nursing and the various specialist roles of those who work within it. There may well be some aspects that you will find more difficult to learn than others and some areas of practice where you will feel more at home. The point here is that you will be exposed to an essential variety of care settings which will facilitate your development and help you make decisions about where you will want to focus your practice when registered.

Your student experience will also be influenced by both local and national developments in policy and practice, for example National Service Frameworks, Clinical Guidelines or Plans for Care and/or Care Pathways (which will be referred to regularly throughout the chapters that follow).

Essentially then, wherever you undertake your learning the adult field will reflect the fact that contemporary adult nursing takes place in various settings where care is often delivered to a diverse client group. This might seem a tall order if you are new to a nursing programme, but you will bring knowledge and experience with you as you start a course of study and gradually you will be encouraged and guided to build and extend that knowledge and understanding over the three years of your programme and beyond, thereby embarking on a lifelong learning journey.

This is where a *professional portfolio or profile* and your skills of *reflective practice* will prove invaluable. Completing a programme of study in a practice discipline such as nursing is akin to learning to walk up hills and mountains. When you first begin doing so the terrain is unfamiliar and you will find yourself concentrating on your feet so you don't fall over. Sometimes you will get out of breath if you try to climb too quickly or if you are trying to keep up with colleagues. At some point you will stop to catch your breath, turn around and admire the view and then realise just how far you have come. This then gives you the confidence to look up and out rather than down as the terrain becomes more familiar. You will build sufficient stamina to keep going and face each new challenge. Occasionally you will have to walk round or even down to be able to carry on climbing. Indeed, professional resilience and resourcefulness are necessary attributes in the pursuit of safe, self-aware practice.

Your professional profile is a comprehensive record of your professional achievements and developing reflective skills. It is a requirement of registration with the Nursing and Midwifery Council that every nurse is able to demonstrate that they have met the requirements for practice and continuing professional development (NMC, 2013). Keeping a professional profile or portfolio will help you adopt a lifelong learning approach to both your professional and personal development.

Within any profile it is important to provide demonstrable evidence of that development. This evidence will help you demonstrate to others that you have achieved the required learning outcomes in practice. During your studies you will acquire both study and practice skills to prepare you for your role as a qualified nurse. These skills will include those that are necessary to become a reflective practitioner, i.e. a professional individual who challenges practice in a constructive and helpful way.

Hence your profile will be a record of your development as a nurse throughout every aspect of your course. It is a means of demonstrating your ongoing achievement and recording your development throughout your course and beyond. It is also a tool to help you develop the skills of *critical awareness, reflective practice, rational decision making* and *clinical judgement*. In summary, your student portfolio is your showcase. It gives value to both the practical and the academic work you have completed.

Reflection is a process by which you can think about and achieve a better knowledge and understanding of your practice, learning from your own experiences in order to improve the care you provide to patients. Reflecting on our experiences and interactions with others enables us as caring professionals to establish what we have learnt and the influence we may have had on others. The key message about reflection here is that it is purposeful and has meaning when it is undertaken and, just as with nursing practice, is constantly evolving.

Reflection is often also referred to as *reflexivity,* which acts as an internal monitor or check for an individual's ever-changing self (Todd, 2002: 62). As individuals we learn and evolve through education and a range of professional, personal and third party experiences; this then influences our behaviours and actions. Reflexivity is an integral part of developing as an effective nurse and is crucial whether we are caring for a dying patient, someone who is suffering from an acute illness or a patient who is in need of additional support to manage a chronic condition.

Schon (1983) suggests that there are two types of reflective practice, *reflection in action* and *reflection on action*, and purports that experienced nurses are able to reflect whilst in action and if necessary change and adapt, whereas the novice reflects retrospectively. However, in reality it is likely that a combination of these actions occur partly due to the evolution of nurse training since the 1980s. Nursing students are introduced to the concept of reflection and are encouraged throughout their course and professional life to apply reflexivity to their practice.

Reflection is an active, purposeful act intended to make us challenge the nursing world around us. It is a lifelong process of learning about ourselves and how things that happen to us can be thought about, deliberated and acted upon. This does not have to be a significant life-changing episode that you may have witnessed with patients (for example a terminal diagnosis), it may be something that has made you stop and consider the impact this has had on you.

There are many different models of reflection that can be used depending on your individual learning style and personal preference. One such example is the Gibbs

Reflective Cycle (1988) illustrated in Figure 1.1: this describes reflection as a process with distinct steps, as a description of what happened and the feelings evoked, followed by your evaluating and analysing the situation, concluding the situation and providing an action plan for future practice.

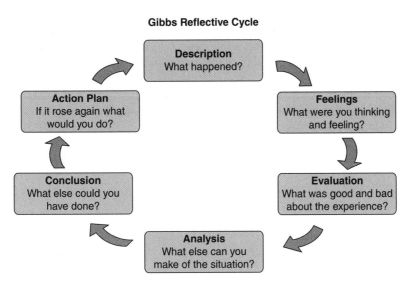

Gibbs Reflective Cycle

Figure 1.1   The Gibbs Reflective Cycle (1988)

By documenting in your student profile the things you have learned, the challenges you have faced (both the good and bad experiences encountered) and the wide range of people you have met in possibly heart-breaking circumstances, you will not only make a record of your student journey and provide evidence of your achievements, you will also build your reflexive aptitude and a capacity for self-awareness which should help you engage more effectively in order to improve patient outcomes. The important thing is that you are able to learn from your experiences and apply what you have learnt to your future practice. By using reflective practice and your profile in this way you should be able to trace the development of your knowledge base and skills for practice, your clinical judgement and decision making and your leadership and management approaches as you prepare to nurse adults irrespective of their age, health status, culture or disability. The ability to reflect upon practice in this way is something that we will revisit in various chapters throughout this book.

'Profession', 'professional' and 'professionalism'

Throughout this chapter we will use the words 'profession' and 'professional' quite liberally. However, it is important to understand the difference between the two.

- What does being professional mean to you?
- Can you describe what professionalism means?

Entering or belonging to a profession means that you have undertaken a specific area of study (mainly at degree level) and the way in which you carry out your work is governed by a set of codes and standards and that is regulated by legislation (law). As a professional, you have a certain level of autonomy and you are both *responsible* and *accountable* for all of your actions.

Belonging to a profession affords a status; being professional describes how you conduct yourself in that status. 'Professionalism' describes a set of values and behaviours which influence not just *what* you do but also *how* and *when* you do it. Professionalism is also framed in terms of awareness, attitudes and behaviours and relates to having sufficient professional judgement to identify the attitude and type of behaviour that are appropriate in any given situation. This is a distinction that may sometimes be missed. In all of the caring professions, professionalism includes the ability to demonstrate the following values:

- Integrity.
- Honesty.
- Transparency.
- A sense of duty.
- Decency.

These values will dictate how you should behave as a professional and therefore will have a direct impact on patient care. Indeed, professional values is the first domain of the NMC Competency Framework (NMC, 2010b) and includes that nurses:

… must practise autonomously and be responsible and accountable for safe, compassionate, person-centred, evidenced based nursing that respects and maintains dignity and human rights. They must show professionalism and high integrity and work within recognised professional, ethical and legal frameworks.

ACTIVITY 1.2

1. Go to the Scottish Government website and access and read the Chief Nursing Officer for Scotland's report below which focuses on professionalism: CNO for Scotland (2012), 'Professionalism in nursing, midwifery and the allied health professions in Scotland: a report to the Coordinating Council for the NMAHP Contribution to the Healthcare Quality Strategy for NHS Scotland' (available at: www.scotland.gov.uk/publications/2012/07/7338).

Write down the key elements which are thought to be important and keep these handy. You will need to compare these later.

2. Now access the Health and Care Professions Council UK (HCPC) website and download the latest report focusing on 'Fitness to practise' cases referred to professional regulators (available at: www.hcpc-uk.org.uk).

3. Make a list of the type of cases the HCPC is likely to consider.
4. Access a copy of the subsequent study commissioned as a result of these findings by going to www.hpc-uk.org and go to 'research publications'. Download the *Professionalism in Healthcare Professionals* document (HCPC, 2011)

In the study outlined in the report on the Scottish Government's website above, you may notice a trend in cases linked to a broad range of behaviours which were distinct from technical capability and generally termed 'professionalism'. The subsequent study carried out by Durham University (Study 2) included students and educators from three different regulated health professions (paramedics, occupational therapists and podiatrists/chiropodists) and provides an excellent summary of what professionalism entails. It also puts this in the context of healthcare in terms of relevant examples.

The key findings of the study were that:

1 The concept of what professionalism is remains common regardless of the professional group, status or training route.
2 Regulations are considered to be basic guidance and signposting on what is appropriate and what is unacceptable behaviour (acting as a baseline for behaviour rather than a specification) (HCPC, 2011).

An appropriate set of moral values and personal qualities must be the foundation to which we add specialist knowledge and clinical skills. The above study supports the view that it is both possible and desirable to 'be professional' before acquiring the necessary knowledge and skills to become a registered professional. This is particularly crucial in the context of healthcare students who, unlike many other undergraduate students, must be professional from day one since they must interact with patients, families and qualified healthcare professionals whilst on placements. Professionalism is the consequence of qualities that an individual brings to the profession – indeed many of those questioned in the study felt that this was an essential part of themselves. Yet how does this manifest itself? Consider the examples in the following Stop and Think.

STOP AND THINK

The way in which we present ourselves is significant as it is the first impression people will get. What does it say about you if:

• you regularly turn up on time for lectures or shifts?
• you often appear dishevelled and unkempt?
• you turn up to pre-arranged meetings with your mentor/tutor having undertaken some preparation before hand?
• you are sometimes rude or brusque?
• you listen carefully and act upon feedback?

How might a patient interpret each of the above behaviours in terms of the standard of care they will receive?

Obviously there will always be the odd occasion when we are running late and even with the very best of intentions our plans can sometimes go wrong. However, turning up on time to meetings, lectures or shifts in practice is one way of demonstrating our ongoing commitment – to patients, colleagues and other professionals. Similarly, being rude to or about our colleagues gives a very poor impression to patients and their families, not only of ourselves as individuals but of the whole team providing care. Faulkner (1998) argues that those who find it difficult to communicate effectively with each other are less likely to be effective when interacting with patients and families. This is also demonstrated by HCPC UK (2011) who found that individuals who are professional have an innate sense of decency towards others and suggest that they are polite, courteous, non-condescending and act honestly and with integrity.

How do legal and ethical principles underpin our professional practice?

The law may be broadly defined as:

> The system of rules which a particular country or community recognises as regulating the actions of its members and which it may enforce by the imposition of penalties. (OED, 2014b)

This is clearly reflected in the NMC's *Standards for Pre-registration Nursing Education* (NMC, 2010a, 2010b: 5), where it states that nurses will 'act with professionalism and integrity and work within agreed professional, ethical and legal frameworks and processes to maintain and improve standards'. As our professional roles develop alongside innovations in healthcare knowledge and practice, associated technologies and increasing public demand, Wheeler (2012: 3) reminds us that ' ... moral values guide our thinking and behaviour and impact on our ethical decision making in relation to caring'. Therefore as a student of nursing you are a developing professional and it is essential that you understand the NMC's *Guidance on Professional Conduct for Nursing and Midwifery Students* (NMC, 2009) and how this relates to The Code (NMC, 2015) to which you ultimately aspire and to all aspects of your everyday life and work.

ACTIVITY 1.3

Access and read a copy of the following documents:

1. NMC Guidance on Professional Conduct for Nursing and Midwifery Students (NMC, 2009) (available at www.nmc-uk.org/Students/Guidance-for-students/).
2. The NMC Code (NMC, 2015) (available at www.nmc-uk.org).

   - What do you consider to be the aims of the guidance and code?
   - Which elements do you consider to be the most important and why?

The *NMC Student Guidance* and *NMC Code* are designed to ensure your practice is safe and that you do not leave your actions open to challenge. However, you are also expected to explore topics such as moral values, ethical theories, attitude development, accountability, confidentiality, integrity and trust, to mention but a few. Each of these will underpin the relationships you form with service users, colleagues, the profession and society in general. Developing your knowledge base to include these aspects will help you increase your appreciation of how legal requirements affect your work and also be alert to situations where you should gain further advice and support.

If an understanding of the law helps us to better understand what is considered to be legally right and wrong within the parameters of our nursing practice then an appreciation of ethical principles helps us determine, through a process of structured reasoning, the morally 'good' course of action from the 'bad'. In both cases the perception of what is right and what is good will be influenced by your personal beliefs and values. For example, in the previous Stop and Think when asked to reflect on why you want to become a nurse, you may have considered that your desire is driven by your own moral compass, including your personal beliefs and values. Is this perhaps related to a belief in the centrality of integrity, compassion and a willingness to be kind and caring and a wish to empathise with those in need? However, what happens if your impulse is not based on a willingness to care? What if you are not empathic or non-judgemental?

It is important that nurses are open-minded and able to care equally for all individuals irrespective of their illness, age, sexuality or religion. As an adult nurse you will be required to adhere to the ethical principles enshrined within The Code (NMC, 2015), including the intention to *do good*, the insight to *do no harm*, the capacity to *ensure justice* and the competence to promote dignity by *respecting autonomy* and *affording participation and choice* (Beauchamp and Childress, 2009). This is a complex and complicated process that relies on commitment and conviction and will require discipline and an enduring capacity to explore your own impulses. You will need to foster an ability to justify and articulate your choices both in terms of your actions and omissions. You will often be called upon to balance your private understandings against public expectations and professional requirements and to promote the best interest of individuals, society and the profession. You will need to accept shared professional parameters and role model professional values. You will also need to understand and be able to articulate your obligations to clients and colleagues alike.

It is vital to your own development – and more specifically to those in receipt of your care – that you are sure of the moral basis of your impetus to nurse. You may remember the answers you gave to the previous Stop and Think above. However, we would invite you to expand on these here and reflect upon the following questions:

- What informs your impulse to care?
- Why have you deliberately opted to work with individuals experiencing illness?
- How would you define nursing?
- What makes a good nurse and what kind of nurse do you want to be?
- As a conduit through which caring is facilitated, what skills do you possess/would you like to foster in order to best enact your nursing role?
- How might these skills be best secured and articulated?
- How can you give yourself the best chance of success?
- What are your goals?
- What are your sources of motivation and inspiration?

STOP AND THINK

When reflecting upon how you might define nursing you may wish to consider the three definitions of nursing that have evolved over the last one hundred and fifty years:

> Nature alone cures ... and what nursing has to do ... is to put the patient in the best condition for nature to act upon him. (Nightingale, 1859: 191)

> The unique function of the nurse is to assist the individual – sick or well – in the performance of those activities contributing to health or its recovery (or to peaceful death) that he would perform unaided if he had the necessary strength, will or knowledge. And to do this in such a way as help him gain independence as rapidly as possible. (Henderson, 1960: 3)

> Nursing is the use of clinical judgement in the provision of care to enable people to improve, maintain, or recover health, to cope with health problems and to achieve the best possible quality of life, whatever their disease or disability, until death. (RCN, 2003: 3)

As an adult nurse you will inevitably face a range of ethical dilemmas during the course of your studies and indeed throughout your professional life. As the conduit of care, your moral compass will dictate your actions and inform your choices. Patients deserve to be nursed at all times by someone who is careful, compassionate and considerate. This calls for purposeful *moral engagement* combined with *emotional intelligence* based upon a deliberate intention to place patients at the centre of all your care, a personal philosophy of nursing as privilege and the facilitation of candour in terms of truthfulness and transparency.

The concept of moral engagement arises from social cognitive theory (Bandura, 1986, 1991) and requires you to stand firm in your moral behaviour, despite the possibility of peer or social pressure to act differently. This takes *moral courage*. Bandura suggests that a sure way to demonstrate this concept is through empathy. This means you must accept responsibility for your behaviours and demonstrate a humane concern for others at all times. This ability to self-govern our behaviours ensures that we are able to consider best practice and best interest for those in our care.

Emotional intelligence (EI) is defined by Vitello-Cicciu (2002) as the ability to perceive and regulate your own emotions and those of others in a way that positively influences communication, motivation, and teamwork. According to Goleman (1995) there are five integrated EI domains: self-awareness, self-regulation, motivation, empathy, and social skill. We will be re-visiting the importance of EI again in subsequent chapters.

The 6Cs of Nursing

We have established that caring and compassion have been fundamental aspects of a nurse's role since nursing's inception and that good moral values and personal qualities are central to who a person is and will ultimately directly impact upon their behaviour towards others. You will note that the title of this chapter begins with values and is followed by knowledge and skills which, in their entirety, underpin nursing practice and ultimately give rise to the best possible patient outcomes. Without the appropriate set of values and personal qualities there is no foundation on which to add the building blocks of clinical skills, education, professional standards, codes and ethics (all of which will be discussed in this and other chapters).

In 2012 and in recognition of the importance of these values, the Chief Nursing Officer of England and the Director of Nursing at the Department of Health launched a new strategy (DH, 2012b) based upon six core values (the 6Cs) which have been adopted as a means to determine effective care. This followed similar standards previously outlined in Northern Ireland (DHSSPS, 2006, 2008). These include moral values, professionalism and aspects of dedication which are used to define the basis of good quality nursing care.

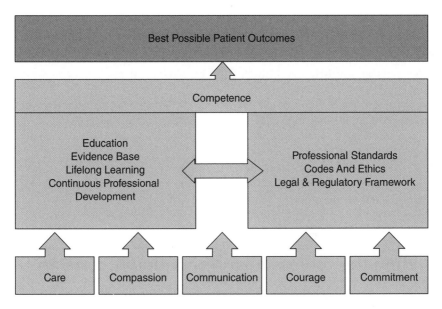

Figure 1.2 The 6Cs – the foundations of professional nursing practice

The key elements identified within this framework are outlined below:

- *Care* – the care we deliver helps the individual person and improves the health of the whole community. Caring defines us in our work. The people receiving care expect it to be right for them consistently throughout every stage of their life.
- *Compassion* – is how the care is given through relationships based on respect.
- *Courage* – relates to us as nurses having the courage to do the right thing for the people we care for, to speak up when we have concerns and to have the personal strength and vision to embrace new ways of working.
- *Communication* – is central to successful caring relationships and effective team working. All successful interactions between individuals are based on good communication, which comes in many formats and encompasses multiple means, such as non-verbal, verbal and written.
- *Competence* – all those in caring roles must have the ability to understand an individual's health and social needs and have the clinical expertise and technical knowledge to deliver effective care and treatments based on research and evidence.
- *Commitment* – to our patients and populations is the cornerstone of what we do and we need to build on our commitment to improve the care and experience of our patients.

As you may realise, the six core values as outlined here are not really new. They are based upon the key fundamental principles of what have always been considered vital to the role of nurse. Florence Nightingale, for example, always tried to strive for accessibility and simplicity of expression and to stress the importance of enacting core values. However, perhaps there is now a need to be more specific and explicit in terms of what these are and how they underpin practice.

ACTIVITY 1.4

Compare the 6Cs Framework above to principles outlined by the CNO for Scotland in the previous exercise, the NHS Constitution (NHS England, 2013) and the Royal College of Nursing Principles of Practice (RCN, 2011).

You can access the *NHS Constitution* document at the following website: www.nhs.uk/choiceintheNHS/Rightsandpledges/NHSConstitution/Pages/Overview.aspx

You can access the *RCN Principles of Practice* at the following website: www.rcn.org.uk

- Make a note of what you consider to be the key elements in each. What are the similarities?
- Are there any differences between the values outlined in each of the documents? If so, what do you think these are?

Upholding the professional reputation of nursing

Thus far we have outlined the fundamental values and principles of nursing practice. However, let's now stop and think about contemporary nursing practice.

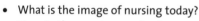

- What is the image of nursing today?
- How is the nursing profession perceived by patients, carers and/or members of the general public?

ACTIVITY 1.5

Follow the link as detailed below which will take you to the personal account of Christina Patterson, a well-known and respected journalist: www.bbc.co.uk/programmes/b01omrzt (this highlights a programme recorded for BBC Radio 4 in 2011, entitled 'Care to be a nurse?' in which she describes her experiences whilst undergoing six operations for breast cancer over a period of eight years at different hospitals).

Whilst listening consider the following questions and make a note of your answers:

- What were the key issues here?
- Why you think this happened?

- How did Christina feel?
- How does this account make you feel?
- As a nurse involved in Christina's care what would you have done differently?
- Were there any barriers – and if so – how might you have overcome them?
- What were the key positive nursing actions important to her?

The NMC Code (NMC, 2015: 15) requires us to 'act with honesty and integrity at all times' to uphold the reputation of our profession and to 'promote professionalism and trust' by being 'models of integrity and leadership'. It would therefore it would be disingenuous if we did not acknowledge the gravity and extent of the challenges to the nursing profession's reputation over the last few years. Whilst it is important to recognise that in some areas there are excellent standards of nursing care we have to acknowledge the evidence which demonstrates that in other areas current opinion of the nursing profession is low. At this point should we perhaps look at events that have brought into question the professional reputation of nurses over the last few years? We need to try to work out why and how these events have been allowed to happen and then create a strategy both of reform and support to ensure that they will not do so again. One of the key aspects that Christina focuses upon is a lack of care, compassion and 'basic human kindness'.

Crucially, before Christina went into hospital the first time she wasn't worried about her care since she didn't think she would have to. Yet she experienced poor care consistently throughout her patient journey. Why was this? Where was the effective *communication*, the *care* and *compassion* for her situation, the *competence* and *commitment* to provide the best evidence-based care and the *courage* to ensure that the nurses who worked with her understood her personal journey through ill health? As her case clearly demonstrates, somewhere along the way the nurses involved in the delivery of her care seemed to have lost sight of the art of nursing.

This example indicates that vulnerability and patient status constitute universal features of the illness experience. Hallett (2012) considers a range of potential factors which may have contributed to Christina's poor experience, including:

- the changing emphasis towards more technical skills and knowledge;
- the shift in roles between what doctors used to have sole responsibility for and the extended role of the nurse;
- the professionalisation of the nursing role;
- the delegation of basic care to healthcare assistants;
- bureaucracy and box ticking given priority over compassion;
- the wider social, economic and political factors.

Christina's account also adds to the wake of revelations from the Care Quality Commission's inspection of over 150 hospitals and care homes (CQC, 2011), the events at Winterbourne View Hospital (BBC, 2012; DH, 2012a), the Princess of Wales and Neath Port Talbot hospitals (Andrews and Butler, 2014) and the publication of the Francis Reports (DH, 2010b, 2013) which described the 'appalling suffering of many patients' between 2005 and 2008 at the Mid Staffordshire Foundation NHS Trust.

ACTIVITY 1.6

Access and read the following documents:

1. The Francis Report (DH, 2013).

You can find this information on the Executive Summary and recommendations at: www.midstaffspublicinquiry.com/report

2. NHS Wales (2013).
3. Care Quality Commission (CQC) and Nursing and Midwifery Council (NMC) responses to the Francis Report, available at:

*   www.cqc.org.uk/content/care-quality-commission-response-francis-report
*   www.cqc.org.uk/content/cqc-highlights-changes-following-francis-report
*   www.nmc-uk.org/About-us/Our-response-to-the-Francis-Inquiry-Report/

Make a list of all factors identified in each report.

The original report into events at Mid Staffs (DH, 2010b) noted that 'it was striking how many accounts related to basic nursing care as opposed to clinical errors leading to injury or death'. Jane Cummings (Chief Nursing Officer for England) noted that 'such poor care is a betrayal of all that we stand for' (DH, 2012b: 7). The Francis Report (DH, 2013) went on to highlight 290 recommendations for stakeholders to consider across a wide and enduring spectrum of concern including the neglect and negligence of individuals along with a wide range of associated factors including organisational structures, staff shortages, management policies, bonus payments for managers and the imposition of targets devoid of any research evidence base. Nor did the CQC emerge from the Francis Report unscathed as it was clear that their criteria for inspection were not sufficiently robust. A response issued by the CQC (2013) acknowledged these shortcomings, highlighting a schedule of changes including the appointment of an Inspector of Hospitals, a more searching assessment process in profiling institutions and an expert base to their inspection teams. They also reaffirmed their remit to monitor the quality of healthcare environments for the people who matter most – service users.

Whilst the vast majority of nurses would find these behaviours and actions to be as abhorrent as they are incomprehensible, you will by now have recognised that nurses have a personal duty of care which includes obligations and promises to adhere to the standards as espoused within The Code (NMC, 2015). This means that we are personally and collectively responsible and accountable for the decisions we make and the actions we take, regardless of the pressures or environment we are working within. This therefore calls upon us to display courage and commitment – acting as advocates for our patients to ensure that we always act in their 'best interest'.

The challenges to contemporary practice

At the outset of this chapter we outlined the challenges faced by nurses, whether they be in the nature of some of the very personal aspects of the work, the issues of gender, the fight for recognition as a profession, the emotional labour involved or the hardships of nursing during wartime (Heaton, 2012). Some of these challenges remain ever-present whilst others will change and evolve. Many of these are covered in more depth in later chapters but this chapter highlights some of the key issues facing nurses today. Perhaps the most significant challenge is that of public perception, namely the image of nursing and the prevailing culture within our profession.

Advances in technology and the changing emphasis in recent years to nurses becoming more technically specialised have been blamed in a number of quarters for the loss of care and compassion (Hallett, 2007; Pearcey, 2008; Law and Aranda, 2010). However, we should consider whether these two need to be mutually exclusive.

We would be failing ourselves and our profession if we did not maintain our competence and continue to develop as techniques and technology improve. Hallett (2007: 430) also suggests that core values are constants whereas technology is 'a tool to be wielded in the services of health'. When people require any kind of medical intervention, it is the level of empathic and compassionate care they receive that makes the difference between a good or bad experience: it is good communication (especially listening carefully), kindness, caring and empathy and not the technical intervention (which is almost taken as a given) that really make the difference. It is also clear that such values, qualities and behaviours are crucial to good nursing. In one study, Smith (1992) found that 44 different words or phrases were used by patients to describe 'ideal' and 'real' nurses. Interestingly, only six of these related to functional attributes such as efficient, observant and capable of doing their job. The caring and emotional aspects of nursing were clearly seen as distinct but complementary to, and more importantly, *underpinning* the functional aspects of everything we do as nurses. *Kindness*, *helpfulness* and *patience* were the attributes most frequently used. *Talking*, *listening*, *showing interest* and *sympathy* also featured heavily as aspects of the ideal nurse. It is clear how these attributes align closely with the 6Cs, but perhaps all of this is best expressed by one patient who concluded:

A nurse has to be aware of the patient's condition and how to tackle it. She has to have a nursing manner which requires a lot of patience and forethought and to try and relieve pain and suffering not by medical means but by compassion. (Smith, 2012: 27)

Furthermore, perhaps as a result of wider access to the internet, the public are much better informed and have access to a huge amount of information and related data about their health. They will often have high expectations in terms of openness and transparency and the right to be included and informed. As a result, as nurses we must work hard to keep our own knowledge up to date and ensure that our practice is firmly based on sound evidence. We must also demonstrate care and compassion not only in how we treat our patients and their families but also in respecting their right to be involved in all the decisions affecting them. Respect, privacy and dignity should feature strongly in every aspect of our care delivery. We must ensure that we listen to their concerns, needs and wants, acting as patient advocates when required. This requires commitment to ensure that we are continually updating our knowledge and that we maintain our competency. It also requires good communication to ensure that we listen to people's concerns and answer their questions, making sure that we explain ourselves clearly and that we have been understood (a topic that will be focused upon in more detail in subsequent chapters).

Fitness to practise

Part of the NMC's role as a professional regulator is to maintain the professional register and ensure the public are protected from poor practice. The NMC takes these aspects of their work most seriously in order to maintain the reputation of the profession and promote public confidence that nurses on the register meet the necessary standards of a competent practitioner. There are procedures in place to guide employers, colleagues and the public who wish to raise concerns about any nurse's *fitness to practise* and the NMC investigates these concerns thoroughly.

So what does the term 'fitness to practise' mean? The current NMC guidance (NMC, 2014) states that a nurse who is fit to practise is one who has successfully completed an approved pre-registration education programme, is registered with the NMC and thereafter maintains that ability to practise safely and independently whilst following the professional code of practice as set out in The Code (NMC, 2015). In practical terms this means that as a nurse you maintain appropriate standards of proficiency, ensure you are of good health and good character, and that you adhere to the principles of good practice that are set out in the various standards, guidance and advice.

The notion of being suitably prepared by your educational programme to undertake the nurse registrant's role and that you should have valid and current registration with the regulatory body is really quite straightforward. Demonstrating that you are of good health and good character is closely linked to the ways in which you work and live and ensuring that these are aligned to The Code (NMC, 2015).

ACTIVITY 1.7

Follow the links on the NMC website (www.nmc-uk.org) and read the current version of the NMC Code (2015) and the information related to *fitness to practise* and *good health and good character*.

Make a note of any questions that occur to you as you read this and consider where or to whom you might go for help in answering your questions.

One of your questions may well be '*How do I prepare for this responsibility?*', or '*What happens if something occurs that means I question my own fitness to practise?*'

It is important that we explore this concept of 'fitness to practise' with you and what it means to be of good health and good character. You will soon appreciate that during your programme of study you will normally be well prepared to face the challenges of professional life and demonstrate the knowledge, skills, behaviours and standards of care that the public would expect from nurses.

One of the first things you should do is to read the guidance the NMC provides for students of nursing and midwifery.

ACTIVITY 1.8

Access the NMC website (www.nmc-uk.org) and follow the required link to read the *Guidance on Professional Conduct for Nursing and Midwifery Students* (NMC, 2011a).

- Compare this guidance with that set out in the current NMC Code.
- What do you note about the information contained within each document?

During your programme of study there will be information and opportunities for discussion which will enable you to develop a better understanding of these concepts and recognise the implications for student nurses who fail to study appropriately and/or fail to abide by the NMC Guidance for Nursing and Midwifery Students (NMC, 2011a) or The Code (NMC, 2015) to which you aspire. While you are not expected to enter your pre-registration education with all of the required professional attributes, it is important to ensure that you are made aware of these concepts, that you understand them and that you grow in competence and confidence with regard to these skills alongside other areas of your development.

We will start with the concept of good health. You may wonder why demonstrating good health is an essential component of a nurse's fitness to practise. Clearly, if we are able to demonstrate that we lead a healthy lifestyle then the benefits of this are that we may be better able to guide those in our care. However, there will be occasions for all of us where we become temporarily incapacitated such that we are unable to work or study. In these circumstances our professional behaviour is to follow the relevant sickness and absence policies. There may be some conditions which challenge our ability to undertake our role safely and competently. At these times it is vital that we seek appropriate support in a timely way to make certain that we have the right help and that we do not endanger our colleagues or service users. Often it is not the event or incidence of ill health that becomes an issue but rather what we have done about it. Have we been honest with ourselves and others? Have we sought appropriate professional support and guidance?

There are four main areas from which an individual's fitness to practise can be called into question. These are *criminal behaviour*, *dishonesty*, *unprofessional behaviour*, and *ill health* (Ellis et al., 2011). Here you will see that honesty and integrity figure highly in the professional equation, i.e. our ability to know right from wrong and thus act appropriately.

Look again at the four main areas that may make us question our fitness to practise:

- Are you able to identify any potential risks to your own or a colleague's fitness to practise, and if so what are they?
- What should you do about any concerns you have noted?

STOP AND THINK

In considering these four areas again it may be that some activities feel easier to identify than others: for example harm to another person; stealing; misuse of or dealing in illegal substances; fraudulent activity; and the abuse of vulnerable people. These are unacceptable behaviours and ones which do not adhere to The Code (NMC, 2015). However, by reading this chapter you should also be aware that unprofessional behaviours (such as ongoing poor time management, rudeness to service users or colleagues, breach of confidentiality, examination cheating or plagiarism and bullying) are equally relevant.

Health issues can also catch us out. We don't want to let the team down so we go to work even though we are not really well enough. A diabetic who does not take regular breaks for food or medication. A student who feels that they never have a hangover so they can drink heavily before going on duty. All these actions demonstrate a lack of insight into our health and well-being.

ACTIVITY 1.9

Visit the NMC website (www.nmc-uk.org) and find a case presented to the Fitness to Practice Committee which related to out of work activities compromising their professionalism.

- How do you feel about these circumstances?
- Which circumstances were work related and which occurred in her personal time?

Perhaps what is particularly significant here is the notion that what happens in your personal life is just as important as events in your professional, registrant and/or student life.

STOP AND THINK

Whether you are a student or a registrant, sit back for a minute and think about the things you do in terms of email correspondence, being out with friends or engaging in online social media:

- How do you speak to people?
- Does this vary depending on who it is?
- Do you use a form of shorthand in text or on social media?
- Is this appropriate?
- Does it matter?

For further guidance on social networking please refer to NMC (2011b) guidelines.

These are the sorts of questions you must be able to answer. Perhaps you can discuss this with fellow colleagues, teachers or line managers. As students we are able to seek advice and feedback from teachers and mentors to support our professional development and, since 2004, we have been asked as students to affirm that we are of good health and good character in line with the NMC requirements for pre-registration courses (NMC, 2004, 2010a).

As registrants we also affirm our good health and character each year when our registration is renewed and it is clearly stated in The Code (NMC, 2015) that we have a duty to inform both our employer and the NMC of any concerns we have about our ability to practise safely or any involvement with the police as soon as possible after a concern is highlighted. Do remember that any caution or conviction recorded by the police remains on your personal record for life and is viewed by employers through the Disclosure and Barring Service (further information about this service can be accessed at the following website: www.gov.uk/government/organisations/disclosure-and-barring-service/about).

ACTIVITY 1.10

What are the processes for investigating fitness to practise in your school of nursing and how are these issues addressed in your programme of study?
   Now visit www.nmc-uk.org/Hearings/How-the-process-works/ and compare your university process with that of the NMC when investigating allegations of professional misconduct.

- What differences have you highlighted?
- Does your university process mirror that of the NMC?

Most students and registrants do not have their fitness to practise challenged in such a way that requires investigation and possible sanction. David and Bray (2009) acknowledge that the percentage of students investigated via these procedures is thought to be low. The reason for this is that although each university is charged with having a fitness to practise procedure for students there is no central collation of the number of students investigated or the outcomes of such investigations. However, from half a million registered nurse and midwives over 4,000 were investigated by the NMC in 2012/13 (NMC, 2014).

David and Lee-Woolf (2010) also point out that student nurses are still learning and therefore the seriousness of any given situation may vary dependent upon the stage reached in the programme of study. However, it is necessary that you are aware of the potential pitfalls that can sometimes catch you unawares and must not close your eyes to the subject. You should be careful to be self-aware and not self-righteous in respect of this concept, ensuring that by safe practice and reflective development you are able to recognise any problems or challenges to your practice and act appropriately. Similarly, as a registrant, whilst there is an expectation that you will adhere to The Code (NMC, 2015), there is also an acknowledgement of varying degrees of experience which may impact on any allegation that questions your fitness to practise as a nurse.

Both student and registrant processes which examine fitness to practise have a number of sanctions that can be applied to any given situation. These can range from there being no case to answer, through varying levels of supervision or suspension, to a student's place on their course being withdrawn or a registrant removed from the register permanently. Whatever the outcome in relation to the sanctions applied there must be robust evidence in support of any allegations made and the probability of the event reoccurring must be balanced against the sanction chosen.

In most cases – as either student or registrant – there will be evidence of mitigation to be considered alongside an allegation. It is important to realise that such mitigation can never condone an unprofessional action but it may be used to determine the outcome and level of sanction imposed.

ACTIVITY 1.11

Visit the NMC website and sample some of the recent hearing records and the outcomes applied: these are available at www.nmc-uk.org/hearings/

- Are you able to see why the NMC reached the decision they did?
- Do you agree with the decision or not and why?

Note that nurses, midwives and members of the public are welcome to observe hearings, so there is an opportunity for you to do this if you wish to though you will have to book your place in advance. See the NMC website for further details.

The importance of evidence-based practice

We have acknowledged growing public awareness and the perennial challenge that nurses should be able to justify their actions. The Code (NMC, 2015) also tells us to ensure that our nursing practice should be based on the best available evidence. Therefore, as adult nurses we must learn how to find this evidence and ascertain whether it is good or not.

Good, evidence-based, patient-centred care is vital to modern healthcare and will underpin the expertise and sensitivity of care strategies, thus demonstrating the quality of care provision (Emanuel et al., 2011). Evidence-based practice is an essential component in defining the efficacy of our nursing practice, though it is perhaps worthwhile realising that we will not find a research base for every aspect of care. However, the increasing breadth of knowledge and technology available to inform our decisions adds weight to the explanations of why we do what we do. Our knowledge base for nursing is influenced by knowledge from other disciplines such as the physical and social sciences, law and ethics. We must be able to work with these different elements and apply them to all the clinical situations we encounter.

The capacity to know what is the right thing to do in any nursing situation relies on our ability to explore the relevant and current knowledge in a certain area, to understand what that is trying to tell us and for us to utilise our research appreciation skills to distil whether or not this knowledge can be applied to a particular situation. Although this is a tall order, we as professional nurses are committed to life-long learning that will facilitate our clinical development over our working lives.

Therefore, during your programme of study or as a registrant you will be expected to learn and develop the skills of research appraisal (see Chapter 7, pp.194–198). These will enable you to reflect critically on research worthiness and not only to understand the implications of research for nursing care but also to play your part in ensuring that appropriate research-based care strategies are implemented in practice.

Developing your nursing skills

We all enter nursing with different levels of life experience and emotional maturity and these can differ widely regardless of age. The concept of emotional intelligence (explored in more detail in Chapter 2) is often associated with experiential learning and learning from the lessons of life and this will evolve as we are exposed to more such experiences and gain experience in the nursing context.

STOP AND THINK

- Are you ready to practise nursing?
- Are you fit to practise?

Pause for moment and reflect on whether these questions are asking the same thing.

- How would you answer these questions if asked?

Chapter summary

Throughout this chapter we have introduced you to a diverse range of information. In doing so we have drawn attention to the evolution of nursing by highlighting the events and people who have helped to shape the profession we have today. We have asked you to consider and reflect upon your motivation to nurse and your own philosophy on caring and we have explored some of the legal, moral and ethical issues that can challenge our fitness to practise. We have also discussed some of the challenges faced by nurses today and the tension that exists between the technical expertise of caring and its softer, yet vital skill counterpart – compassion.

As you begin your life-long journey in the profession we trust that this chapter has helped you to share our passion and has stimulated your interest to read and explore the concepts and issues highlighted in subsequent chapters of this book.

Suggested further reading

Cullum, N., Ciliska, D., Haynes, B. and Marks, S. (2007) *Evidence Based Nursing: An Introduction*. Chichester: Wiley.
Dimond, B. (2011) *Legal Aspects of Nursing*. Harlow: Pearson Education.
Timmins, F. and Duffy, A. (2011) *Writing your Nursing Portfolio: A Step by Step Guide*. Maidenhead: Open University Press.

Professor Christine Hallett is director of the UK Centre for the History of Nursing and Midwifery and chair of the UK Association for the History of Nursing. She was also the founding chair of the European Association for the History of Nursing. Professor Hallett's current work focuses on the nurses of the First World War:

Hallett, C. (2014) *Veiled Warriors: Allied Nurses of the First World War*. Oxford: Oxford University Press.

The following clips of Professor Hallett talking about her research are available at: www.youtube.com/watch?v=DznpSeb6wM4
and

 Nursing: The Lost Art at https://mediasite.uit.no/Mediasite/Play/152d249a450941f9bf6b770cf9 ba30581d

References

Alexander, Z. and Dewjee, A. (1984) *The Wonderful Adventures of Mary Seacole in Many Lands.* Bristol: Falling Wall Press.

Andrews, J. and Butler, M. (2014) *Report of the External Independent Review of the Princess of Wales Hospital and Neath Port Talbot Hospital at Abertawe Bro Morgannwg University Health Board.* Cardiff: WAG.

Baly, M. (1997) *Florence Nightingale and the Nursing Legacy.* London: Whurr.

Bandura, A. (1986) *Social Foundations of Thought and Action: A Social Cognitive Theory.* Englewood Cliffs, NJ: Prentice-Hall.

Bandura, A. (1991) 'Social cognitive theory of self-regulation', *Organizational Behavior and Human Decision Processes*, 50: 248–87.

BBC (2011) Radio 4 - Four Thought Series 2: Christina Patterson: *Care To Be A Nurse?* Available at: www.bbc.co.uk/programmes/b010mrzt (last accessed 5 March 2015).

BBC (2012) *The Hospital that Stopped Caring.* Available at: www.bbc.co.uk/programmes/ b01nqn4d

Beauchamp, T. and Childress, J. (2009) *Principles of Biomedical Ethics*, 6th edition. Oxford: Oxford University Press.

Bostridge, M. (2008) *Florence Nightingale: The Woman and her Legend.* London: Penguin.

Bulmer Smith, K., Profetto-McGrath, J. and Cummings, G.G. (2009) 'Emotional intelligence and nursing: an integrative literature review', *International Journal of Nursing Studies*, 46: 1624–36.

Care Quality Commision (2011) *Dignity and Nutrition Inspection Programme: National Overview.* Newcastle upon Tyne: CQC. Available at: www.cqc.org.uk (last accessed 31 January 2014).

Care Quality Commission (2013) *Care Quality Commission Response to Francis Report.* Available at: www.cqc.org.uk/content/care-quality-commission-response-francis-report (last accessed 19 November 2014).

Commission on Funding of Care and Support (2011) *The Report of the Commission on Funding of Care and Support: Fairer Care Funding.* London: Crown. Available at www.ilis.co.uk/ uploaded_files/dilnott_report_the_future_of_funding_social_care_july_2011.pdf (last accessed 5 March 2015).

David, T.J. and Bray, S.A. (2009) 'Healthcare student fitness to practise cases: reason for referral and outcomes', *Education Law Journal*, 196–203.

David, T.J. and Lee-Woolf, E. (2010) 'Fitness to practise for student nurses: principles, standards and procedures', *Nursing Times*, 106(39): 23–6.

Department of Health (2010a) *Preceptorship Framework for Newly Registered Nurses, Midwives and Allied Health Professionals.* London: DH.

Department of Health (2010b) *Independent Inquiry into Care Provided by Mid Staffordshire NHS Foundation Trust, January 2005–March 2009.* London: HMSO. Available at: www. midstaffspublicinquiry.com (last accessed 5 March 2015).

Department of Health (2012a) *Transforming Care: A National Response to Winterbourne Hospital.* London: HMSO. Available at: www.gov.uk/government/uploads/system/uploads/ attachment_data/file/213215/final-report.pdf (last accessed 5 March 2015).

Department of Health (2012b) *Compassion in Practice: Nursing, Midwifery and Care Staff: Our Vision and Strategy.* London: HMSO.

Department of Health (2013) *Report of the Mid Staffordshire NHS Foundation Trust Public Inquiry*. London: HMSO. Available at: www.midstaffspublicinquiry.com

Department of Health, Social Services and Public Safety (2006) *Modernising Nursing Careers: Setting the Direction*. Belfast: DHSSPS.

Department of Health, Social Services and Public Safety (2008) *Improving the Patient and Client Experience*. Belfast: DHSSPS.

Ellis, J., Lee-Woolf, E. and David, T. (2011) 'Supporting nursing students during fitness to practise hearings', *Nursing Standard*, 25 (32): 38–43.

Emanuel, V., Day, K. and Diegnan, L. (2011) 'Developing evidence-based practice amongst students', *Nursing Times*, 107 (49/50): 21–3.

Faulkner, A. (1998) 'The ABC of palliative care: communication with patients, families and other professionals', *British Medical Journal*, 316 (7125): 130–2.

Gibbs, G. (1988) *Learning by Doing, A Guide to Teaching and Learning Methods*. Oxford: Further Education Unit, Oxford Brookes University.

Goleman, D. (1995) *Emotional Intelligence*. New York: Bantam.

Griffon, D.P. (1995) "Crowning the edifice": Ethel Fenwick and state registration', *Nursing History Review*, 3: 201–12.

Griffon, D.P. (1998) "A somewhat duskier skin": Mary Seacole in the Crimea', *Nursing History Review*, 6: 115–27.

Hallett, C.E. (2007) 'Editorial: A "gallop" through history: nursing in social context', *Journal of Clinical Nursing*, 16(3): 429–30.

Hallett, C.E. (2012) 'Nursing: The lost art?'. Conference paper presented at The International History of Nursing Conference, Kolding, Denmark, 11 August.

Hawkins, S. (2010) *Nursing and Women's Labour in the Nineteenth Century*. London: Routledge.

Haycock-Stewart, E., James, C., McLachlan, A. and MacLaren, J. (2014) *Identifying Good Practice in Fitness to Practise Processes in Higher Education Institutes in Scotland*, Report to NHS Education Scotland. Available at: www.nes.scot.nhs.uk/media/2731991/identifying_good_practice_in_fitness_to_practise_processes.pdf (last accessed 17 September 2014).

Health and Care Professions Council UK (2011) *Research Report: Professionalism in Healthcare Professionals*. London: HCPC.

Health and Social Care Information Centre (2013) *Hospital Episode Statistics: Emergency Readmissions to Hospital within 28 Days of Discharge. Financial Year 2011/12*. Leeds: HSCIC. Available at: www.hscic.gov.uk/catalogue/PUB12751/hes-emer-read-hosp-28-days-disc-2002-2012-rep.pdf (last accessed 5 March 2015).

Heaton, A.J. (2012) 'Female nurses in the First World War'. Unpublished dissertation, University of Salford.

Helmstadter, C. (1993) 'Old nurses and new: nursing in the London teaching hospitals before and after the mid-nineteenth century reforms', *Nursing History Review*, 1: 43–70.

Helmstadter, C. (1996) 'Nurse recruitment and retention in the 19th century London teaching hospitals', *International History of Nursing Journal*, 2 (1): 58–69.

Henderson, V. (1960) *Basic Principles of Nursing Care*. London: ICN.

Hockey, L. (2001) *Oral History Interview by Jane Brooks in Edinburgh on 8 August*. UK Centre for the History of Nursing and Midwifery, School of Nursing, Midwifery and Social Work, University of Manchester.

Law, K. and Aranda, K. (2010) 'The shifting foundations of nursing', *Nurse Education Today*, 30: 544–7.

Mann Wall, B. (1998) 'Called to a mission of charity: the sisters of St Joseph in the Civil War', *Nursing History Review*, 6: 85–113.

Mason, K. (2005) *Dr Lisbeth Hockey, 1918-2004: Biography*. Available at: www.nursing.manchester.ac.uk/ukchnm/archives/nurseleaders/lisbethhockey/biography/ (last accessed 5 March 2015).

McFarlane, J.J. (1970) *The Proper Study of the Nurse*. London: Royal College of Nursing. Available at www.rcn.org.uk/__data/assets/pdf_file/0016/235420/Series_1_Introduction.pdf (last accessed 5 March 2015).

Moore, R. (2012) *Professionalism in Nursing, Midwifery and the Allied Health Professions in Scotland: A Report to the Coordinating Council for the NMAHP Contribution to the Healthcare Quality Strategy for NHS Scotland*. Edinburgh: Scottish Government.

NHS Education for Scotland (2006) *Flying Start NHS: Developing Confident, Capable Practitioners*. NHS Education for Scotland. Available at: www.flyingstart.scot.nhs.uk/ (last accessed 28 September 2014).

NHS Employers (2014) *Simplified Knowledge and Skills Framework* (KSF). Available at: www. nhsemployers.org/SimplifiedKSF (last accessed 17 September 2014).

NHS England (2013) *The NHS Constitution*. London: DH.

NHS Wales (2012) *Preceptorship Foundation Policy For Newly Qualified Nurses*. Available at: www.wales.nhs.uk/sitesplus/documents/862/112PreceptorshipFoundationPolicyForNewlyQu alifiedNursesv1.pdf (last accessed 28 September 2014).

NHS Wales (2013) *Delivering Safe Care: Compassionate Care. Learning for Wales from The Report of the Mid Staffordshire NHS Foundation Trust Public Inquiry*. Cardiff: WAG.

Nightingale, F. (1859) *Notes on Nursing: What It Is and What It Is Not*. London: Harrison.

Northern Ireland Practice Education Council (NIPEC) (2013) *Preceptorship Framework for Nursing, Midwifery and Specialist Community Public Health Nursing*. Belfast: NIPEC.

Nursing and Midwifery Council (2004) *Standards of Proficiency for Pre-Registration Nursing Education*. London: NMC.

Nursing and Midwifery Council (2010a) *The NMC Standards for Pre-registration Nursing Education*. London: NMC. Available at: http://standards.nmc-uk.org (last accessed 19 November 2014).

Nursing and Midwifery Council (2010b) *Standards for Competence for Registered Nurses*. Available at: www.nmc-uk.org/Documents/Standards/Standards%20for%20competence.pdf (last accessed 19 November 2014).

Nursing and Midwifery Council (2011a) *Guidance on Professional Conduct for Nursing and Midwifery Students*. London: NMC.

Nursing and Midwifery Council (2011b) *Regulation in Practice – Social Networking Sites*. London: NMC. Available at: www.nmc-uk.org/Nurses-and-midwives/Advice-by-topic/A/Advice/Social-networking-sites/ (last accessed 5 March 2015).

Nursing and Midwifery Council (2013) *Draft Revalidation Strategy*. London: NMC.

Nursing and Midwifery Council (2014) *Fitness to Practice Activity 2012–2013*. Available at www. nmc-uk.org/Hearings/restrictions-and-sanctions/Actions-we-took-in-2012-2013/ (last accessed 17 September 2014).

Nursing and Midwifery Council (2015) *The Code: Professional Standards of Practice and Behaviour for Nurses and Midwives*. London: NMC.

O'Brien D'Antonio, P. (1993) 'The legacy of domesticity: nursing in early nineteenth-century America', *Nursing History Review*, 1: 229–46.

Oxford English Dictionary (2014a) Available at: http://dictionary.reference.com/browse/nurse (last accessed 28 September 2014).

Oxford English Dictionary (2014b) Available at: www.oxforddictionaries.com/definition/english/ law (last accessed 5 March 2015).

Pearcey, P. (2008) 'Shifting roles in nursing: does role extension require role abdication?', *Journal of Clinical Nursing*, 17 (10): 1320–26.

Petrides, K.V. and Sevdalis, N. (2010) 'Emotional intelligence and nursing: comment on Bulmer Smith, Profetto-McGrath and Cummings (2009)', *International Journal of Nursing Studies*, 47: 526–8.

Reverby, S. (1987) *Ordered to Care: The Dilemma of America Nursing*. New York: Cambridge University Press.

Reynolds, W., Scott, B. and Jessiman, C.W. (1999) 'Empathy has not been measured in clients' terms or effectively taught: a review of the literature', *Journal of Advanced Nursing*, 30 (5): 1177–85.

Rolfe, D., Freshwater, D. and Jasper, M. (2011) *Critical Reflection in Practice: Generating Knowledge for Care*, 2nd edition. Basingstoke: Palgrave.

Royal College of Nursing (2003) *Defining Nursing*. London: RCN. Available at: www.rcn.org.uk (last accessed 5 March 2015)

Royal College of Nursing (2011) *The Principles of Nursing Practice*. London: RCN.

Smith, P. (1992) *The Emotional Labour of Nursing: How Nurses Care*. Basingstoke: Palgrave Macmillan.

Smith, P. (2012) *The Emotional Labour of Nursing Revisited*, 2nd edition. Basingstoke: Palgrave Macmillan.

Todd, G. (2002) 'The role of the internal supervisor in developing therapeutic nursing'. In D. Freshwater (ed.), *Therapeutic Nursing*. London: Sage. pp. 58–82.

Vitello-Cicciu, J.M (2002) 'Exploring emotional intelligence: implications for nursing leaders', *Journal of Nursing Administration*, 32 (4): 203–10.

Weir, R.I. (2004) *Educating Nurses in Scotland: A History of Innovation and Change, 1950–2000*. Penzance: The Hypatia Trust.

Wheeler, H. (2012) *Law, Ethics and Professional Issues for Nursing: A Reflective and Portfolio Building-Approach*. London: Routledge.

White, R. (1978) *Social Change and the Nursing Profession: A Study of the Poor Law Nursing Service, 1848-1948*. London: Henry Klimpton.

2 Nursing Therapeutics

CAROLINE JAGGER, HEATHER ILES-SMITH AND JULIA JONES

The term 'nursing therapeutics' encompasses the therapeutic relationship that exists between nurse and patient and the key elements which influence that relationship. Influencing factors include the notion of *person-centred care* and the use of *systematic approaches* in planning, implementing and evaluating nursing care provision. The application of effective interpersonal skills and an ability to critically reflect upon the care we have provided, along with consideration of the underpinning professional values and the legal and ethical frameworks outlined in the previous chapter are also of utmost importance.

Nursing therapeutics is not a new concept. It has been an integral part of nursing throughout history although it has not always been clearly defined or its importance been articulated in the nursing literature.

Throughout this chapter the concept of a therapeutic nurse–patient relationship and the associated concepts above will be explored in more depth. The overarching aim of this chapter is to define what we deem to be a therapeutic relationship, to identify the components of such a relationship and to explore how this can be developed through the use of frameworks and reflection. Examples from practice will be used to highlight how a therapeutic relationship is established and maintained in practice.

After reading this chapter you should be able to:

- Explain underpinning theories which are used to define a *therapeutic approach* in nursing.
- Identify key communication skills which assist in the development of a therapeutic relationship.
- Discuss the importance of person-centred care.
- Consider how systematic approaches can be used to enhance patient-centred care.
- Appreciate how the use of 'reflection' can positively impact upon your own practice.

Related NMC competencies

The overarching NMC requirement is that all nurses must:

... use excellent communication and interpersonal skills. Their communications must always be safe, effective, compassionate and respectful. They must communicate effectively using a wide range of strategies and interventions, including the effective use of communication technologies. Where people have a disability, nurses must be able to work with service users and others to obtain the information needed to make reasonable adjustments that promote health and enable equal access to services. (NMC, 2010a: 15, 2010b: 9)

─────────────── To achieve entry to the register as an ───────────────
adult nurse you should be able to:

- Build partnerships and therapeutic relationships through safe, effective and non-discriminatory communication, responding warmly and positively to people of all ages who may be anxious, distressed or facing problems with their health and taking account of individual differences, capabilities and needs.
- Practise autonomously, compassionately, skilfully and safely, and must maintain dignity and promote health and wellbeing.
- Use therapeutic principles to engage, maintain and, where appropriate, disengage from professional caring relationships, always respecting professional boundaries.
- Use a range of communication skills and technologies to support person-centred care and enhance quality and safety.
- Use the full range of communication methods including verbal, non-verbal and written to acquire, interpret and record your knowledge and understanding of people's needs.
- Demonstrate the ability to listen with empathy.
- Ensure that people receive all of the information they need in a language and manner that will allow them to make informed choices and share decision making.
- Recognise when language interpretation or other communication support is needed and know how to obtain it.
- Take into account the many different ways in which people communicate and how these may be influenced by ill health, disability and other factors, recognising and responding effectively when a person finds it hard to communicate.
- Recognise when people are anxious or in distress and respond warmly and positively to people of all ages effectively, using therapeutic principles to promote their well-being, manage personal safety and resolve conflict.
- Use effective communication strategies and negotiation techniques to achieve best outcomes, respecting the dignity and human rights of all concerned.
- Be aware of your own values and beliefs and the impact these may have on your communication with others.
- Carry out comprehensive systematic nursing assessments that take account of relevant physical, social, cultural, psychological, spiritual, genetic and environmental factors, in partnership with your patients and others through interaction, observation and measurement.

(Adapted from the NMC Standards of Competence for Adult Nursing, 2010a, 2010b.)

Therapeutic relationships

A therapeutic relationship in nursing involves nurse and patient working in partnership to help speed up the recovery process and enhance the patient experience (Peplau, 1991). However, due to the complexity of disease processes and the human body's resourcefulness it is important to acknowledge that patients may recover despite what we do rather than because of what we do. Nevertheless, the therapeutic relationship enables us to maximise the likelihood that an individual will recover because we have helped them in some way.

There is no single definition of a therapeutic relationship. Likewise there is no single means of defining the role of a nurse, other than a fundamental wish to make a positive difference to the patient's or service user's life. However, there are numerous models detailing the key elements of a therapeutic relationship.

Therapeutic relationship models

- **Travelbee**'s (1966) Human to Human relationship model: '... caring involves the dynamic, reciprocal, interpersonal connection between the nurse and the client developed through communication and the mutual commitment to perceive self and other as unique and valued'.
- **Paterson and Zderad** (1976) described humanistic nursing theory as a metatheory: 'a systemised body of knowledge formulated for the purpose of making something else possible' (Paterson, 1978: 50).
- **Watson** (1979) suggested that the therapeutic relationship is seen as a two-way reciprocal relationship between nurse and patient and that each 'grows' and learns from the other. She considers the mind, body and soul to be interlinked and describes ten factors that could provide a framework for nursing care: formation of an altruistic system of values; instillation of faith-hope; cultivation of sensitivity to self and others; development of a help–trust relationship; acceptance of positive and negative feelings; use of the scientific problem-solving method for decision making; promotion of interpersonal teaching–learning; provision for a supportive, protective and/or corrective mental, physical, socio-cultural and spiritual environment; assistance with the gratification of human needs and the allowance of existential–phenomenological forces.
- **Benner** (1984) explained that the nurse should view the patient with an unconditional positive regard, also known as 'mutuality'.
- **Peplau** (1987) identified three essential attitudes of the therapeutic relationship: genuineness, respect and empathy.
- **Muetzel**'s (1988) model of activities and factors in the therapeutic relationship includes intimacy, reciprocity and a partnership between patient and nurse. Intimacy includes 'spirit' closeness, vulnerability and atmosphere such as security and freedom with dynamics such as control, contact and communication.
- **Rogers** (1996) suggested five client-related outcomes of nursing presence: achievement of client goals, satisfaction with nursing care, comfort, growth, and enhancing care. These all encompass what is viewed as the therapeutic relationship.
- **Sundeen et al.** (1998) suggested four key stages:

  ○ A pre-interaction stage – requires planning and includes a review such as patient notes, past medical history and social circumstances.
  ○ An orientation stage – first meeting with the patient laying down the foundation of the relationship where good communication is imperative. A 'contract' is developed and this can be either formal or informal: it is the foundation of the relationship.
  ○ A maintenance phase – both the nurse and patient are progressing towards the agreed goal, each of which involves good communication and leads to 'feelings' being exchanged.
  ○ A termination phase – the ending of the relationship.

A therapeutic relationship is considered to be two-way, with both the patient and the nurse positively benefiting from the experience (McKlindon and Barsteiner, 1999). This falls within the notion of *reciprocity*, a theory underpinned by sociological concepts down the ages. Reciprocity can be defined as a positive act being returned via another positive deed between two individuals. Sociological studies have shown that such positive or 'kind' endeavours lead individuals to behave in a more friendly and cooperative way (Ernst and Gächter, 2000). A nurse's acts of kindness can give rise to feelings of well-being for both patient and nurse, which are likely to help build trust and aid the development of a positive therapeutic relationship.

Muetzel (1988) developed a theory of partnership, intimacy and reciprocity which enveloped three circles with the patient at the centre.

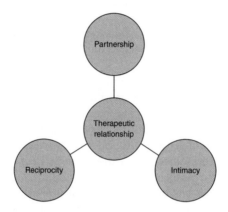

Figure 2.1   Meutzel's model of activities and factors in the therapeutic nurse-patient relationship (adapted from Meutzel 1988)

Intimacy includes *spirit closeness, vulnerability* and *atmosphere* such as security and freedom encompassing dynamics such as control, contract and communication. Although Muetzel's theory may seem dated it is still reflected in some government policies today. For example the *No Decision About Me, Without Me* (DH, 2012) proposals are aimed at ensuring that patients and their families are involved in the decision-making aspects of care provision. Similarly, an independent review of the use of the Liverpool Care Pathway (a multidisciplinary patient-centred tool for all health professionals involved in the terminal stage of life) highlighted concerns regarding instances where relatives had not been informed of the decision to end active treatment and where care decisions were taken without the consent of the families involved (Neuberger et al., 2013). (This is discussed further on p.404.)

The therapeutic relationship is concerned with both the *science* and *art* of nursing and how we transfer our knowledge and skills into meaningful exchanges with patients, service users and carers. The science of nursing is conceptualised by a scientific understanding of the human body (including normality and symptoms) and knowledge of the latest medications, treatments and evidence-based care. Conversely, the art of nursing includes the practitioner's high levels of emotional intelligence, expert interpersonal and communication skills and values-based care, which encompass the notions of compassion, empathy, trust, dignity and respect. The ability to engage in judiciously intimate interactions with patients is a key part of the therapeutic relationship (Williams, 2001). Nursing is dependent on a thorough understanding of its science and a mastery of its art. Factors such as experience and additional learning will influence the ease at which you are able to build effective therapeutic relationships with your patients. Yet compassion, empathy, emotional intelligence and good communication skills are at times far more important than experience. Adult nursing requires commitment, intellectual intelligence, emotional intelligence and the inherent capacity to care (see Figure 2.2).

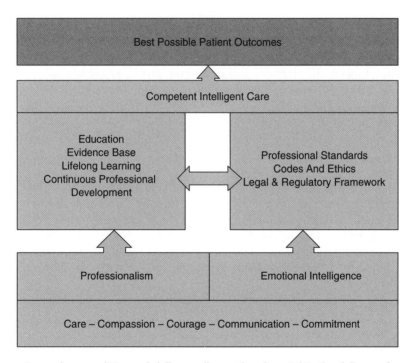

Figure 2.2   Core values, qualities and skills are all considered crucial to the delivery of competent, intelligent care

Moral dimensions of nursing care

By previously focusing on nursing history and the development of professional nursing in Chapter 1 you will have already explored the societal expectation that all nurses will possess characteristics associated with the strong moral virtues or values – sometimes being referred to by patients, public and the media as 'angels'. This was highlighted by Caroline Aherne (a sufferer of retina, bladder and lung cancer) who described her nurse as an 'angel' and someone who was 'able to answer all her questions, and laugh with her' (BBC News, 2014).

The expectation to do good; to be compassionate at all times, express empathy and sympathy and treat patients and their families with dignity and respect – these qualities are a fundamental requirement of the adult nursing role. They lie at the heart of delivering good nursing care and are the foundation of a therapeutic relationship (Von Dietze and Orb, 2000).

Compassion is a complex concept and is often discussed alongside associated notions such as empathy, sympathy, respect and dignity (Dewar et al., 2011; Nouewn et al., 1982). In fact, it is often difficult to separate these concepts as they are all inter-connected, resulting in ill-defined definitions of compassion. The *Oxford English Dictionary* (2014) describes compassion as 'sympathetic pity and concern for the sufferings or misfortunes of others'. However, Schantz (2007) believes that compassion goes further than purely sympathy and pity and involves actions to relieve distress. Other authors suggest that compassion is a basic human-to-human understanding and a need to receive and give comfort and alleviate someone's suffering, distress or pain (Nussbaum, 1996; Straughair, 2012). A great deal of emphasis has been placed on the integral part compassion plays in the delivery of good nursing care and effective therapeutic relationships by both government and professional bodies. Indeed, the NHS Constitution (DH, 2013), Northern Ireland's Strategy for Nursing (DHSSPS, 2000), The Scottish Government's Quality Strategy (2010) and NHS Wales's Quality Delivery Plan (2012) all outline pledges that patients, service users and carers can expect to be treated with compassion, humanity and kindness by all healthcare professionals. Likewise, compassion is a consistent thread throughout the Nursing and Midwifery Council's (NMC, 2010a, 2010b, 2015) competencies.

Empathy, often described as 'the ability to walk in another's shoes', has also been widely accepted as an essential part of effective nursing care and is at the heart of the therapeutic nurse/patient relationship. Empathy is a key component of compassion and the therapeutic relationship. It is an essential attribute – not only to have an understanding of a patient's emotional state but also to have the ability to remain professional. Empathy is different from sympathy as sympathy is more emotionally charged (Peplau, 1987).

According to Kunyk and Olson (2001), there are five conceptualisations of empathy:

- A human trait.
- A professional state.
- A communication process.
- A caring relationship.
- A special relationship.

That is not to say that when patients receive bad news as a professional you should remain stoic and motionless, but as an adult nurse you will still need to be able to function and support patients and their emotional needs, having an ability to put the needs of patients above your own.

Presence can also be linked with empathy as it entails sensitivity along with other traits such as holism, intimacy, vulnerability and the ability to adapt to unique circumstances (Finfgeld-Connett, 2006). Paterson and Zderad (1976) viewed nursing as an inter-subjective dialogue and transaction that involved meeting, relating and presence in a world of people, things, time and space. Further to this, Finfgeld-Connett (2006) suggests that there are six features of presence:

- Uniqueness.
- Connecting with the patient's experience.
- Sensing.
- Going beyond the science.
- Knowing.
- Being with the patient.

Fredriksson (1999) argues that the value of presence lies in a nurse's ability to create a space where a patient can be in deep contact with their suffering, thereby allowing that patient to share with a caring individual and assisting the patient in finding their own way forward. Rogers (1996) suggests five client-related outcomes of nursing presence: achievement of client goals; satisfaction with nursing care; comfort; growth and enhanced healing. The act of being present with a patient allows that individual to perceive a meaningful exchange. Boeck (2014) clearly illustrates the meaning and value of 'presence' in contemporary nursing practice (see Figure 2.3).

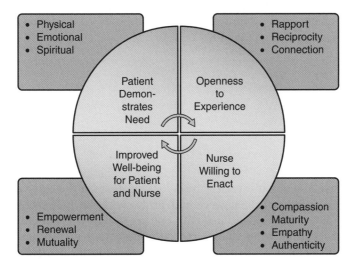

Figure 2.3   Presence: a concept analysis

Source: Boeck (2014)

Emotional intelligence (EI) is a concept that has been widely researched (though generally within psychology literature) and was made popular by psychologist and journalist Daniel Goleman (1995). However, EI is a relatively new concept to nursing even though emotions are perceived as vital to genuine, authentic and compassionate relationships. The importance of reflective practice has also already been established (see Chapter 1, pp.12–13). The use of reflection enables a therapeutic relationship to be developed and sustained through the assessment of our behaviours and our impact on patient care.

STOP AND THINK

Review the section in Chapter 1 which outlines the concept of EI if necessary (see p.18) before considering the following:

- What personal qualities would you associate with emotional intelligence?
- How might you use these positively to develop therapeutic relationships with patients?
- Consider how emotional intelligence links to the concept of professionalism and the 6Cs framework.

As nurses our work is clearly set within a rollercoaster of human emotions whether these be fear, pain, sadness and despair, or at the other end of the spectrum, joy, relief and hope. It is understandable that patients want empathic and emotionally competent nurses but it is equally clear that patients' perceptions suggest that these aspects are often lacking along with effective communication skills (Reynolds et al.,1999; Williams and Stickley, 2010).

A defining quality in being able to establish a therapeutic relationship is the ability to recognise what others are feeling. While this in part is being able to empathise, we must first recognise that there are some concerns or problems. As described below, in terms of communication, more than 90% of messages are transmitted non-verbally and as a result we must use our emotional intelligence to identify those feelings. The previous Stop and Think might have prompted you to include some of the following:

- Sensitivity.
- Awareness.
- Perceptive.
- Thoughtful.
- Anticipatory.
- Intuitive.
- In tune.
- Insightful.

You may also have noted that it is clear from looking again at the core values of the 6Cs in the context of emotional intelligence and professionalism that there are significant overlaps. Many of the values associated with one are also associated with the others and thus are many sides of the same thing – the *art* of nursing that is so fundamental to the therapeutic relationship. It is often through the application of these attributes and skills that we are able to identify the real issues faced by our patients. By having a sensitive awareness and/or intuition or by simply 'being interested', we can often pick up that something is wrong. Our own life experience of the same or similar situations enhances our ability to do this. However, previous experience in a similar situation that we have observed, reflected upon and learnt from also provides us with increasing perceptiveness or anticipation of what may occur. By listening carefully to what is being said, the tone or verbal expression that is used – and perhaps more importantly what is not said (along with facial expressions and body language) – can reveal more information to us.

The importance of effective communication

It is widely accepted that words form only a small percentage of our communication (Hargie et al., 2004; Sherman, 1993). Over 90% of communication is via non-verbal messages transmitted through our body language, tone and facial communication.

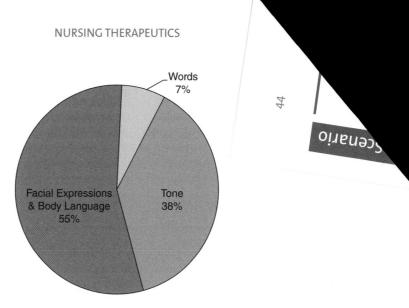

Figure 2.4 It's not just what you say, it is very much how you say it

Reflecting on the role that we ourselves play in our interactions is integral in understanding how effective we are as practitioners at communicating with others. Awareness of our own values and beliefs and how these influence our behaviours can also lead to us being more attentive to patients' needs and assist us to develop productive therapeutic relationships. To make our interactions with patients, service users and carers meaningful we must consider what we wish to achieve. For example, if we intend to advise how to take a medication this is likely to be achieved by using a more formal, verbal interaction with written information supplied to aid *concordance*. How we transmit information which is meaningful and that our patients are able to process and understand is crucial to prevent misunderstanding, misinterpretation and confusion. This is dependent on our ability to combine non-verbal and the most appropriate verbal communication through the use of jargon-free language coupled with active listening, questioning, clarification and summarising the conversation to ensure that we have been understood.

Active listening is defined by Mobley (2005) as the primary way of conveying empathy as it demonstrates that we are giving individuals our full attention. According to Webb (2011), active listening is important for several reasons. When people are worried they will often experience difficulties in communicating their ideas or problems clearly. It can help people who are in a stressful situation to get their ideas across so that their problems can be resolved more easily. Active listening is as much to do with body language as it is with verbal skills and such skills are particularly useful when people are angry or highly emotional. The skills of active listening include the following:

- *Attending and acknowledging* – e.g. providing verbal or non-verbal awareness of the other person.
- *Restating and paraphrasing* – e.g. responding to the person using their basic verbal message.
- *Reflecting* – e.g. feelings, experiences or content that have been heard or perceived through cues.
- *Summarising* – e.g. bringing together feelings and experiences to provide a focus.
- *Checking perceptions* – i.e. are your perceptions and interpretations accurate?
- *Being quiet* – e.g. giving the other person time to think as well as to talk.

HILDA

Hilda, an elderly lady under your care in hospital, is very upset. She is both tearful and fractious. She has mislaid her wedding ring but she doesn't tell you as she doesn't want to trouble you. You think she is a little agitated because she is due to undergo an operation in the morning.

- Consider how you would respond to this situation.

Freshwater (2003: 93) asserts that 'One sigh may be communicating a lifetime of emotions'. Having picked up that something is wrong, we then have to engage and this can be achieved very simply. It is the emotionally intelligent practitioner who hears the sigh, makes eye contact, communicates understanding and demonstrates human care. This very basic human contact – achieved through engaging with the eyes together with perhaps a knowing look or a smile – could in that moment have the most profound and healing effect (Freshwater and Stickley, 2004).

As an emotionally intelligent nurse in this situation you would speak to Hilda and try to elicit the reason for her distress. You might also consider that there could be another reason behind this (other than the obvious one) and would then actively explore the possibility. One way of earning Hilda's trust and respect would be by demonstrating genuine interest and care or as Rogers (1961) describes it 'being present'. Active listening requires a nurse to listen very carefully to what is being said so they are able to understand the position from the patient's point of view. More than this though, Egan (2002, 2006) argues that it also requires an ability to convey to the patient that they understand what has been said, not by repeating their words but to be present – *psychologically, socially,* and *emotionally*.

Hilda is far more likely to open up to you if she knows she will be actively listened to. By taking the time and care to find out more you might learn for example that Hilda had lost her wedding ring and that her husband of more than forty years had died only three months previously. You would therefore have a deeper understanding that the emotions expressed by Hilda were manifested in her raw grief. As an emotionally intelligent nurse you would perhaps use the whole spectrum of communication and interpersonal skills to allow Hilda to talk about and express her feelings and emotions, taking into account that she may be afraid of the impending surgery but that this has been compounded by the loss of her husband and now, further compounded, by not having the comfort of her wedding ring and all that it represented with her. Demonstrating this understanding could have a profound impact – even if the ring could not be found.

TIM AND STEFAN

Tim (a newly qualified staff nurse working on an orthopaedic ward) is providing post-operative care for Stefan, a young man who has fractured (broken) his tibia and fibula (lower leg). Stefan has returned from the operating theatre with a plaster of paris cast to his lower leg. During his early post-operative care, Tim checks Stefan's observations including his blood pressure. As Tim applies the blood pressure cuff he ascertains that Stefan seems uncomfortable, agitated and pale. Wanting to help comfort Stefan and on speaking to him further, Tim realises that he is experiencing intense pain around the site

of the plaster yet Stefan's blood pressure is only slightly raised. Tim
doctor to review Stefan who is quickly diagnosed with *acute compr*
medical emergency – and subsequently undergoes urgent surgery

(Note: Acute compartment syndrome is most likely to occur after a fracture
a crush injury and involves increased pressure due to either swelling or bleedin.
muscle bundle. Fascia surrounds the muscle bundles; it does not contain any elasticity a
unable to expand. Therefore, during bleeding or swelling, pressure increases due to the inelas-
ticity within the muscle. Additionally, the presence of a plaster of paris increases the pressure
further. Late diagnosis of compartment syndrome can lead to the loss of a limb or even life.)

In the above scenario, although Tim had little experience in the field of orthopaedics, good verbal and non-verbal communication skills coupled with compassion led to an accurate assessment of the patient's symptoms and condition. Tim concluded that Stefan's condition had deteriorated and consequently sought help. The therapeutic relationship between Tim and Stefan, in addition to the good working relationship between Tim and the doctor, resulted in quick and appropriate action being taken. Perhaps it is important here to also consider Tim's relationship with the doctor. Tim described Stefan's symptoms clearly to the doctor and coupled with the urgency in Tim's voice the doctor understood the need to attend the ward and review his patient.

Verbal communication

Communicating effectively through verbal discourse enables a nurse to establish whether a patient is confident and if they have understood what their care involves.

This is also clearly illustrated in the scenario below.

 HARSHA AND PETER

Harsha (the district nurse) is undertaking one of her weekly visits to her patient Peter. Peter's HBA1c blood glucose readings have been consistently higher than normal over the past six months despite being prescribed medication to control his diabetes. Harsha suspects that this might be due to the fact that Peter has stopped taking his medication regularly.

In order to understand if Peter takes his medication at a certain time of day, in a certain way, or has stopped taking it altogether further information is required. In nursing there are different purposes for our questioning and so we must use a series of open, closed or searching/probing questions. If we consider whether Peter is taking his medication as prescribed we may use closed questions such as 'Have you taken your diabetes *medication* today?' This is factual and can be used in an emergency situation or to give structure to a conversation. However, leading questions are generally considered to be unhelpful as the question may prompt and influence the question. This in turn may skew the information given by Peter when replying to the question. Open questions on the other hand are a way to allow him to give additional information. For example, asking what time of day he normally takes his medication allows for further discussion. searching or probing question would allow him time and help Harsha develop a deeper understanding of his perceptions. Therefore questioning in the right format is crucial to successfully communicating with patients and their carers.

Questioning styles

The types of questions Harsha may use during her interaction with Peter about his medication may include closed or open questions such as the following:

Example of a *closed* question: 'Do you understand how to take your medication?' (Peter's response would probably be 'yes' or 'no').

Example of an *open* question: 'What do you understand about taking your medication?'

Example of a *searching* question: 'How are you feeling today?'

Paralanguage is concerned with the way something is said such as the pitch and tone, the softness or loudness of words, all of which can support or contra-indicate what is being said (Thompson, 2011). Therefore it is important to consider not only what you are going to say but also how you are going to say it (see Figure 2.4). Of equal importance is the environment in which the communication takes place. The need to consider the scene for an interaction also plays a part in successful communication. In a study undertaken by Swayden et al. (2012), patients perceived that a doctor spent more time with them when he/she had sat down next to their bedside than when they had stood up, demonstrating how the perception of the time can be affected and lead to an increased satisfaction with the information received.

Non-verbal communication is concerned with anything that is communicated without the use of verbal language, such as the way we nod appropriately. In fact, Argyle (1988) suggested that non-verbal communication is up to five times more effective than verbal communication. During any interaction it is crucial that we consider how we are positioned in relation to a patient. Egan (2002) suggests using the acronym SOLER:

S = sit squarely in relation to the patient.

O = in an open position.

L = lean slightly towards the patient (at approximately 45 degrees).

E = maintain eye contact.

R = remain relaxed.

Applying the SOLER framework during a clinical interview when breaking bad news or during any other communicative contact with patients and/or relatives will help set the scene and put individuals at ease. If managed well it can also help us transmit empathy and compassion to those we are interacting with.

STOP AND THINK

Can you think of a conversation you have had with someone who has not given you their full attention or there is a contrast between what they are saying and what they are doing?

• How did it make you feel?

Consider a vulnerable patient who feels that they have not been listened to:

- How could you make this different?
- How could the environment, your body language, vocabulary, pitch and tone, as well as the content of your conversation affect the outcome of the situation?
- What could you do to show you are attentive to their needs?
- Does this interaction help to build a positive mutual relationship?

It may be that the inferences made through inflections in the voice or body language or the lack of eye contact were the main elements that led to your dissatisfaction. Professional communication is a skill that can be enhanced by being aware of your own interactions: it differs from social communication as it is purposeful, ethical and has boundaries. Good communication is an important component in any workplace and professional role. Moreover in nursing, excellent communication and advanced interpersonal skills are crucial for successful interactions with carers, other healthcare professionals and patients. They are the bedrock for formulating and maintaining therapeutic relationships. Effective communication is essential to ensure the best outcomes occur for our patients. However, unfortunately 18% of all hospital complaints arise from communication difficulties (Patient and Client Council, 2013) and therefore the use of communication as an effective tool should never be underestimated.

It is important to recognise that there are many potential barriers to effective communication. These include the following:

- Use of jargon, slang terms or abbreviations.
- Use of foreign languages, dialect or difficulties with speech.
- Sensory deprivation (i.e. blindness, deafness, or difficulty hearing).
- Cultural differences.
- Emotional difficulties, anxiety or distress.
- Environmental issues (i.e. poor lighting, noisy environments or physical barriers).

 GLADYS

Some years ago as a student I was encouraged, as part of my learning, to attend the 'ward round', whereby the nurse, the consultant and junior doctors went round the ward to receive an update on patients. This included examining each patient, ordering blood tests and confirming diagnoses with patients. We arrived at the end of Gladys's bed (an 85-year-old female patient) who was sat on the commode behind the curtains drawn around her bed. Apparently oblivious to her predicament, the consultant opened the curtains, proceeded to ask how she was and then informed her that she had a growth on her liver. Gladys thanked the doctor as he quickly left ... leaving Gladys still sat on the commode.

Case Scenario

This episode highlights the need for improvement in many areas, including lack of effective communication but perhaps more importantly a serious lack of respect for a patient's privacy and dignity is demonstrated. Gladys was very grateful and thanked the doctor for coming to see her. However, she clearly had not understood that she had a diagnosis of liver cancer and this illustrates very clearly the consultant's inability to deliver 'bad news' appropriately as well as his insensitivity and apparent lack of empathy and compassion. It is never easy to give bad news and perhaps this particular consultant found it extremely stressful to give a terminal diagnosis. According to Ptacek and MacIntosh (2009), delivering bad news can psychologically affect doctors due to the fact that they are sometimes unable to make a positive difference and as such this is often a source of heightened stress. Certainly in this scenario there are ways in which the breaking of bad news to Gladys could have been improved upon.

Delivering good news is easy: delivering bad news should be framed around all of the 6Cs outlined previously in Chapter 1. In the first place, and as professionals we must have the *courage* to deliver bad news. We must *carefully* and *compassionately* explain what is and is not possible and the reasons for this. We must also be credible and this is demonstrated through our *competence* and in how we *communicate* this in terms of what we say and how we say it and crucially, how we demonstrate that we have listened to and understood a patient's concerns. How we communicate is determined not least by our compassionate approach, demonstrating that we care for and are *committed* to our patient and their family (the topic of 'breaking bad news' is explored in more depth in Chapter 13, pp.401–403).

The use of therapeutic touch

Consideration should be given to the use of *therapeutic touch* as a means of non-verbal communication. There are formal ways of using touch (such as massage and Reiki) but the act of laying hands on a patient (such as hand holding) can also have a positive effect; it is a means of communication at a very basic human level. As children we are often nurtured and given lots of hugs by our parents and families. As adults, generally speaking, there are fewer opportunities to continue with this with the loss of partners and grown-up children. The *appropriate* use of touch can cut through culture, race and nationalities and can help us to connect with patients. It can be considered a visible sign of caring (Busch et al., 2012), although as healthcare professionals it is important to remain cognisant of cultural differences, certain settings and particular circumstances where touch is not appropriate (David Hizar and Giger, 1997). For example, a study carried out by Muliira and Muliira (2013) found that Muslim patients preferred to be asked before being touched (we will visit the topic of *cultural competence* later in this chapter). They proposed the use of an acronym 'TOUCH' that should be considered before using a therapeutic touch:

- T: Talk to patients and identify preferences and comfort levels before touch.
- O: Observe a patient's verbal and non-verbal cues to guide their preference, such as avoiding eye contact.
- U: Understand and show understanding when touch is rejected.
- C: Care provider (e.g. if the same sex it is more acceptable to the patient).
- H: Handedness (e.g. touch with the right hand is preferred as some Muslim patients believe the left hand is unclean).

Whilst Clark and Clark (1984) argue that empirical support for the use of therapeutic touch is weak some studies have shown that patients have benefited from the use of touch. These benefits can show a reduction in anxiety, a decrease in perceived pain and a reduction in heart rate and blood pressure (Blankfield et al., 2001; Denison, 2004; Woods et al., 2005).

Maslow, a humanist psychologist who examined animal and human behaviour, suggested that humans have a hierarchy of needs and also argued that unless we have our physiological needs fulfilled we cannot move further up the hierarchy (Maslow, 1943).

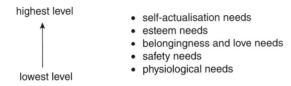

highest level

- self-actualisation needs
- esteem needs
- belongingness and love needs
- safety needs
- physiological needs

lowest level

Figure 2.5   A representation of Maslow's hierarchy of needs

Maslow's model considered five levels of need whereby individuals were able to move up to the next level. He suggested that our needs commence with basic physiological needs (e.g. food, water, warmth, rest), followed by safety needs (e.g. security), then belonging and love needs (e.g. having friends and intimate relationships), esteem needs (e.g. prestige, feelings of accomplishment and self-respect), and finally self-actualisation (e.g. achieving one's full potential and creative activities). The role of the adult nurse in any setting is to empower and educate our patients to try and achieve their goals.

Person-centred care

In recent years there has been a shift from the doctrine of the patient being at the mercy of healthcare professionals to one where the patient is now the centre of all decisions. *Person-centred care* (PCC) is considered the bedrock of good patient care and the opposite of disease- or task-based care, something that has been extensively implemented throughout nursing and medical history. PCC plays a key role in developing and maintaining a therapeutic relationship as it enables both patient and nurse to establish trust and understanding. Although there are numerous definitions of PCC and also differing terminologies for similar outcomes-based care, Rogers (1961) was one of the first to develop a form of PCC known as 'client-centred therapy'. This is not a technique but an approach based on a small set of core conditions that are required to facilitate therapeutic relationships, requiring high-level skills of emotion, intellect, attitudes and behaviour which encapsulate the concept of emotional intelligence discussed earlier. These conditions are:

- empathy;
- unconditional positive regard;
- congruence.

Unconditional positive regard is having an attitude that enables us to be non-judgemental and to act without bias or prejudice. Congruence relates to sincerity, genuineness, and 'being present' in the relationship because you genuinely care. It is the difference between caring *for the patient* and *caring about the person*. Corbin (2008) describes this as putting caring into practice through behaviours which address the specific needs of patients by getting 'in touch' with the person behind the patient to discover and understand those needs.

The overarching goal of PCC is to include patients or service users in the assessment and planning of their care to meet their agreed physical and psychological needs, ensuring that they feel valued, listened to and included. This method elicits trust between the nurse and patient and empowers the patient to make decisions about their own care and future health requirements, thereby fostering a productive therapeutic relationship. During PCC the *locus of control* or power between nurse or healthcare professional and patient is likely to be equally distributed (Parley, 2001).

Conversely, disease- or task-based care involves a nurse delivering care according to a patient's disease or symptoms. In such cases assumptions of a patient's requirements can often be made by those delivering care. Task-based care was constructed around Parsons' (1951) 'sick role' which theorised that a patient was dependent on a nurse, doctor or carer who was the most knowledgeable participant in the relationship. The power of the relationship was firmly within the remit of the healthcare professional and patients were often discouraged from asking about or questioning the care delivered by nurses or doctors.

Historically task- or disease-based nursing care was often delivered according to a nurse's schedule, focused around their need to 'get the job done' by the end of the shift rather than based on the needs of individual patients. This kind of care often involved the allocation of basic nursing care tasks as separate duties, with nursing staff focusing on a task or several tasks during their shift (such as observations, toileting, changing dressings, escorting patients to theatre). Unfortunately there are still elements of task-based nursing care in modern day nursing, particularly where time pressures are prevalent. Even recently, some NHS Trusts have asked nurses to introduce hourly interactions with patients to check that they have all that they require in terms of drinks and toileting. In some areas this has been translated into a cyclical routine exchange with each patient in turn and is sometimes referred to as 'rounding'. The method has been reported to demonstrate safe practice and protect patients from unnecessary harm (Dix et al., 2012). However, Snelling (2013) questions the validity of the evidence presented and suggests that further high quality research is required to fully evaluate the effectiveness of this method.

In general PCC is the care model of choice in mainstream nursing, with its advantages leading to effective relationships between patients and healthcare professionals. However, whilst the approach is more challenging to implement when patients or service users have diminished cognitive abilities or reduced capacity, there is some evidence that patients do better. For example, Edvardsson and Innes (2010) conducted a literature review related to PCC in patients with dementia. This suggested that implementing PCC reduced agitation and patients appeared calmer. The care of patients with dementia is discussed further in Chapter 12.

Case Scenario

 SONIA

Fifty-five year old Sonia (a female patient with terminal cancer) is admitted to hospital. Her mobility has reduced and her pain has increased. Outwardly she is a very positive person and is busily trying to arrange her wedding whilst on the ward. Her care plan is focused upon priorities agreed with her on admission, mainly to provide supportive care and mini-mise her pain to ensure she can attend her wedding venue. All of the staff are caught up in the excitement of the wedding and Sonia's positively upbeat attitude.

However, whilst walking past Sonia in her side room, a nurse asked how she was feeling. Sonia replied that she felt 'awful' but then quickly corrected herself and stated that she was fine. The nurse stopped what she was doing, sat down beside her and taking her hand asked

Sonia if she would like to talk. Sonia started crying and spoke of her fears of dying and questioned her decision to get married: 'Why should I be going to all this trouble when I know I am going to die anyway?' She also questioned whether she would live long enough to get married and how she would cope with the ceremony. The nurse held her hand throughout this time as Sonia relayed all her fears without interrupting or reassuring her that everything would be fine or offering false hope. During Sonia's stay, the nurse ensured that she did everything possible to keep her comfortable.

Sonia managed to get married and was discharged home after two weeks. She died peacefully at home.

This example encompasses not just the science but also the art of nursing and highlights the essential elements of the therapeutic relationship. The patient received timely patient-centred care based upon a clear understanding of the issues identified by utilising effective communication. The nurse demonstrated empathy and compassion with the use of therapeutic touch to alleviate her patient's distress. The presence of the nurse *just being there* made a difference, enabling the patient to open up and share her fears.

The importance of cultural competence in nursing

Cultural competence can be defined as having the attitude, knowledge and skills necessary for providing quality care to diverse populations: ensuring that the needs of all patients and service users are addressed irrespective of their ethnicity or cultural background (Seeleman et al., 2009). The term 'cultural competence' is often used to describe an ability to consider how social and cultural factors influence individual attitudes towards health and healthcare (Black and Purnell, 2002). At an interpersonal level, this includes having an ability to bridge cultural differences in order to build an effective therapeutic relationship. The key features of cultural competence are outlined by Saha et al. (2008) below:

- The ability of the healthcare organisation to meet the needs of diverse groups of patients. For example:

  o A diverse workforce which reflects the patient population
  o Healthcare facilities which are convenient for the community
  o Language assistance is available for patients with limited English proficiency
  o Ongoing staff training regarding the delivery of culturally and linguistically appropriate services

- The ability of a healthcare provider to bridge cultural differences in interpersonal interactions and to build an effective patient relationship. For example:

  o Exploring and respecting patient beliefs, values, preferences and their understanding of the meaning of illness
  o Building rapport and trust
  o Finding common ground
  o Being aware of own biases/assumptions
  o Being knowledgeable of other cultures

o   Being aware of disparities and discrimination affecting minority groups
o   Using an interpreter when needed (Saha et al., 2008).

As with a patient-centred approach, the essence of cultural competence lies in a nurse's ability to see a patient as an individual. In that sense Saha et al. (2008) suggest that there is some degree of overlap between the two and as cultural context and effective communication are relevant to the care of patients, cultural competence has the capacity to enhance patient centeredness and improve quality for all patients and not just those from a different ethnic, racial or cultural background to our own.

Think carefully about how you might demonstrate cultural competence in your daily nursing practice.

•   What will this involve?
•   How does this influence the outcome of the care that you deliver?

First and foremost you will need the ability to learn about yourself (i.e. be *self-reflective*).

Cultural awareness is defined as having the ability to acknowledge one's own culture, but also to recognise the potential for prejudice, bias and stereotyping. To recognise and reflect upon how our own culturally specific beliefs, customs and values influence not only our practice but also the behaviours of our patients and service users is crucial. Having the capacity to alter our behaviour in response to this deeper understanding is defined as *cultural sensitivity*. Matteliano and Street (2012) describe this as learning about different cultures and then adapting the way we deliver care to account for these differences.

It perhaps also goes without saying that you will need to draw upon most of the skills outlined earlier by:

•   building trust and conveying unconditional positive regard by never making assumptions about cultural practices or beliefs and showing respect for a patient's support group (e.g. their family, friends, religious leaders)
•   asking questions about cultural practices in a professional and thoughtful manner if necessary
•   addressing any communication or language barriers (e.g. using interpreter services if appropriate).

Patient-centred care and holistic assessment

It is crucial that nurses are able to deliver person-centred, evidence-based nursing care in a sensitive and compassionate manner. Care planning is a highly skilled process. Applying a systematic approach to this process is a way of encouraging us to think clearly about what we do for patients and why we do certain things rather than carrying out nursing tasks in a ritualistic fashion. It also provides us with opportunities to plan, implement and evaluate care effectively, taking into account all of the factors that can impact upon health. The *nursing process* was first conceived by Orlando (1961) as a cyclical way of focusing upon patient-centred nursing problems, setting agreed measureable and realistic goals intended to improve health. The modern-day process ASPIRE (Barrett et al., 2012) includes the following:

- *Assessment:* Find out what the patient can or cannot do.
- *Systematic diagnosis:* Make a nursing diagnosis – identify the health and nursing care needs of the patient.
- *Plan:* In discussion with the patient, come to an agreement about how their identified health and nursing needs can be met, setting mutually agreed goals.
- *Implement:* Deliver evidenced-based nursing interventions.
- *Recheck:* Consider if the interventions above are helping to meet the agreed goals.
- *Evaluate:* Measure and carefully document whether agreed interventions and approaches have been successful or not.

Following the evaluation of nursing interventions the cycle begins again with a re-assessment and evaluation of the effectiveness of the care undertaken in close collaboration with the patient. The cycle ensures that patient needs are constantly re-evaluated using the latest *evidence-based care.*

The assessment of patient needs and their care requirements can also involve the use of other nursing models, for example the Roper, Logan and Tierney model (2000) which encompasses 12 activities of daily living (see Figure 2.6).

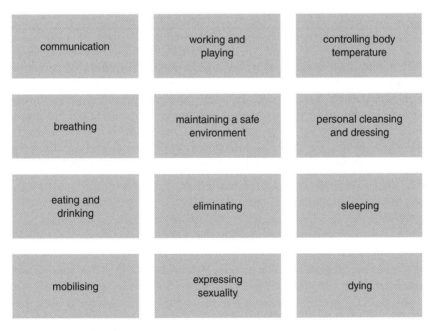

Figure 2.6   Activities of Daily Living

Source: Roper et al. (2000)

The Activities of Daily Living Framework (Roper et al., 2000) is one tool or framework that nurses can use to carry out an holistic assessment of patient need. The model respects the need to provide a 'cradle to the grave' nursing service that looks at the life continuum from birth until death and is applicable to patients irrespective of the disease or problems they are experiencing. However, care must be taken to ensure that the 'list' of ADLs is not merely used as a checklist. Instead, the process should involve nurse *and* patient setting short- and long-term goals for the actual and potential problems identified. To illustrate this further, we will consider a patient with Chronic Obstructive Pulmonary Disease (COPD).

RUTH

Ruth (a 67-year-old patient) has been admitted with an exacerbation of COPD. She is very breathless and finding it difficult to hold a conversation. She normally lives alone in a house with a bathroom upstairs. Her past medical history includes coeliac disease, osteoporosis and arthritis.

Consider the scenario above:

- How would you assess Ruth's needs?
- What frameworks or tools might help you in this process?
- What could you do to facilitate the development of a nurse-patient therapeutic relationship in this scenario?
- Will Ruth's condition improve because of what we do or in spite of what we do?

The NMC Code (2015:) states that we should 'put the interests of people using or needing nursing services first'. Therefore we will need to assess Ruth, ensuring that the care received is patient-centred, holistic, timely and safe promoting trust through professionalism. The depth of the assessment will depend on a variety of factors such as nurse expertise, the time available and the client's expectations, priorities and cooperation (Dowling, 2006). We would also need to assess Ruth's risk of developing pressure sores and/or falling due to her reduced mobility and malnutrition together with possible anxiety or depression.

ACTIVITY 2.1

Using some of the suggested Further Reading material at the end of the chapter undertake the following:

- Identify some of the various other models and frameworks than can be used to support a nurse in assessing, planning and evaluating care (including any other assessment tools that might help you with this process).
- Which of these (if any) you are currently using in your placement area.
- Determine the supporting evidence base for use of these tools.

The systematic nursing process which incorporates the Roper, Logan and Tierney model is useful in ensuring that a person-centred approach to care planning is adopted although as you will have recognised there are a number of other models and approaches also available. As a nurse you will find that using one single approach does not always fit every situation, and you may sometimes need to 'mix and match' tools and frameworks to ensure the best approach is adopted. Additional assessment tools you might use could include:

- a pressure ulcer risk assessment tool (e.g. Waterlow, 2008)
- a falls risk assessment tool (e.g. National Institute for Health and Care Excellence, 2013)
- a nutritional assessment tool (e.g. Malnutrition Universal Screening Tool (MUST), British Association for Parental and Enteral Nutrition, 2011)
- a depression and anxiety assessment tool (e.g. Patient Health Questionnaire 9PHQ-9, Kroenke et al., 2001).

We will be introducing you to various other assessment frameworks, models and tools in subsequent chapters.

Meeting the needs of a difficult/unpopular patient

The unpopular patient was originally described by Stockwell (1972) who concluded that people who behave in a certain manner (e.g. grumbling, complaining or otherwise demanding attention) could at times be considered by nursing staff to be difficult or unpopular. Certainly there are times that for whatever reason some patients project challenging behaviour and this may be due to many complex reasons. It could be that they are in pain, anxious or distressed; that they may be incapacitated, or feel that they have a lack of control due to their illness. Nevertheless it is the nurse's role to reflect on their own behaviours and find a way to develop a therapeutic relationship and remain professional.

 ALICE

Alice (a 76-year-old patient) was admitted to a four-bedded bay on a medical ward for routine investigations. Several days following her admission she became increasingly demanding, and in particular (during the nursing handover) kept on pressing the buzzer for various things she needed; for example fresh water, her pillows were uncomfortable and the duvet was not 'sitting right' on the bed. Because of this 'demanding' behaviour Alice became known as an 'unpopular' patient. A newly qualified nurse who had recently started working on the ward was caring for her. He spoke with Alice giving her his full attention, disregarded the comments made by other members of staff and found Alice to be very pleasant once he had engaged with her. It took some time to find out that previously she had been a nurse and liked to use the technical terms for things. He also established that she was very anxious and at times in acute discomfort. He explained to Alice that whilst he was caring for her he would do his utmost to ensure that she had what she required and was comfortable, but that he also needed to review other patients and offer them the same level of treatment. He also explained that he would return regularly to ensure that she remained comfortable. In doing so, he managed to build a rapport with Alice. She enjoyed and appreciated the regular contact and extra reassurance as she did not get many visitors.

Case Scenario

ANDRE

Case Scenario

Andre (a 42-year-old man) was admitted on to a surgical ward directly from theatre. Information given to the nurse at handover was that he had suffered deep lacerations from a knife injury. He was placed in a side ward and the nurse took his observations and completed a nursing assessment. He had many wounds to his abdomen and when checking his wound dressings the nurse asked Andre how he had sustained his injuries. Andre described how he had opened his front door to be confronted by a man wielding a knife who then tried to stab him, resulting in the numerous lacerations. It later transpired that Andre had been stabbed by his brother for allegedly raping his young niece.

STOP AND THINK

Consider the above scenarios and ask yourself the following:

- How would you feel towards Alice or Andre?
- How would you manage each situation?
- What are the challenges you would face?
- How would you develop a therapeutic relationship with patients who exhibit challenging behaviour or are unpopular? For example, would you be able to ensure your body language remained unchanged?
- How could the culture on the ward influence the reactions of members of staff to these patients?
- How might these affect each patient's recovery?

Roger's (1961) core condition of *unconditional positive regard* is simply having an attitude which enables us to be non-judgemental and to always act without bias or prejudice. In this way, the emotionally intelligent practitioner will not see or pre-judge either of these patients. Indeed, the NMC (2010a: 13, 2010b: 4) makes it clear that 'all nurses must practice in a holistic non-judgemental caring and sensitive manner that avoids assumptions, supports social inclusion, recognises and respects individual choice and acknowledges diversity. Where necessary you must provide the highest standard of practice and person-centered care possible at all times, additionally you must put aside your own personal and cultural preferences when considering the needs of those in your care.

STOP AND THINK

Either reflect on a situation that you may have already experienced or try to imagine that you are in the same situation as the nurse in each of these scenarios:

- Who could you talk to about this?

Look at the Gibbs model of reflection provided previously (p. 13):

- Can you use this model to help you to reflect on this or your chosen similar situation?

Consider the 6Cs introduced in Chapter 1: how would each of the these inform your approach?

It is very clear that compassionate care is central to nursing practice. As an adult nurse you will no doubt be faced with many challenging situations in the future that you will need to reflect upon and then consider how these experiences might influence or change your future practice. As healthcare professionals we learn to put the needs of others before ourselves. Nurses will often spend their working day exposed to the emotional strain of dealing with people who are sick or dying and those who have extreme physical and/or emotional needs. However, with an ever-increasing workload and an unprecedented demand on resources, nurses can often feel 'stressed' and begin to suffer from physical and mental fatigue. One American physician (Remen, 2006), suggests that '… the expectation that we can be immersed in suffering and loss daily and not be touched by it is as unrealistic as expecting to be able to walk through water without getting wet'. This emotional strain, coupled with other stress factors inherent in the healthcare work environment, results in healthcare professionals being especially vulnerable to stress and *burnout* and is more likely to occur when a nurse struggles with their work–life balance, job uncertainty, a lack of control in the workplace and feeling undervalued (Garosa et al., 2011).

ACTIVITY 2.2

Access the following articles and then write down your answers to the questions that follow:

- www.compassionfatigue.org/pages/RunningOnEmpty.pdf

- Wright. S. (2013) 'The differences between stress, burnout and compassion fatigue', *Nursing Standard*, 28(5): 34–35.

- Thompson, A (2013) 'How Schwartz rounds can be used to combat compassion fatigue', *Nursing Management*, 20(4): 16–20.

What is 'compassion fatigue'?

1. Who does it affect?
2. How might we recognise it in ourselves and/or our colleagues?
3. What are the contributory factors?
4. What can we do about it?

It is important to develop some strategies to cope with such stressors. Maytum et al. (2004) found that both short- and long-term coping strategies, such as taking part in self-care activities (for example, going to the gym, walking and having a sense of humour and a positive mental attitude) were useful. Longer-term strategies included having an awareness of the various triggers and developing coping strategies, for example having supportive relationships that are both professional and personal.

Summary

Contemporary nursing practice demands an ability to build therapeutic relationships with all of our patients. The development of an effective therapeutic relationship, the ability to demonstrate empathy, compassion and caring, foster reciprocity and uphold the professional values of nursing are what remain central to the delivery of good nursing care. To do this well you will need to be able to communicate effectively with all of your patients, putting them at the heart of your decision-making processes, listening to their views and involving them in decisions that are taken about their care (so long as they are willing and able to do so). Systematic approaches to nursing care and nursing models offer processes that can guide the delivery of high quality person-centred nursing care. However, as health services continue to evolve it is essential that our practice is based upon sound nursing values and principles. The use of reflection enables us to continue to build upon and learn from the interactions we have with patients, carers and colleagues. Additionally, the use of empathy and the 6Cs, encompassing care and compassion, is a vital element of nursing therapeutics that should be realised and put into practice by all nurses.

Suggested further reading

Arnold, E. and Underman-Boggs, K. (2011) *Interpersonal Relationships: Professional Communication Skills for Nursing*, 6th edition. St Louis, IL: Elsevier Saunders.

Barrett, D., Wilson, B. and Woollands, A. (2012) *Care Planning: A Guide for Nurses*, 2nd edition. Harlow: Pearson.

Freshwater, D. (2002) *Therapeutic Nursing: Improving Patient Care through Self Awareness and Reflection*. London: Sage.

Holland, K., Jenkins, J., Solomon, J. and Whittam, S. (2008) *Applying the Roper-Logan-Tierney Model in Practice*, 2nd edition. Edinburgh: Churchill Livingstone.

NHS Education for Scotland (2009) *Spiritual Care Matters. An Introductory Resource for All NHS Scotland Staff*. Edinburgh: NHS Scotland

Orem, D.E. (2001) *Nursing: Concepts of Practice*. St Louis, IL: CV Mosby.

Smith, P. (2011) *The Emotional Labour of Nursing Revisited: Can Nurses Still Care?*, 2nd edition. Basingstoke: Palgrave Macmillan.

Stockwell, F. (1972) *The Unpopular Patient*. London: RCN.

References

Argyle, M. (1988) *Bodily Communication*, 2nd edition. London: Methuen.

Arnold, E. and Underman-Boggs, K. (2011) *Interpersonal Relationships: Professional Communication Skills for Nursing*, 6th edition. St Louis, IL: Elsevier Saunders.

BAPEN (British Association for Parental and Enteral Nutrition) Available at: www.bapen.org.uk (last accessed 12 September 2014).

Barrett, D., Wilson, B. and Woollands, A. (2012) *Care Planning: A Guide for Nurses*, 2nd edition. Harlow: Pearson.

BBC News (2014) *Caroline Aherne: Humour Helps Deal with Cancer*. Available at: www.bbc.co.uk/news (last accessed 26 June 2014).

Benner, P. (1984) *From Novice to Expert: Excellence and Power in Clinical Nursing Practice*. Menlo Park, CA: Addison-Wesley.

Benner, P. (1998) 'Nursing as a Caring Profession'. Paper presented to the American Academy of Nursing, Kansas City, MO.

Black, J.D. and Purnell, L.D. (2002) 'Cultural competence for the physical therapy professional', *Journal of Physical Therapy Education*, 16: 3–10.

Blankfield, R.P., Sulzmann, C., Geotz Fradley, L., Artim Tapolyai, A. and Zyzanski, S.J. (2001) 'Therapeutic touch in the treatment of Carpal Tunnel syndrome', *Journal of the American Board of Family Practice*, 14(5): 335–42.

Boeck, P.R. (2014) *Presence: A Concept Analysis*. doi: 10.1177/2158244014527990 2014 4: SAGE Open.

Busch, M., Visser, A., Eybrechts, M., Komen, R., Oen, I., Olff, M., Dokter, J. and Boxma, H. (2012) 'The implementation and evaluation of therapeutic touch in burn patients: an instructive experience of conducting a scientific study within a non-academic nursing setting', *Patient Education and Counselling*, 89: 439–46.

Carper, B. (1978) 'Fundamental patterns of knowing in nursing', *Advances in Nursing Science*, 1(1): 13–23.

Clark, P.E. and Clark, M. J. (1984) 'Therapeutic touch: is there a scientific basis for the practice?', *Nursing Research*, 33 (1): 37–41.

Corbin, J. (2008) 'Guest Editorial: is caring a lost art in nursing?', *International Journal of Nursing Studies*, 45: 163–5.

David Hizar, R. and Giger, J.N. (1997) 'When touch is *not* the best approach', *Journal of Clinical Nursing*, 6: 203–6.

Denison, B. (2004) 'Touch the pain away: new research on therapeutic touch and persons with fibromyalgia syndrome', *Holist Nurs Pract*, 18: 142–51.

Department of Health (2012) *Liberating the NHS: No Decision About Me, Without Me*. Available at: www.gov.uk/government/uploads/system/uploads/attachment_data/file/216980/Liberating-the-NHS-No-decision-about-me-without-me-Government-response.pdf (last accessed 22 June 2014).

Department of Health (2013) *The NHS Constitution*. Available at: www.nhs.uk/choiceintheNHS/Rightsandpledges/NHSConstitution/Pages/Overview.aspx (last accessed 29 September 2014).

Department of Health, Social Services and Public Safety (2000) *A Partnership for Care, Northern Ireland Strategy for Nursing and Midwifery 2010 - 2015*. Belfast: DHSSPS.

Dewar, B., Pullin, S. and Tocheris, R. (2011) 'Valuing compassion through definition and measurement', *Nursing Management*, 17 (9): 32–7.

Dix, G., Phillips, J. and Braide, M. (2012) 'Engaging staff with intentional rounding', *Nursing Times*, 108(3):14–16.

Dowling, M. (2006) 'The sociology of intimacy in the nurse patient relationship', *Nursing Standard*, 20: 48–54.

Edvardsson, D., Winblad B. and Sandman P.O. (2008) 'Person-centred care of people with severe Alzheimer's disease: current status and ways forward', *Lancet Neurology*, 7(4): 362–367

Edvardsson, D. and Innes, A. (2010) 'Measuring person centred care: a critical comparative review of published tools', *The Gerontologist*, 50(6): 834–46.

Egan, G. (2002*) The Skilled Helper: A Problem Management and Opportunity Development Approach to Helping*, 7th edition. Pacific Grove, CA: Brooks Cole.

Egan, G. (2006) *Essentials of Skilled Helping: Managing Problems, Developing Opportunities*. Pacific Grove, CA: Brooks Cole.

Ernst, F. and Gächter, S. (2000) 'Fairness and retaliation: the economics of reciprocity', *Journal of Economic Perspectives* 14(3): 159–81.

Finfgeld-Connett, D. (2006) 'Meat-synthesis of presence in nursing', *Journal of Advanced Nursing*, 55(6): 708–14.

Fredriksson, L. (1999) 'Modes of relating in a caring conversation: a research synthesis on presence, touch and listening', *Journal of Advanced Nursing*, 30(5): 1167–76.

Freshwater, D. (2003) *Counselling Skills for Nurses, Midwives and Health Visitors*. Buckingham: Open University Press.

Freshwater, D. and Stickley, T. (2004) 'The heart of the art: emotional intelligence in nurse education', *Nursing Enquiry*, 11(2): 91–8.

Garrosa, E., Moreno-Jimenez, B., Rodriguez-Munoz, A. and Rodriguez-Carvajal, R. (2011) 'Role stress and personal resources in nursing: a cross-sectional study of burnout and engagement', *International Journal of Nursing Studies*, 48(4): 479–489.

Gibbs, G. (1988) *Learning by Doing: A Guide to Teaching and Learning Methods*. Oxford: Further Education Unit, Oxford Polytechnic.

Goleman, D (1995) *Emotional Intelligence*. New York: Bantam.

Green, J. and Tones, K. (2010) *Health Promotion: Planning and Strategies*, 2nd edition. London: Sage.

Hargie, O., Dickson, D. and Tourish, D. (2004) *Communication Skills for Effective Management*. Basingstoke: Palgrave.

Inzucchi, S.E., Bergenstal, R.M., Buse, J.B., Diamant, M., Ferrannini, E., Nauck, M., Peters, A.L., Tsapas, A., Wender, R. and Matthews, D.R. (2012) Management of hyperglycaemia in type 2 diabetes: a patient-centered approach: Position statement of the American Diabetes Association (ADA) and the European Association for the Study of Diabetes (EASD), *Diabetologia*, 55:1577–96.

Kaye, P. (1996) *Breaking Bad News*. Northampton: EPL.

Kroenke, K., Spitzer, R.L. and Williams, J.B. (2001) 'The PHQ-9: validity of a brief depression severity measure', *J Gen Intern Med*, 16(9): 606–13.

Kunyk, D. and Olson, J.K. (2001) 'Clarification of conceptualizations of empathy', *Journal of Advanced Nursing*, 35(3): 317–25.

Maslow, A.H (1943) 'A theory of human motivation', *Psychological Review*, 50(4): 370–96. Available at: http://psychclassics.yorku.ca/Maslow/motivation.htm (last accessed 5 March 2015).

Matteliano, M.A. and Street, D. (2012) 'Nurse practitioners' contributions to cultural competence in primary care settings', *Journal of American Academy of Nurse Practice*, 24(7): 425–35.

Maytum, J.C., Heiman, M.B. and Garwick, A.W. (2004) 'Compassion fatigue and burnout in nurses who work with children with chronic conditions and their families', *Journal of Pediatric Health Care*, 18(4): 171–17.

McKlindon, D. and Barnsteiner, J.H. (1999) 'Therapeutic relationship', *American Journal of Maternal and Child Health Nursing*, 5: 237–43.

Mobley, J. (2005) *An Integrated Existential Approach to Counseling Theory and Practice*. Lewiston, NY: Edwin Mellon.

Muetzel, P.A. (1988) 'Therapeutic nursing'. In A. Pearson (ed.), *Primary Nursing: Nursing in the Burford and Oxford Nursing Development Units*. Beckenham: Croom Helm.

Muliira, J. and Muliira, R. (2013) 'Teaching culturally appropriate therapeutic touch to nursing students in the sultanate of Oman: reflections on observations and experiences with Muslim patients', *Holist Nurs Practice*, 27(1): 45–8.

National Institute for Health and Care Excellence (2013) *Falls: Assessment and Prevention of Falls in Older People, Guideline [CG161]*. Available at: www.nice.org.uk/guidance/cg161 (last accessed 22 November 2014).

Neuberger, J. (2013) *More Care, Less Pathway: A Review of the Liverpool Care Pathway*. Independent review of the Liverpool Care Pathway (Executive Summary). Available at: www. gov.uk/government/uploads/system/uploads/attachment_data/file/212450/Liverpool_Care_Pathway.pdf (last accessed 23 July 2014).

NHS Wales (2012) *Achieving Excellence: The Quality Delivery Plan for the NHS in Wales*. Cardiff: Welsh Assembly Governement.

NHS Wales (2014) *Education Programmes for Patients*. Available at: www.wales.nhs.uk/sites3/home.cfm?orgid=537 (last accessed 23 July 2014).

NICE (2013) *Fall Assessment and the Prevention of Falls in Older People*. Available at: http://pathways.nice.org.uk/pathways/falls-in-older-people (last accessed 23 September 2014).

Nouwen, H., McNeill, D. and Morrison, D. (1982) *Compassion: A Reflection on the Christian Life*. London: Darton, Longman and Todd.

Nursing and Midwifery Council (2010a) *Standards for Pre-Registration Nursing Education*. London: NMC. Available at: http://standards.nmc-uk.org/PublishedDocuments/ (last accessed 5 March 2015).

Nursing and Midwifery Council (2010b) *Standards for Competence for Registered Nurses*. Available at: www.nmc-uk.org/Documents/Standards/Standards%20for%20competence. pdf (last accessed 5 March 2015).

Nursing and Midwifery Council (2015) *The Code: Professional Practice and Behaviour: Standards of Nurses and Midwives*. London: NMC.

Nussbaum, M. (1996) 'Compassion: the basic social emotion', *Social Philosophy and Policy Foundation*, 13(1): 27–58.

Orlando, I.J. (1961) *The Dynamic Nurse-Patient Relationship: Function, Process And Principles.* New York: G.P. Putman's Sons. [Reprinted 1990, New York: National League for Nursing.]

Oxford Dictionaries (2014) *Oxford English Dictionary.* Available at: www.oxforddictionaries. com/definition/english/compassion (last accessed 21 June 2014).

Parley, F. (2001) 'Person-centred outcomes: are outcomes improved where a person-centred care model is used?', *Journal of Intellectual Disabilities,* 5(4): 299–308.

Parsons, T. (1951) *The Social System.* London: Routledge & Kegan Paul.

Paterson, J. and Zderad, L. (1976) *Humanistic Nursing.* New York: NLN.

Patient and Client Council (2013) *Annual Complaints.* Report 212/2013. ISBN 978-0-9576919-40.

Peplau, H.E (1987) 'Interpersonal constructs for nursing practice', *Nurse Education Today,* 7: 201–8.

Peplau, H.E. (1991) *Interpersonal Relations in Nursing.* New York: Springer. (Original work published 1952.)

Ptacek, J. and MacIntosh, E. (2009) 'Physician challenges in communicating bad news', *J Behav Med,* 32: 380–7.

Rathert, C., Wyrwich, M.D. and Boren, S.A. (2012) 'Patient-centered care and outcomes: a systematic review of the literature', *Medical Care Research and Review,* 70(4): 351–79.

Remen, R.N. (2006) *Kitchen Table Wisdom: Stories that Heal* (10th anniversary edition). London: Penguin.

Reynolds, W., Scott, B. and Jessiman, C.W. (1999) 'Empathy has not been measured in clients terms or effectively taught: a review of the literature', *Journal of Advanced Nursing,* 30(5): 1177–85.

Rogers, C. (1961) *On Becoming a Person: A Therapist's View of Psychotherapy* Wiltshire: Redwood Books.

Rogers, C. and Farson, R. (1987) 'Active listening'. In R.G. Newman, M.A. Danzinger and M. Cohen (eds), *Communicating in Business Today.* Washington, DC: Heath and Co.

Rogers, S. (1996) 'Facilitative affiliation: nurse-client interactions that enhance healing', *Issues in Mental Health Nursing,* 17 (3): 171–84.

Roper, N., Logan, W.W. and Tierney, A.J. (2000) *The Roper-Logan-Tierney Model of Nursing: Based on Activities of Living.* London: Churchill-Livingstone.

Roper N., Logan W.W. and Tierney A.J. (1980) *The Elements of Nursing.* Churchill Livingstone.

Saha, S., Beach, M.C. and Cooper, L.A. (2008) 'Patient centeredness, cultural competence and healthcare quality', *Journal of Natural Medicine Association,* 100 (11): 1275–85.

Schantz, M. (2007) 'Compassion: a concepts analysis', *Nursing Forum,* 42: 48–55.

Schon, D. (1983) *The Reflective Practitioner.* London: Temple Smith.

Schon, D. (1991) *The Reflective Practitioner: How Professionals Think and Act.* Aldershot: Avebury.

Seeleman, C., Suurmond, J. and Stronks, K. (2009) 'Cultural competence: a conceptual framework for teaching and learning', *Med Educ,* 43(3): 229–37.

Sherman, K.M. (1993) *Communication and Image in Nursing: Behaviours that Work.* New York: Delmar.

Snelling, P. (2013) 'Intentional rounding: a critique of the evidence', *Nursing Times,* 109 (20): 19–21.

Stockwell, F. (1972), *The Unpopular Patient. The Study of Nursing Care Project Reports.* London: Royal College of Nursing.

Straughair, C. (2012) 'Exploring compassion: implications for contemporary nursing, Part 2', *British Journal of Nursing,* 21(4): 239–44.

Sundeen, S.J., Stuart, G.W., Rankin, E.A.D. and Cohen, S.A. (1998) *Nurse–Client Interaction: Implementing the Nursing Process,* 6th edition. St Louis, MO: Mosby.

Swayden, K., Anderson, K., Connelly, L., Moran, J., McMahon, J. and Arnold, P. (2012) 'Effect of sitting versus standing on perception of provider time at bedside: a pilot study', *Patient Education and Counselling,* 86(2): 166–71.

The Scottish Government (2010) *The Healthcare Quality Strategy for NHS Scotland.* Edinburgh: The Scottish Government.

Thompson, N. (2011) *Effective Communication: A Guide for People Professions*, 2nd edition. Basingstoke: Palgrave Macmillan.

Todd, G. (2002) 'The role of the internal supervisor in developing therapeutic nursing'. In D. Freshwater (ed.), *Therapeutic Nursing*. London: Sage. p.62.

Travelbee, J. (1966) *Interpersonal Aspects of Nursing*. Philadelphia: F.A. Davis.

Von Dietze, E. and Orb, A. (2000) 'Compassionate care: a moral dimension of nursing', *Nursing Inquiry*, 7(3): 166–74.

Waterlow, J. (2008) *Pressure Ulcer Risk Assessment and Prevention*. Available at: www.judy-waterlow.co.uk/waterlow_score.htm (last accessed 23 September 2014).

Watson, J. (1979) *Nursing: The Philosophy and Science of Caring*. Colorado: University of Colorado Press.

Watson, J. (2003) 'The Attending Nurse Caring Model: Integrating theory, evidence and advanced caring-healing therapeutics for transforming professional practice', *Journal of Clinical Nursing*, 12: 360–65.

Webb L., (2011) *Nursing: Communication Skills in Practice*. Oxford: Oxford University Press.

Williams, A. (2001) 'A literature review on the concept of intimacy in nursing', *Journal of Advanced Nursing*, 33(5): 660–7.

Williams, J. and Stickley, T. (2010) 'Empathy and nurse education', *Nurse Education Today*, 30: 752–5.

Willis Commission (2012) *Quality with Compassion: The Future of Nursing Education*. Available at: www.williscommission.org.uk/ (last accessed 21 June 2014).

Woods, D.L., Craven, R.F. and Whitney, J. (2005) 'The effect of therapeutic touch on behavioral symptoms of persons with dementia', *Alternative Therapies in Health and Medicine*, 11(1): 66–74.

3 Interprofessional and Multidisciplinary Team Working

JEAN ROGERS

So far, the previous chapters have focused on the knowledge and skills required to be an adult nurse as well as the concept of safe and effective person-centred care. However, often this cannot be achieved by one individual: it takes a team of healthcare professionals to deliver truly effective quality patient care. The aims of this chapter therefore are to explore how *interprofessional* and *multidisciplinary working* have the potential to positively impact upon the health needs of patients and identify factors that contribute to the development of therapeutic partnerships.

After reading this chapter you should be able to:

- Define the terms interprofessional and multidisciplinary working.
- Reflect upon and identify the factors that contribute to the development of a therapeutic partnership and team work considering how you can develop these skills.
- Identify and reflect upon factors that can prevent a collaborative partnership and team working.
- Explore strategies for overcoming the barriers to interprofessional working and consider how you can develop these skills.
- Explore the benefits of effective team working in the provision of effective healthcare and consider how you can apply these within a contemporary healthcare setting.

Related NMC competencies

The overarching NMC requirement is that:

> All nurses must work effectively across professional and agency boundaries, actively involving and respecting the contribution of others to the provision of integrated person-centred care. They must know when and how to communicate with and refer to other professionals and agencies in order to respect the choices of service users and others, promoting shared decision making, to deliver positive outcomes and to co-ordinate smooth, effective transition within and between services and agencies. (NMC, 2010: 21, 2010b: 7)

To achieve entry to the register as an adult nurse you should be able to:

- Work independently as well as in teams.
- Understand the roles and responsibilities of other health and social care professionals and seek to work with them collaboratively for the benefit of all who need care.
- Maintain accurate, clear and complete records (including the use of electronic formats) using appropriate and plain language.
- Respect individual rights to confidentiality and keep information secure and confidential in accordance with the law and relevant ethical and regulatory frameworks, taking into account local protocols.
- Actively share information with others when the interests of safety and protection override the need for confidentiality.

(Adapted from the NMC Standards of Competence for Adult Nursing, 2010.)

Real examples and case studies will be used throughout the chapter so that you are able to gain a wider perspective of interprofessional and multidisciplinary working. However, before exploring interprofessional and multidisciplinary working further it would be useful to define what each term means.

STOP AND THINK

What do the terms 'multidisciplinary' and 'interprofessional' working mean to you?

Multidisciplinary working describes the mechanism by which holistic care for patients is ensured and a seamless service is delivered across the boundaries of primary, secondary and tertiary care (Jeffries and Chan, 2004). However, it is about the task and not necessarily the collective working process and therefore it does not imply collaboration. There are some distinct advantages and disadvantages to multidisciplinary working.

Table 3.1 Advantages and disadvantages of multidisciplinary working

Advantages	Disadvantages
Patient receives better all-round care	Differing professions work together but keep their defined role (working in their silos)
All plans can be discussed so that all pros and cons can be considered	Takes more time to come to conclusions
Less likely anything is missed	Information not always shared properly
Team members aware of progress in case anyone becomes ill	Communication can be a challenge
Best use of resources	Erodes professional identity
Reduces the number of people to whom the patient needs to relate	

Alternatively, Pollard et al. (2005:4) define *interprofessional working* as 'when two or more professions/or agencies work and/or learn together collaboratively to provide integrated health and/or social care for the benefit of the patient'. This is supported by Day (2006: 9) who believes it is about 'professions relating to and among each other for the mutual benefit of those involved'. Similarly there are also some clear advantages and disadvantages to interprofessional working which will be discussed later in the chapter.

Barrett et al. (2005) believe the prefix *multi* indicates the involvement of personnel from different professions and does not imply collaboration, whereas *inter* implies collaboration. Therefore, it is judicial to define collaboration.

What does collaboration mean to you?

STOP AND THINK

Biggs (1997) defines *collaboration* as working together to achieve something that no profession could achieve alone. Barrett et al. (2005) agree and describe collaboration as a common purpose that develops mutually negotiated goals with agreed plans and procedures. Individual knowledge and expertise are brought together to facilitate decision making that is undertaken jointly with shared viewpoints from a number of professions for the benefit of patients. So as Barrett et al. (2005) maintain, collaborative practice is the same as interprofessional working.

The terms 'interprofessional' and 'multidisciplinary' are often used interchangeably and thus for the purposes of this chapter we will be using the term *interprofessional working*. To understand these concepts further it is judicial to look at the background to interprofessional working.

Background to interprofessional working

Interprofessional team working is a key driver in any contemporary healthcare setting. Working interprofessionally is seen by all professional bodies as essential in promoting effective patient care. However, it is not a new concept (Lavin et al., 2001) as team working has been an integral part of healthcare from the 1960s onwards (Baldwin, 1993). Prior to this, staff from various disciplines worked in distinct professional teams (silos) and had no real knowledge of what each other's roles entailed. This often resulted in the multiple duplication of documentation which often resulted in patients being asked for the same details over and over again. Patient care was also fragmented. Ongoing developments in approaches to service delivery also resulted in high levels of specialisation. Irvine et al. (2002) maintain this often meant that it was not possible for any one professional to have the knowledge and skills to respond appropriately to patient need, particularly where the complex needs of communities or individuals are required.

What do you think are the key strengths of interprofessional working?

STOP AND THINK

One of the key strengths of interprofessional working is that the combined expertise of a range of health professionals is used to deliver seamless, comprehensive care to individual patients. The World Health Organization (WHO, 2010) suggest that interprofessional collaboration is an essential component of satisfactory service delivery. Barrett et al. (2005) argue that the quality of service received is dependent on how effectively different professions work together. This is supported by Baker et al. (2006) who believe that the modernisation of healthcare delivery has initiated a move towards the collaborative delivery of care and that this effective teamwork links to more positive patient outcomes (Grumbach and Bodenhiemer, 2004).

1997 saw massive and radical changes in health and social care policy, with UK governments advocating collaboration and clear partnership working across the public sector, and placing a strong emphasis on collaborative working and its importance in meeting patients' needs by bringing together health and social care professionals across a range of organisations. It was clear that in order for health service modernisation to be effective, robust and integrated, professional working was required. In England this was promoted further in the NHS Plan (DH, 2000a), a ten-year plan to reform practice which was instrumental in shaping the way we view and adopt interprofessional working today. Indeed UK healthcare provision has changed radically and rapidly in the last decade and this is reflected in political and policy decisions at all levels, regionally, nationally and internationally (Furlong and Smith, 2005).

ACTIVITY 3.1

Within NHS settings, what recent changes are you aware of that have impacted upon the delivery of patient care?

• Make a list of these.

Now access one of the following websites below and identify the relevant government health policy documents which highlight the changing context in which healthcare is delivered in your area:

England: www.gov.uk/government/organisations/department-of-health

Scotland: www.scotland.gov.uk/

Northern Ireland: www.dhsspsni.gov.uk/

Wales: www.wales.gov.uk

In England several documents highlight the changing context in which healthcare is delivered: these include the *NHS Plan* (DH, 2000a), *Modernising Nursing Careers: Setting the Direction* (DH, 2006), *Nursing Towards 2015* (NMC, 2007), *Pre-registration Education: Phase 1* (NMC, 2007), *High Quality Care for All: Next Stage Review* (DH, 2008) and the *Berwick Report* (DH, 2013). Additionally, the *Health and Social Care Bill* (HoL, 2011), *Health and Social Care Act* (HoC, 2013) and Willis Commission Report (2012) all highlight the changing context in which healthcare is delivered. These documents emphasise the increasingly busy environment in which care takes place, the constantly changing staff population, the growing use of technology, the increasing acuity of the patient population, an ageing population and the move to more community nursing with limited resource availability. Such changes will continue and there is now more than ever a realisation of the importance of holistic patient-centred care and a wider recognition that no one person has the knowledge and skills to deliver high quality care (Atwal and Caldwell, 2005). Thomas (2005) also maintains that the active contribution of patients to the decision-making process will make working together truly collaborative. This has currently become more crucial than ever with the general public becoming increasingly aware of highlighted examples of poor NHS care, for example in Bristol (DH, 2001), the Royal Liverpool Children's Enquiry (Redfern et al., 2001) and the Mid Staffordshire NHS Foundation Trust (2013).

Socially and politically there is a demand for service-user involvement in planning and prioritising service delivery, with UK governments promoting the principle of choice for users and working in partnership. For example, in 2006 the Department of Health stressed the importance of effective interprofessional and multidisciplinary working when planning services for people with long-term needs (DH, 2006). The aim was to establish joint health and social care teams, using joint case-notes and/or records to support people with the most complex needs, and thereby ensuring that care was truly multidisciplinary. Indeed, there are some excellent examples where teams have been able to work effectively and collaboratively together (e.g. some multidisciplinary teams working with people with severe and long-term mental health problems in their own homes have demonstrated real benefits: see Thornicroft and Tansella, 2002). Healthcare professionals working in interprofessional teams communicating and addressing the complex needs of the patients, as well as combining expertise, perspectives and resources, are able to form a common goal to restore, maintain and improve outcomes for patients.

Reflect on the teams you have previously worked within.

- Has your experience been a positive or negative one?
- Why do you think this might be?

STOP AND THINK

Over the last decade significant progress has been made towards creating environments where interprofessional working can thrive and be a positive experience, but in some practice areas it appears this is not so easy to achieve (Hanson et al., 2008). There have been numerous examples where difficult and challenging interprofessional working has been reported (Glasby et al., 2008). Atwal (2002) argues this is because power, status, autonomy and expert knowledge have become challenges. Weiss and Welbourne (2008) agree, stating that the characteristics of some professions bring about distinct occupational identities and exclusionary market shelters (domination) which set occupations apart and often in opposition. Kell and Owen (2008) maintain that this is as a result of creating boundaries so tight that only one profession can deliver that activity (e.g. medicine) which can then make them static. This strong group bonding legitimises participants and ensures they have negative attitudes to people outside of their group.

You may remember that in Chapter 1 we highlighted that until late in the twentieth century some groups - predominantly male occupations (e.g. medicine) - were identified as professions, with distinct characteristics of completing a course of education to at least graduate level, having autonomy and self-regulation and remaining free from managerial control. Alternatively, other predominantly female occupations (e.g. nursing, midwifery) were seen as semi professions that in contrast received 'training' and were regulated and overseen by other occupational groups (Barrett et al., 2005).

Kesby (2002) maintains that the current drive towards interprofessional working will help to give the semi professions power to raise their status. Jeffrey and Trowman (2009) however disagree and state that professions are losing their position of prestige and trust. Medicine and other professions are also 'under attack'. The development of Clinical Commissioning Groups (CCGs) has seen new NHS organisations set up to organise the delivery of NHS services in England underpinned by the *Health and Social Care Act* (DH, 2012), thus giving other clinicians as well as GPs the power to influence commissioning decisions for their patients.

A PRISON

A large male prison sends prisoners with medical problems for scans on an individual basis to the local hospital. Only one prisoner is able to attend at a time for security reasons and has to be accompanied at a cost of £250 a visit. Therefore waiting times for these patients are vast. There are also further problems in that prisoners have to be handcuffed, resulting in a high failure rate for scans (for security reasons the prisoners are not told in advance the day or time of the scan). This has often meant that they are not prepared properly, for example having eaten when they should not have done so. In response to the issues identified above, the prison service and CCG aimed to develop a more collaborative approach to meet patient need. The local CCG commissions a GP-led ultrasound team who visit the prison once a week, working with and alongside the prison healthcare team, scanning seven or eight prisoners at any one time. This saves local money, improves efficiency and provides dignity for the prisoners (Bradford, 2008), thus streamlining their care.

The above scenario provides a good example of how money can be saved in the NHS. However, it is not just about saving money but utilising precious resources more efficiently and effectively in order to achieve a better standard of patient care. This may require greater involvement and collaboration between the private sector and charities as well as healthcare providers. On the other hand though, media scandals such as the Shipman Enquiry (Smith, 2002), the Bristol Enquiry (DH, 2001) and failures at the Mid Staffordshire NHS Trust (Francis, 2013) have changed the public perception of professions, thereby increasing law suits. The public have become much more knowledgeable through the increase in technology and education, making knowledge more accessible. However, sometimes that knowledge is incorrect or limited and does not provide the full evidence. It can therefore be much more challenging to negotiate and compromise with members of the public. This has also had an effect on policy, creating turbulence where policy is formulated in order to achieve political goals, address systemic failings, and produce rapid fire responses to public disillusionment (Bradford, 2008). Healthcare professionals working within these environments are then left to make sense of new ways of working and demands, i.e. what they do and how they should go about it (Baxter, 2011).

List the reasons why people/patients may lose faith in the NHS.

- What effect do you think this might have on the healthcare professionals working within this service?

Across the United Kingdom (UK) poor interprofessional collaboration has been identified as a contributing factor in very high profile cases with poor outcomes (DH, 2001, 2003; Laming, 2009; Francis, 2013). Following such criticisms people lose faith with the NHS because they are concerned with carelessness in services, long waits and poor communication. For health professionals this can cause disillusionment with the profession and lower morale. There are assumptions that interprofessional working will prevent such tragedies as well as poor practice, however as yet there is no real research or evidence to support this assumption. This is mainly due to the complex nature of the research, the funding available, and the collaboration needed across practice and Higher Education Institutions to execute meaningful research studies (Barr et al., 2005).

There are however some advantages to interprofessional working. What do you think these are?

There are distinct advantages to interprofessional working which include the following:

- Enhancing personal and professional confidence. For example, Chloe, a nursing student on her first placement, has been on the ward for a few weeks. A doctor asks her to take some blood samples from a lady who was going to theatre. Chloe had met the doctor at an interprofessional education (IPE) session and felt able to inform the doctor that she could not do this as she had not been taught how to. The doctor therefore proceeded to undertake this with Chloe observing the procedure.
- Promoting mutual understanding of all the professions and their roles.
- Promoting interprofessional communication and breaking down barriers to communication.
- Recognising and respecting each professional role and their contribution to patient care.
- Contributing to job satisfaction: working together in harmony makes working life much better.
- Sharing information and knowledge to provide improved decision making regarding patient care (Spry, 2006).
- Problem sharing: as the old adage goes 'a problem shared is a problem halved'. Just talking through patient care problems with another professional colleague can sometimes help to provide the solution to a problem.

Case Scenario

 SANJIT

Sanjit suffered a spinal injury and after many months of rehabilitation he was more or less ready to go home. Members of the multidisciplinary team had been involved in his care. Physiotherapists had got him to a stage where he could transfer himself from his wheelchair to a bed or toilet. The occupational therapist had assessed him as being able to make simple drinks and food. The nursing staff had ensured he remained motivated and had included his family in his care. The doctors had monitored him and ensured he had recovered and the pharmacist had ensured his medication met his new needs. Sanjit was going on a home visit with a view to staying at home if all was okay. Two hours later he returned to the ward very subdued. The occupational therapist explained to the team that when Sanjit arrived at his home he was unable to get into the house as the doors were not wide enough: she also advised that it could take up to two weeks for the adaptation service to resolve this. One small thing was therefore keeping Sanjit in hospital and damaging his morale which could affect his future. On further discussion one staff member suggested that she would contact the facilities staff and ask them for a favour. She rang them and explained the situation and they promised to carry out the alterations in the next hour 'although it was not part of their remit'. The occupational therapist agreed to stay on in order that Sanjit could be safely discharged as planned. The doors were widened and the patient was discharged that day much to his and the team's delight.

The case scenario above illustrates multiprofessional working at its best with all disciplines working together to achieve streamlined quality patient care that helped Sanjit to return back to his own home as soon as possible.

Case Scenario

 GEORGE

George was admitted to hospital following a stroke which resulted in him suffering a left-hand side weakness and speech difficulties. A case conference was held to agree a discharge plan (attended by the social worker, an occupational therapist, a physiotherapist, a speech and language therapist, one of the nursing team and a medical colleague). The physiotherapist was concerned that George's wife, Gloria, may not manage. The occupational therapist offered to carry out a home assessment visit prior to discharge to ensure that she could. The team devised a mobilisation programme to enhance George's mobility, a social work assessment to see if he needed any more help and a speech and language assessment to ensure that his nutrition remained at an optimum level. The speech and language therapist also helped Gloria to communicate with her aphasic husband. George was discharged home three weeks later.

- Referring to the above scenario, what do you think went well?
- What could have been improved and how?

This scenario displays good interprofessional working, although this could have been improved further by including of the patient and his wife in the discussions!

Barriers to effective team working

While acknowledging there are some real advantages to interprofessional working we must also admit that there are some real barriers. Lymbery (2006) maintains that not acknowledging barriers to interprofessional working is, in itself, a cause of failure and that it is crucial to recognise all the stumbling blocks encountered. Some of the common barriers to interprofessional working might include the following:

- *Suspicion of the motives behind collaboration* (e.g. is this about improving patient care or is there a different agenda?).
- *A lack of confidence in one's own professional knowledge base for fear of being wrong.* For example, a newly qualified nurse might not challenge a newly qualified doctor because of fears she might be wrong and does not want to appear as if she is not sure what she is talking about.
- *Traditional professional cultures.* For example, joint working is difficult where there are perceived status differences between occupational groups. Some practitioners view this as a threat to their professional status, autonomy and control when asked to participate in more democratic decision making.
- *Mistrust of other professions* due to a lack of knowledge leading to stereotyping.
- *Lack of training and preparation to work in teams.*
- *Lack of shared values, visions and principles.*
- *Lack of investment on an individual, professional and organisational level.*

Consider your current or recent placement and the teams you have worked in:

- Did the teams work well together or not?
- Why do you think this was the case?
- Try to identify all of the potential barriers to effective team working. How do you think these might be overcome?

STOP AND THINK

Greater communication, problem solving and sharing common values and goals would be a starting point. Humphries and Hean (2004) also believe that the high profile cases already mentioned previously highlight not only the need to move towards collaborative team working but also a need to review professional education and training in the UK, with a view to making this interprofessional as well as driving the interprofessional agenda within health and social care organisations (something that we will discuss again later in the chapter).

Team working

Working in health and social care settings usually involves some aspect of team working. Effective team working does not just happen when a team of people work together – in fact team work could be really poor in a group of people working together or could be really effective.

Katzenbach and Smith (1993) define team work as a small number of people who have skills that are complementary and are committed to a common purpose, performance goals and approaches, generating synergy through their co-ordinated effort. Within a healthcare setting, team working is vital in delivering high quality care. The best outcomes are achieved when professionals work and learn together, as well as engaging in clinical audits and generating innovative ways of moving the practice and service forward together. In order to do this effectively there are some key factors that encourage team work (Reeves et al., 2009; Salas et al., 2009).

These include the following:

- *Personal commitment* – this comes from individuals who are committed to the success of the team and also requires that the leader of the team allows members to ask questions. In teams where this occurs, all the members will have an idea about what best practice is and staff are not expected to go beyond their level of competence unsupported. Their weaknesses however are minimised and their strengths maximised, thereby releasing their true potential.
- *A common goal or vision* – all teams need to develop a common goal or vision. When teams are working towards a common goal they are committed and this inspires people to learn and gain confidence. In fact within healthcare teams there may need to be two visions: one for the team and one for the organisation.
- *Clarity of roles* – staff need to be clear about their various roles within a team as this will maintain their motivation. It is also important that they are clear about the roles of other team members. In today's environment we are increasingly working with members from different organisations and professional groups. It is thought that this understanding encourages a team approach to patient need, where information and knowledge are shared to enable improved decision making regarding patient care (Spry, 2006). This will also encourage mutual trust and respect within teams.
- *Communication* – effective communication between team members is crucial for patient safety. It encourages joint problem solving and the provision of excellent interprofessional patient-centred care. The team will adopt two-way information giving rather than unidirectional pathways, thus ensuring information is shared with the whole team.
- *Support* – the best teams work most effectively where there is a framework to support interprofessional working. Pirrie et al. (1998) however believe the degree of support can be variable.

Interprofessional working can be really effective if all of the above occur. However there are some advantages and barriers to such team working.

STOP AND THINK

Consult the views of current members of the team in which you are working.

- What do they think are the advantages and disadvantages of team working?

There are some clear advantages to team working in a healthcare setting (Clements et al., 2007; Leggat, 2007). In the Stop and Think above your colleagues may have identified some or all of these:

- *Improvements in the quality of patient care* – when the team communicates effectively and work together as a unit the quality of patient care increases. They have a clear commitment to excellence of care. This increases co-ordination, especially in complex cases. Imagine what would happen in the following scenario if the team did not work together efficiently.

PATRICK

A patient is admitted to the emergency department following a road traffic accident where he has been knocked off his bike. He is unconscious and has serious life-threatening injuries. The trauma team (i.e. nurses and doctors) are on stand-by and the radiographer has also been called on stand-by in case she is needed. When the patient arrives he is being resuscitated: the nurses and doctors quickly assess the situation, call the radiographer, the orthopaedic surgeons and the chest surgeons, and the patient is quickly (once stabilised) taken to theatre. He survives and goes home six weeks later.

- *Improvements in patient safety* – if team work is effective the patient becomes an active partner in their own care. The patient is listened to and monitored and procedures are based on feedback. This has the potential to reduce medication errors and unnecessary procedures, thereby creating a safer environment for the patient.
- *Improvements in staff satisfaction*– teams that work efficiently and effectively brainstorm and problem solve together. The workload tends to be distributed more evenly and stress is reduced.
- *Improvements in communication* – because the team members regularly interact with each other they are able to contribute to the decision making in the team, thus making their shared goals and visions achievable.
- *Improved knowledge of each person's role* – a team working well together will learn about each person's role and limitations. This strengthens relationships and builds unity in the team.
- *Enhanced reflection* – efficient and effective teams regularly reflect on how they work together and how effective they are being.
- *More innovative approach to work* – a team that works well together can potentially be more innovative in their outlook. There is verbal and practical support for new ideas, thus moving the team forward.
- *Improved problem solving* – an effective team bounces ideas off each other. Each person offers their unique perspective on a problem and comes up with the best solution.
- *Enhanced skills* – no one person is the same as another and so teams need to use each person's unique skills to improve one other and be more productive in the future.

Disadvantages of team working

As you can see, there are many advantages to team working which are often talked about but there are some disadvantages here too (Day, 2006; Sim et al., 2014). These include the following:

- *Unequal participation* – sometimes some members of the team will sit back and let others do most of the work. This can have an adverse effect by causing resentment which can then cause conflict and affect morale.

- *Members who are not team players* – some people do not function well as part of a team and prefer to work alone. They can be excellent workers in the right situation but have difficulty fitting into a team, thus causing dissatisfaction and disharmony.
- *A lack of constructive conflict* – once a team works well together members may become reluctant to argue or dispute a point. If all conflict is avoided resentment can build up and team members can become lazy and apathetic, thus stifling creativity.
- *Traditions and professional cultures* – for some this can cause split loyalties between the team and their own discipline. Some team members may be reluctant to accept suggestions from other professions and become very defensive, particularly if they are used to assuming sole responsibility.
- *Personality clashes* – not all people can get on all of the time and personality clashes can occur. These can then cause unwanted conflict in a team and even split the team.

STOP AND THINK

You will no doubt have come across some of the barriers identified above in some of your practice placements.

- How do you think these could be overcome? (Before reading on note down your ideas.)

Overcoming the barriers to team work

Barriers can be overcome with time and patience and by undertaking the following:

- *Choosing the right members of the team* – although this is not always possible in a healthcare setting as far as is practicable this should be done. Some team players may have to move to another area if they cannot work in the team.
- *Team building* – allow time for the team to get to know each other and each person's role and unique contribution to the team. This allows team members to develop respect for one another.
- *Develop an atmosphere of trust and respect in the team members* – this takes time and effort and actions speak louder than words.
- *Ensuring clarity of team goals* – ensuring members of the team understand the team's common goal and vision. These should include specific and measurable outcomes.
- *Encouraging a supportive environment* – make sure that all members are aware how their action or inaction might impact upon their patients and other team members.
- *Encourage debate and constructive challenges* – this can help the team to keep improving and coming up with their own ideas. Mechanisms need to be developed to review goals and roles over time.
- *Dealing with conflict* – this needs to be dealt with and resolved right away otherwise it can prove detrimental to the team.

The importance of record keeping and team work

There is no denying that record keeping is crucial in healthcare and each member of a team has personal responsibility and accountability for good record keeping (NMC, 2010a, 2010b, 2010c, 2015) including students. Patient record keeping is one of the most basic clinical tools that we can use to ensure that our patients receive the best possible clinical care. This helps us communicate with each other and is essential for ensuring that an individual's assessed needs are met in a timely and efficient manner.

The principles of good record keeping apply to all types of patient records (e.g. electronic, hand-held or written) and include the following:

- Handwriting should be legible.
- All entries to records should be signed. In the case of written records, the person's name and job title should be printed alongside the first entry.
- In line with local policy, there should be a date and time on all records. This should be in real time and chronological order, and as close to the actual time as possible.
- Records should be accurate and recorded in such a way that their meaning is clear.
- Records should be factual and not include unnecessary abbreviations, jargon, meaningless phrases or irrelevant speculation.
- Professional judgement should be used to decide what is relevant and what should be recorded.
- All details of any assessments should be recorded and reviews undertaken and provide clear evidence of the arrangements made for future and ongoing care. This should also include details about information given with regard to care and treatment.
- Records should identify any risks or problems that have arisen and show the action taken to deal with them.
- All entries should communicate fully and effectively with colleagues, ensuring that they have all the information they need about the people in our care.
- Team members must not alter or destroy any records without being authorised to do so.
- In the unlikely event that we need to alter our own or another healthcare professional's records, we must give our name and job title and sign and date the original documentation. We should make sure that the alterations we make, and the original record, are clear and auditable.
- Where appropriate, the person in our care, or their carer, should be involved in the record-keeping process.
- The language used should be easily understood by the people in our care.
- Records should be readable when photocopied or scanned.
- Coded expressions of sarcasm or humorous abbreviations to describe the people in our care should not be used.
- Records should not be falsified.

What can you do as a student nurse to ensure that you are involved in effective record-keeping processes?

STOP AND THINK

As a student it is important that you are involved in all aspects of a patient's record keeping. You will need to discuss with your mentor the best ways you can do this within the placement. However, your record keeping should clearly differentiate between facts, opinion and judgements.

The way in which record keeping is undertaken is generally set out by the employer and in the past each discipline within a multiprofessional team would have maintained their own separate records. However, with an ever-increasing focus on improving the quality of care for patients, *clinical governance* is now a driver to maintaining and improving the delivery of quality care to patients. One of the main components of clinical governance is the use of high quality systems to effectively monitor clinical care for clinical record keeping and the collection of relevant information (DH, 1998). This has led to many employers looking towards integrating their record keeping for all disciplines. The NMC (2010c) support the use of the same documentation within agreed protocols by all members of the team providing patient care because this can enhance collaborative working. The advantages of having one document for all patient notes are:

- improved communication;
- reduction in the duplication of information;
- reduction in the recording of irrelevant data;
- maintains the continuity of a patient's journey;
- it encourages deeper discussion about a patient and their care.

More recently electronic record keeping has become more prevalent as national programmes for the use of information communication technology and electronic record keeping are introduced throughout the UK. Electronic records that are complete, integrated and legible offer added value as they can be accessed from multiple sites and can be used to generate risk alerts and prompts indicating that new information is available (Pullen and Loudon, 2006). However, this can sometimes causes issues for students in the practice area as they need to be able to obtain a password in order to access the systems. Despite this paper records will not be made obsolete for some time and the principles of good record keeping must be adhered to regardless of how records are held.

Confidentiality

Confidentiality is as crucial in record keeping as it is in all aspects of healthcare and is identified in Article 8 of the European Convention of Human Rights (European Court of Human Rights, 1990). It is not acceptable for any member of staff **including students** to discuss patients or their care outside of the clinical setting (e.g. in public where they could be overheard or on social media) or to leave records unattended where they could be seen. All of this is covered by the *Data Protection Act* (1998) which governs the processing of information that can identify individuals. Patients need to be assured and have confidence in all staff that their data are protected. This is covered by legislation from common law and statute law.

STOP AND THINK

What is the difference between the terms 'common law' and 'statute law'?

Common law refers to decisions made by a court of law; *statute law* is passed in parliament. Under these laws every patient can expect that any information given to a healthcare practitioner (including students) will only be used for the purpose given. It also encompasses a person's right to control access to their health information. Therefore if a relative was to ask for information on a patient that patient would have to be consulted. In fact confidentiality also continues following the death of a patient.

Consider how a person's confidentiality can be broken.

- How might this occur?
- What would you do if you suspected that there had been a breach in confidentiality?

If you believe there has been a breach of confidentiality you must raise your concerns with someone in authority. A risk or breach of confidentiality may be due to individual behaviour or as a result of organisational systems or procedures. The NMC Code (NMC, 2015: 8) is clear on this and states that 'You must be supportive of colleagues who are encountering health or performance problems. However, this support must never compromise or be at the expense of patient or public safety'. We have a professional duty to take action to ensure the people in our care are protected and failing to take such action could amount to professional misconduct. There are however certain circumstances where records can be disclosed.

Disclosure

In all circumstances and if at all possible, patients should be consulted and access to their records given with consent. They need to know why and with whom the information is being shared and give their consent freely. The only time that information about patients can be shared without consent is 'when the interests of patient safety and public protection override the need for confidentiality' (NMC, 2015: 6). This includes the detection and prevention of serious crime and to prevent abuse or serious harm to others. As healthcare professionals we need to be aware that disclosures of this nature need to be justified to the courts and the NMC, so clear and accurate decision trails (i.e. documentation) need to be kept.

Contrary to popular belief, the police do not have an automatic right to access to patients records and must obtain a warrant to do so. However, if a person is at risk of serious harm then it is acceptable but must be discussed with your management team and/or your union or NMC and patient consent should be sought.

Record keeping in healthcare is a potential minefield. Therefore you need to ensure that you abide by the NMC Code (2015) and the local policies of the organisation you are working within.

Developing your team working skills

Team work and interprofessional working are crucial to the future of the NHS and nursing. The 'hub and spoke model' to facilitate student learning has been adopted in some placement areas. This model involves the main practice area that a student is allocated to being termed the 'hub' and the 'spokes' being the other disciplines that are associated with that speciality. This then guides students to who they should seek to work with and also to explore how a team approach contributes to the patient experience in this area.

An example of a hub and spoke placement

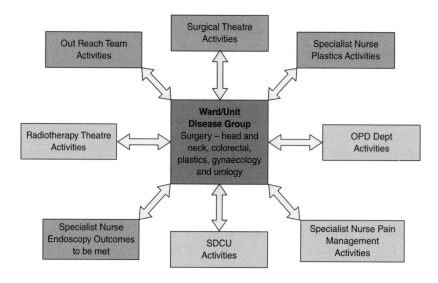

Figure 3.1   Hub and spokes model

How might you use the above model on your placement to help you develop key team-working skills?

Key skills which could be achieved by applying this model include:

- developing a better understanding of the roles and responsibilities of other professionals;
- building partnerships and therapeutic relationships through safe, effective and non-discriminatory communication;
- working effectively across professional and agency boundaries, actively involving and respecting others' contributions to integrated person-centred care.

As a student nurse you could start by speaking to your mentor and exploring the other services or departments that are connected to that placement: in doing so you can really start to develop a deeper understanding of the roles of others. For example, if you are working on an elderly care ward, it would be useful to spend some of your time with the discharge coordinator. You can then reflect on their role:

- What is the discharge policy and how does it work in practice?
- Who do they need to liaise and collaborate with to ensure the discharge goes smoothly?

Under supervision you could then go on to plan a discharge of your own. This will help you become more confident and competent in your role and your future role as a trained member of staff.

As a student nurse (or even as a newly qualified nurse moving into another area of practice), consider how you might integrate into a new team.

- What could you do to enhance the integration process?

Integrating into teams

Wherever you are working it is essential that you try and integrate into the teams you will work with as soon as possible. Here are some suggestions:

1. Do a little detective work and find out about the team you are joining (even if only for a short while) before you get there. This might involve visiting the organisation's website or calling the placement area to ask them a little about the services they provide. If you are near enough, try to arrange to pop in for a short visit. This can often make a good first impression (though consideration should always be given to the demands on staff, particularly in a very busy environment!).
2. Once you are on the placement, find out who the key members of the team are and arrange to go and see them in collaboration with your mentor. Refer to the hub and spoke model mentioned previously and try to fill in the diagram as it relates to your placement area. This could help you identify relevant learning opportunities.
3. Be proactive rather than reactive as this really helps in the placement area. If you just stand around waiting to be told what to do you and who to meet with this will not make a good impression.
4. Know what you want to learn about the specialism and the team before you go on placement and discuss this also with your mentor/educator. So long as this plan meets the related learning outcomes of your placement the team should help you achieve these.
5. Demonstrate a willingness to work as part of the team in all aspects of patient care.
6. Ask questions – learn as much as you can about all the professionals working to provide holistic patient care. Do not be afraid to ask any member of the team what they contribute to the care of the patient (no question is a silly question!).

There are many challenges and opportunities in healthcare today. You will definitely need to plan and identify your experience and needs before you get to the placement and once there it is a good idea to let your mentor/educator know what these are.

Interprofessional Education (IPE)

At this point it is judicious to define and explore the concept of interprofessional education further as it does have an impact on interprofessional working. CAIPE (2002: 19) define IPE as 'when two or more students of different professions within health and social care engage in learning from and about each other'. In the past nurses, doctors and allied health professionals (AHPs) were always educated separately and there were no real opportunities for learning together. Therefore cohesive team working in everyday practice did not always occur. However, the delivery of the NHS's modernisation agenda requires interprofessional practice that is underpinned by robust and integrated working and learning (DH, 2000, 2001).

Therefore, the context of healthcare policy and the nature of healthcare itself have both had a major influence on educational developments in relation to interprofessional teaching and learning. The World Health Organization (WHO) began to promote IPE and following their lead some countries developed organisations that were dedicated to IPE. At the forefront in the UK is CAIPE (The Centre for Advancement of Professional Education). Numerous other drivers include relevant professional bodies: the Nursing and Midwifery Council (NMC, 2009), the General Medical Council (2006), and the Health and Care Professions Council (2014).

It is suggested that interprofessional education should take place as early as possible to help to break down the artificial walls that separate professional training and help to reinforce the silo working that we know exists (Rafter et al., 2006). Reynolds (2005) recommends this is best executed in practice placements and in Higher Education Institutions (HEIs). In fact it is recommended that interprofessional curricula be implemented where students from all disciplines can meet and collaborate before they enter practice settings in order that they can build the basic values of working in interprofessional teams. The WHO (1988) recognises that if healthcare professionals are taught together and learn to collaborate throughout their student years, there is much more of a chance that they will work together in their professional lives. Lloyd Jones et al. (2007) advocate that this will ensure practitioners are equipped with effective team-working skills to enhance patient care. The face-to-face interaction of different professionals should help to prevent stereotyping and inform and challenge outdated beliefs. Although this is the ideal it is not always possible in practice and can prove very difficult to achieve logistically.

ACTIVITY 3.2

Reflecting upon your current and any previous placements, identify all of the potential/actual opportunities available to you for interprofessional learning:

- Have these been arranged by your employing organisation or your educational provider?
- Is there potential for you to be able to arrange individualised/bespoke/informal IPE for yourself (i.e. bespoke or experience days with other professionals)?

Write down/make a list of all the potential opportunities available to you. Discuss the practicalities and possibilities of these with your mentor.

As an individual nurse you can often find creative ways for interprofessional learning to occur throughout your career so that you are able to continuously develop the skills you will need to work with other professions. Whilst IPE does takes place in practice on a day-to-day basis, Lloyd Jones et al. (2007) maintain it is not easily recognised or acknowledged by staff. If it does occur it is usually very sporadic and ad hoc, with a lack of planning for specific experiences and a reliance on opportunistic experiences. Miers et al. (2008) agree and also believe that even if staff do value the importance of IPE they choose to prioritise profession-specific skills.

However, it is perhaps important here that we differentiate IPL and IPE from 'shared learning' (e.g. where professionals sit in the same lecture theatre), recognising that some key skills that all health professionals could be taught together (for example communications skills, e.g. listening, gathering information and building a rapport with patients) would help students challenge discriminatory statements about other professions (Pecukonis et al., 2008). Yet IPL and IPE should also include the opportunity to collaborate, discuss and learn about each other, with the aim being to improve patient care. The aims of IPE are to enhance the sharing of skills and knowledge between healthcare professions, which in turn allows for a better understanding of each other, sharing values, and respecting each other's role. If this can be established then the quality and safety of patient care can be optimised. We have already seen in the high profile cases identified earlier how poor healthcare team working and communication can have a very negative impact on patient outcomes.

IPE can work well if all professions are able to work together to make this happen (both in practice and academic settings). There are some excellent examples of how this works well within the UK (Oandason and Reeves, 2005; Reeves et al., 2007).

 ## AN OCCUPATIONAL THERAPIST

Case Scenario

A community Occupational Therapist (OT) attended a Trust's 'Interprofessional Learning (IPL) Champions' Forum' (a forum that has been developed to enable IPL Champions from all disciplines to meet together). Another member of the group (a podiatrist) shared information about some new drop-in sessions that she was holding in her area, and was surprised that the OT was unaware of these as the information had been distributed on flyers to all the clinics. However the OT was based in another building which had not been included in the distribution. Additionally, due to the hectic pace of NHS work, flyers and distribution information were often missed. The IPL Forum allowed time for the podiatrist and OT to liaise and learn more about each other's services and remit, and the specific changes that were being implemented locally to improve patient care. The OT immediately started to refer patients to the drop-in, which led to much more timely treatment being provided for her patients. The podiatrist also became much more aware about the necessity for effective communication and the need to ensure that all appropriate colleagues were aware of any new services.

Whittington (2003) maintains that some centres are developing and piloting IPE programmes. However, this can be difficult as traditional classroom settings are known to be limited in what can be delivered and the setting often does not reflect the complexities that arise from interprofessional working. Nevertheless, there are some good examples of innovative teaching that do address this issue.

EXAMPLE   QUEEN MARY'S HOSPITAL

Saint George's, Kingston and Brunel and the University of London have developed a training ward at Queen Mary's Hospital, Roehampton, to facilitate students from various disciplines to learn together. It was designed collaboratively as an innovative way of enabling different professions to work together in teams and develop their communication skills, learning about each person's role and responsibilities whilst caring for patients.

EXAMPLE   STOCKPORT NHS FOUNDATION TRUST

Stockport NHS Foundation Trust uses simulation scenarios (SIM) to encourage students from different professions to work together in problem solving complex patient issues. This is undertaken in the SIM suite where students can work together in a safe environment and make mistakes without causing any harm to patients. It involves recreating a real-life patient event so that learners can experience that event through use of a high fidelity environment, thereby gaining new skills, knowledge and attitudes (Mackinnon, 2011).

However, in some areas HEIs have yet to pursue this fully, possibly due to a lack of understanding of its nature, context and purpose. In the past some have argued that there has been a lack of research as to the effectiveness of interprofessional education, suggesting that the cost, the amount of labour required, a general lack of support and timetabling difficulties have helped to fuel the reluctance to operationalise IPE (Cooper et al., 2001). For example, even simple differences such as terms, length and different assignment requirements can often cause a problem and make it logistically very difficult to achieve. However, in the UK evidence is now growing that IPE enables the knowledge and skills necessary for IPE to be learnt (Hammick et al., 2007), has a positive impact on communication between professionals (Lefebvre et al., 2007) and sustains positive attitudes towards collaborative working (Pollard and Miers, 2008).

In 2006, the Health Education England (HEE), formally the Strategic Health Authority (SHA), recognised the need for extra support for learning in practice and developed the role of the Practice Education Facilitator (PEF). Originally this role was developed to primarily support nursing mentors in practice and assist them in supporting nursing students. However, whilst initially slow to develop (Wright and Lindqvist, 2008), the role has since been instrumental in the practice setting for supporting and managing practice-based *multi-professional* student learning. As the PEF role has developed and the need for IPE has become more widely recognised, the role of the PEF has now expanded to assist and support mentors/educators, supervisors and students *across all disciplines*. Indeed some heath care organisations have really embraced the notion of IPE and developed structures to support it.

EXAMPLE   STOCKPORT

Stockport NHS Foundation Trust developed an interprofessional learning (IPL) forum in partnership with Pennine Care NHS Foundation Trust and Stockport Metropolitan Borough

Council (SMBC). This forum brings together key staff interested in education and learning and together they can work towards integrated learning in practice. This involves having IPE Champions at all levels in the organisation to help promote IPE in practice. The patient is seen as being at the centre of their care and the IPL forum promotes the importance of partnership working between all practitioners and their patients. It keeps IPE firmly in mind when working with students, so that they are encouraged to consider interprofessional issues in all aspects of their placements. The Trust has also developed IPL sessions for students from all disciplines. Specific themes or topics are chosen which are of interest to all parties (for example dementia). Participants are then given the opportunity to work in groups, learning about each others' roles and how they would approach the patient scenario from the perspective of all their different disciplines. This gives them time to work together outside of practice and has had some beneficial effects in practice and on patient care. For example, a student nurse and a medical student discussing the care plan of an elderly patient by their bedside and a physiotherapist adding in some practical advice to try to enhance the patient discharge process.

However, as yet there is little formal evaluation or research on the impact of IPL in practice. Most of the available literature focusing upon IPE programmes simply give a descriptions of the programme which provide opinion on its value rather than formal evaluation, with most having been undertaken in the USA. Evaluations that are available lack methodological rigor and have poorly developed outcome measures (Cooper et al., 2001). This does not mean that IPE is not effective, it just means there is still no clear evidence to say it is. Freeth et al. (2002) argue that we need to invest more in evaluating IPE with a small number of high quality, comprehensive evaluations. Humphris and Hean (2004) agree and recommend the need to generate high quality evidence in relation to the dynamic of generating true interprofessional learning.

STOP AND THINK

Make a list of the advantages and challenges of IPE.

- How do you think these could influence your learning as a student nurse?

Advantages of IPE

There are some key advantages to IPE. These include:

- understanding the theoretical principles of team working and collaboration early in a student's career;
- understanding all the roles involved in the patient experience;
- an ability to communicate appropriately and understand the language of different healthcare professionals;
- an understanding of the professional responsibilities, values and accountability of healthcare professionals in meeting the needs of patients;
- being able to work effectively in an interprofessional team;
- understanding how different professions make decisions about patient care;

- understanding how IPE produces better team work, which in turn improves patient care;
- removal of the fear of other professions;
- the ability to challenge professionals for the good of patient care.

As well as these advantages there are some challenges to IPE.

Challenges to IPE

These challenges include:

- difficulty in mapping the curricula for different professions;
- recognising that there needs to be a commitment from all stakeholders to effective planning of IPE;
- recognising that time and opportunity need to be given for professions to address differences;
- allowing for logistics and resource difficulties as learning in small groups is often labour intensive and costly;
- a lack of evaluation of the IPE that has already been implemented: rigorous and robust evaluation is essential;
- a lack of preparation and support for the IPE teachers;
- a lack of student involvement in planning the IPE. Freeth et al. (2005) maintain students should be actively involved in steering their IPE.

Looking into the future of the healthcare service, Ramswammy (2010) believes that we must change the way we educate professionals and also change the milieu in which they work. Silo working and training cannot continue and the development of an integrated interprofessional multi-dimensional workforce is critical. For all of this to happen team work is also crucial.

Chapter summary

Interprofessional working and learning are not new concepts, however it is clear that interprofessional working and learning are essential to the future of healthcare and adult nursing. Indeed, the NMC (2010b) are clear that nursing students must be given opportunities and chances to learn with other professionals, and as far as is reasonably possible with students from other professions. However, for this to occur, all professions need to show a commitment to learning and working together to provide the best high quality patient care. This often involves breaking down traditional boundaries and barriers and working flexibly. It also requires clear leadership and a commitment to ongoing collaborative education for all which should help to build sustainable relationships with mutual understanding, respect and communication that occur through influencing and negotiation. This will involve breaking down hierarchical structures and taking a leap of faith and commitment in order to work proactively for true collaboration.

The key challenges have been identified here and the need for commitment to work through these challenges and develop effective policies is apparent (Barrett et al., 2005). For adult nurses teamwork is key and therefore every opportunity should be taken during the course of your programme to join in all teamwork activities.

Suggested further reading

Stockport IPL Champions Forum (2011) *The IPL Toolkit for Educators and Mentors*. Stockport: Stockport IPL Champions Forum (unpublished). The toolkit includes hints, tips, activities and ideas to help promote a minimal level of interprofessional working with students and ensure a collaborative approach. It can be used to help students in a practice setting develop interprofessional working skills. The ideas and activities can be used at the mentor's/educator's discretion and are not prescriptive. For further information contact the PEF team at Stockport NHS Foundation Trust (Sarah Booth, Practice Education Facilitator – sarah.booth@stockport.nhs.uk or www.stockport.nhs.uk).

References

Atwal, A. (2002) 'A world apart: how occupational therapists, nurses and care managers perceive each other in acute healthcare', *British Journal of Occupational Therapy*, 65: 446–52.

Atwal, A. and Caldwell, K. (2005) 'Do all health and social care professionals interact equally? A study of interactions in multidisciplinary teams in the United Kingdom', *Scandinavian Journal of Caring Sciences*, 19: 268–73.

Baker, D., Day, R. and Salas, E. (2006) 'Teamwork as an essential component of high reliability organisations', *Health Services Research*, 41(4): 1576–98.

Baldwin, D. (1993) 'Development of health professionals to maximise health provider resources in rural areas'. National Rural Health Association HRSA contract. Washington, DC: Bureau of Health Professions.

Barr, H., Koppel, I., Reeves, S., Hammick, M. and Freeth, D. (2005) *Effective Interprofessional Education: Argument, Assumption and Evidence*. Oxford: Blackwell.

Barrett, G., Sellman, D. and Thomas, J. (2005) *Interprofessional Working in Health and Social Care: Professional Perspectives*. Basingstoke: Palgrave Macmillan.

Baxter, J. (2011) *Public Sector Identities: A Review of the Literature*. Maidenhead: Open University Press.

Biggs, S. (2006 [1997]) 'Interprofessional collaboration: problems and prospects'. In J. Day (ed.), *Interprofessional Working* (Expanding Health and Social Care Series, edited by L. Wiggins). Cheltenham: Nelson Thornes.

Bradford, S. (2008) 'Practices, policies and professionals: emerging discourses of expertise in English youth work, 1939–51', *Youth and Policy*, 97(1): 13–26.

Bridges, D.R., Davidson, R.A., Odegard, P.S., Maki, I.V. and Tomkowiak, J. (2011) 'Interprofessional collaboration: three best practice models of interprofessional education', *Medical Education on line*.

CAIPE (2007) *Creating an Interprofessional Workforce: An Education and Training Framework for Health and Social Care*. London: CAIPE (supported by the Department of Health).

Centre for the Advancement of Interprofessional Education (2002) *Definition of Interprofessional Education*. Available at: www.caipe.org.uk/about-us/defining-ipe/ (last accessed 6 June 2014).

Clements, D., Dault, M. and Priest, A. (2007) 'Effective teamwork in healthcare: research and reality', *Healthcare Papers*, 7(Special Issue): 26–34.

Cooper, H., Carlisle, C., Gibbs, T. and Watkins, C. (2001) 'Developing an evidence base for interdisciplinary learning: a systematic review', *Journal of Advanced Nursing*, 35(2): 228–37.

Day, J. (2006) *Interprofessional Working*. Cheltenham: Nelson Thornes.

Department of Health (1998) *A First Class Service: Quality in the New NHS*. London: DH.

Department of Health (2000a) *NHS Plan: A Plan for Reform*. London: DH.

Department of Health (2000b) *A New NHS: Modern and Dependable*. London: HMSO.

Department of Health (2001) *Learning from Bristol: The Report of the Public Inquiry into Children's Heart Surgery at the Bristol Royal Infirmary*. London: HMSO.

Department of Health (2003) *The Victoria Climbié Inquiry*. London: HMSO.

Department of Health (2006) *Modernising Nursing Careers*. London: DH.

Department of Health (2008) *High Quality Care For All the NHS: Next Stage Review*. London: DH.

Department of Health (2012) *Health and Social Care Act*. London: HMSO.

Department of Health (2013) *Berwick Report into Patient Safety*. London: DH.

European Court of Human Rights (1990) *Article 8 of the European Convention on Human Rights*. Available at: www.echr.coe.int/documents/convention_eng.pdf (last accessed 23 September 2014).

Francis, R. (2013) *Report of the Mid Staffordshire NHS Foundation Trust Public Inquiry: Executive Summary*. London: Crown Copyright.

Freeth, D., Hammick, M., Koppel, I., Reeves, S. and Barr, H. (2002) *A Critical Review of Evaluations of Interprofessional Education*. London: Learning and Teaching Network Support Centre for Health Sciences and Practice/CAIPE.

Freeth, D., Hammick, M., Reeves, S., Koppel, I. and Barr, H. (2005) *Effective Interprofessional Education: Development, Delivery and Evaluation*. Oxford: Blackwell.

Furlong, E. and Smith, R. (2005) 'Advanced nursing practice: policy, education and role development', *Journal of Clinical Nursing*, 14(9): 1059–1066.

General Medical Council (2006) *Review of Tomorrow's Doctors*. London: GMC.

Glasby, J., Martin, G. and Regen, E. (2008) 'Older people and the relationship between hospital services and intermediate care: results from a national evaluation', *Journal of Interprofessional Care*, 22(6): 639–49.

Grumbach, K. and Bodenheimer, T. (2004) 'Can healthcare teams improve primary healthcare practice?', *Journal of the American Medical Association*, 291(10): 1246–51.

Hammick, M., Freeth, D., Koppel, I., Reeves, S. and Barr, H. (2007) 'A best evidence systematic review of inter professional education', BEME guide No. 9, *Medical Teacher*, 29(8): 735–51.

Hanson, A., Friberg, F., Segesten, K., Gedda, B. and Mattsson, B. (2008) 'Two sides of the coin: general practitioners' experience of working in multidisciplinary teams', *Journal of Interprofessional Care*, 22(1): 5–16.

Health and Care Professions Council (2014) *Standards of Education and Training*. London: HCPC.

Health and Social Care Directorate (2011) *Transforming Your Care: A Review of Health and Social Care in Northern Ireland (Executive Summary)*. London: HMSO.

Health Professional Networks Nursing and Midwifery Human Resources for Health (2010) *Framework for Action on Interprofessional Education and Collaborative Practice*. Switzerland: World Health Organization.

House of Commons (2013) *The Health and Social Care Act*. Available at: www.legislation.gov.uk/ukpga/2014/23/contents/enacted (last accessed 6 March 2015).

House of Lords (2011) *Health and Social Care Bill*. Available at: www.services.parliament.uk/bills/2014-15/healthandsocialcaresafetyandquality.html (last accessed 6 March 2015).

Humphries, D. and Hean, S. (2004) 'Educating the future workforce: building the evidence about interprofessional learning', *Journal of Health Services Research and Policy*, 9(1): 24–7.

Irvine, R., Kerridge, I., McPhee, J. and Freeman, S. (2002) 'Interprofessionalism and ethics: consensus in clash of cultures?', *Journal of Interprofessional Care*, 16: 199–210.

Jeffrey, R. and Trowman, G. (2009) 'Developing a performative identity'. Paper presented at the European Conference on Educational Research: Theory and Evidence in European Educational Research.

Jeffries, N. and Chan, K.K. (2004) 'Multidisciplinary team working: is it both hostile and effective?', *International Journal of Gynaecological Cancer*, 14(2): 210–11.

Katzenbach, J.R. and Smith, D.K. (1993) *The Wisdom of Teams: Creating the High-performance Organisations*. Boston, MA: Harvard Business Press.

Kell, C. and Owen, G. (2008) 'Physiotherapy as a profession: where are we now?', *International Journal of Therapy and Rehabilitation*, 15(4): 158–64.

Kesby, S. (2002) 'Nursing care and collaborative practice', *Journal of Clinical Nursing*, 11: 357–66.

Laming, W. (2009) *The Protection of Children in England: A Progress Report*. Norwich: HMSO.

Lavin, M.A., Ruebling, I., Banks, R., Block, L., Counte, M. and Furman, G. (2001) 'Interdisciplinary health professional education: a historical review', *Advances in Health Sciences Education: Theory and Practice*, 6(1): 25–47.

Lefebvre, H., Pelchat, D. and Levart, M.J. (2007) 'Interdisciplinary family intervention program: a partnership among health professional, traumatic brain injury patients, and caregiving relatives', *Journal of Trauma Nursing*, 14(2): 100–13.

Leggat, S.G. (2007) 'Effective healthcare teams require effective team members: defining team work competencies', *BMC Health Service Resources*, 7: 17.

Lloyd-Jones, N., Hutchings, S. and Hobson, S.H. (2007) 'Interprofessional learning in practice for pre-registration health: interprofessional learning occurs in practice – is it articulated or celebrated?', *Nurse Education in Practice*, 7(1): 11–17.

Lymbery, M. (2006) 'United we stand? Partnership working in health and social care and the role of social worker in services for older people', *British Journal of Social Work*, 36: 1119–34.

Miers, M., Rickaby, C. and Pollard, K. (2015) *Making the Most of Interprofessional Learning Opportunities: Professionals' and Students' Experience of Interprofessional Learning and Working*. Bristol: The Higher Education Academy and University of England.

Nursing and Midwifery Council (2007) *Consultation: The Future of Pre-registration Nurse Education*. London: NMC.

Nursing and Midwifery Council (2009) *Standards of Pre-registration Education*. London: NMC.

Nursing and Midwifery Council (2010a) *Standards for Pre-Registration Nursing Education*. London: NMC.

Nursing and Midwifery Council (2010b) *Standards for Competence for Registered Nurses*. Available at: www.nmc-uk.org/Documents/Standards/Standards%20for%20competence.pdf (last accessed 5 March 2015).

Nursing and Midwifery Council (2010c) *Record Keeping: Guidance for Nurses and Midwives*. London: NMC.

Nursing and Midwifery Council (2015) *The Code: Professional Practice and Behaviour Standards of for Nurses and Midwives*. London: NMC.

Oandasan, I. and Reeves, S. (2005) 'Key elements for interprofessional education. Part 1: the learner, the educator and the learning context', *Journal of Interprofessional Care*, May, 21–38.

Pecukonis, E., Doyle, O. and Leigh Bliss, D. (2008) 'Reducing barriers to interprofessional training: promoting interprofessional cultural competence', *Journal of Interprofessional Care*, 22(4): 417–28.

Pirrie, A., Wilson, V., Elsegood, J., Hall, J., Hamilton, S., Harden, R., Lee, D. and Stead, J. (1998) *Evaluating Multidisciplinary Education in Healthcare*. Edinburgh: SCRE.

Pollard, K., Sellman, D. and Senior, B. (2005) In G. Barrett, D. Sellman and J. Thomas (eds), *Interprofessional Working in Health and Social Care: An Introductory Text*. Basingstoke: Palgrave Macmillan.

Pollard, K.C. and Miers, M.E. (2008) 'From students to professionals: results in a longitudinal study of attitudes to pre-qualifying collaborative learning and working in health and social care in the United Kingdom', *Journal of Interprofessional Care*, 22(4): 399–416.

Pullen, I. and Loudon, J. (2006) 'Improving standards in clinical record keeping', *Advances in Psychiatric Treatment*, 12: 280–6.

Rafter, M.E., Persun, I.J., Herren, M., Linfante, J.C., Mina, M. and Wu, C.D. (2006) 'A preliminary study of interprofessional education', *Journal of Dental Education*, 70(4): 417–27.

Ramswammy, L. (2010) 'Interprofessional education and collaborative practice', *Journal of Interprofessional Care*, 24(2): 131–8.

Redfern, M., Keeling, J. and Powell, E. (2001) *The Royal Liverpool Children's Inquiry Report*. London: The Stationery Office.

Reeves, S., Goldman, J. and Oandasan, I. (2007) 'Key factors in planning and implementing interprofessional education in healthcare settings', *Journal of Allied Health*, 36(4): 231–5.

Reeves, S., Goldman, J. and Zwarenstein, M. (2009) 'An emerging framework for understanding the nature of interprofessional interventions', *Journal of Interprofessional Care,* 23 (5): 539–42.

Reynolds, F. (2005) *Communication and Clinical Effectiveness in Rehabilitation.* Edinburgh: Elsevier/Butterworth Heinemann.

Salas, E., DiazGranados, D., Klein, C., Burke, C.S., Stagl, K.C., Goodwin, G.F. and Halpin, S.M. (2009) 'Does team training improve team performance? A meta-analysis', *Human Factors,* 50(6): 903–933.

Sims. S., Hewitt, G. and Harris, R. (2014) 'Evidence of collaboration, pooling of resources, learning and role blurring in interprofessional healthcare teams: a realistic synthesis', *Journal of Interprofessional Care,* 25(1): 20–25.

Spry, E. (2006) 'All together for health?', *Student British Medical Journal,* 14: 1–44.

Stockport IPL Champions Forum (2011) 'IPL toolkit for educators and mentors'. Stockport: Stockport IPL Champions Forum (unpublished).

The Scottish Government (2000) *Our National Health: A Plan for Action, A Plan for Change.* Edinburgh: The Scottish Government.

Smith, J. (2002) *The Shipman Inquiry. Death Disguised: First Report.* (Chairman: J. Smith.) Norwich: HMSO.

The Willis Commission (2012) *Quality with Compassion: The Future of Nurse Education.* London: RCN.

Thomas, J. (2005) 'Issues for the future'. In G. Barrett, D. Sellman and J. Thomas (eds), *Interprofessional Working in Health and Social Care: An Introductory Text.* Basingstoke: Palgrave Macmillan.

Thornicroft, G. and Tansella, M. (2002) 'Balancing community based and hospital based mental healthcare', *World Psychiatry,* 1(2): 84–90.

Weiss, G.I. and Welbourne, P. (2008) 'The professionalisation of social work: a crossnational exploration', *International Journal of Social Welfare,* 17: 281–90.

Whittington, C. (2003) *Learning for Collaborative Practice with Other Professions and Agencies.* London: DH.

World Health Organization (1988) *Learning Together to Work Together for Health.* Geneva: WHO.

World Health Organization (2010) *Framework for Action on Interprofessional Education and Collaborative Practice.* Geneva: WHO.

Wright, A. and Lindqvist, S. (2008) 'The development, outline and evaluation of the second level of an interprofessional learning programme – listening to the students', *Journal of Interprofessional Care,* 22(5): 475–87.

4 Medicines Management

JULIE GREGORY

This chapter will highlight the importance of medicines management for adult nurses. Specifically, it will examine your role and responsibilities as an adult nurse in ensuring the safety of your patients in relation to medication. Adult nurses are responsible for the safe and effective management of medication and as such medicines management is a major aspect of professional practice (Downie et al., 2008). Indeed it is suggested that approximately 16 hours a week of a registered nurse's clinical time is spent in the management of medicines (Leufer and Cleary-Holdforth, 2013). Therefore the administration of medication is a key element of nursing care.

As an adult nurse therefore, you will need to have a comprehensive knowledge base and access to information to identify and prevent adverse reactions and errors associated with the management of medicines. This chapter aims to examine some of these aspects to ensure patient safety.

After reading this chapter you should be able to:

- Identify the adult nurse's roles in medicines management.
- Describe the skills required for medicine management, in particular the administration of medicines.
- Be aware of some of the factors that may increase the risk of medication errors.
- Understand some of the legal and ethical issues relating to medicines management.
- Relate how pharmacological knowledge is applied to patient care.

Related NMC competencies

The overarching NMC requirement is that all nurses:

> ... practise safely by being aware of the correct use, limitations and hazards of common interventions, including nursing activities and treatments. The nurse must be able to evaluate their use, report any concerns promptly through the appropriate channels and modify care where necessary to maintain safety. (NMC, 2010a: 18, 2010b: 6)

Additionally, all nurses need to meet the competencies outlined within the NMC Skills Clusters (2010c). For further information please see Chapter 5, p.128.

───────── To achieve entry to the register as an adult ─────────
nurse you should be able to:

- Safely use current pharmacological interventions, providing information and taking account of individual needs and preferences (2010a: 18, 2010b: 9) in accordance with the NMC (2007) *Standards for Medicine Management.*
- Contribute to the collection of local and national data and formulation of policy on risks, hazards and adverse outcomes.

(Adapted from the NMC Standards of Competence for Adult Nursing, 2010a, 2010b, 2010c)

Background

In the previous chapter we highlighted the importance of interprofessional working and this is a particularly relevant aspect of medicines management. In order to ensure that the medication taken by your patients is safe and effective, you will be required to work collaboratively with a team of healthcare professionals *and* the patient. For example, a careful and detailed history and assessment of the patient is undertaken by a *prescriber* (usually but not always a doctor), before a written direction or prescription is produced. The *pharmacist* dispenses the medication after checking the accuracy of the prescription. Within a hospital setting the *nurse* may administer the medication to the patient with their consent, although in other settings *patients* will self-administer. You will therefore need to frequently liaise with other members of the team and your patient, as well as account for your actions and be confident that the *correct drug* has been administered to the *correct patient* at all times.

An experienced nurse may make the administration of medicines appear straightforward but this is not a mechanistic task. It requires knowledge, thought, dexterity and the exercise of professional judgement. Your main responsibility as an adult nurse is to ensure that medicines are managed safely. This includes the accurate interpretation of a prescription: you must know the reason for the medication, its action and usual dose, you should be able to question a possible mistake by the prescriber and when in doubt should ask for advice or help. The administration of medicines involves ensuring that the right medicine, correct dose and right route are used and that the medication is given to the right patient at the right time. In addition, you will need to record that the drug has been given or provide reasons for its omission and observe the patient's response (Greenstein and Gould, 2009).

All medicines are potent substances that are used to promote health and to prevent, control and treat disease: they benefit individuals generally by saving and prolonging life and enhancing lifestyles (Downie et al., 2008). However, they can also have potentially life-threatening effects on individuals if not correctly managed. Safely managing medicines is important for adult nurses because approximately 70% of the adult population take prescribed medication. This increases to an estimated 80% of people over the age of 75 years (Baileff et al., 2012).

Definition of medicines management

Medicines management encompasses the entire way in which nurses select, procure, provide, prescribe, supply, administer and review a patient's medicine. Optimal medicine management enables patients to get the maximum benefit from the medicines they need. This is achieved through concordance and teamwork, by placing the patient as the primary focus and by ensuring that nursing interventions are cost-effective, and that any associated risks are identified, communicated and carefully managed. (Baileff et al., 2012: 379)

The adult nurse's role in medicines management

Preventing medication errors is a key aspect of your role as an adult nurse since 20% of clinical negligence litigation arises from errors linked to prescribed medication. The Audit Commission (2001) estimated that these cost the NHS about £500 million a year and increase the hospital stay by approximately 8.5 days.

Medication error is defined as 'any preventable event that may cause or lead to inappropriate medication use or patient harm while the medication is in the control of a health professional, patient or consumer' (National Coordianting Council for Medication Error Reporting and Prevention, 2015).

Medication errors can have several potential impacts:

- *On the patient* (ranging from minor to fatal consequences).
- *On the nurse* (for example, being involved in a medication error can significantly impact upon your self-esteem, confidence, and possibly your professional registration).
- *On the organisation* (for example, this could significantly impact upon an organisation's reputation: organisations will need to instigate an investigation, report, and learn from errors, and this takes time and uses resources that could be channelled towards other aspects of care).

ACTIVITY 4.1

Access the National Patient Safety Agency website at the following address: www.nrls. npsa.nhs.uk/

- Take a note of the details of patient safety incidents that occurred across England between 1 April 2013 and 30 September 2013.
- Now access the report that links to one of the NHS Trusts or organisations and determine how many of these involved drug or medicine administration.

Reports and headlines in the media over recent years have led to an increased awareness of medication errors. This is, in part, as a result of the introduction of various policies such as the NHS Code of Openness (NHS Management Executive, 1995) and the *Freedom of Information Act* (2000). At the same time organisations have often encouraged staff to report errors and near misses and this may have increased the number of errors. However, medication error is not a new phenomenon: a review by Tully (2012) found that there has been concern about medication errors for over fifty years. The majority of reported errors (90%) are associated with *no harm* or *low harm*, and include time errors where a medication may have been given one hour early or one hour late (Tully, 2012). This is also clearly illustrated by a report by the National Patient Safety Agency (NPSA, 2010) which examined instances of omitted medication. A total of 18,527 incidents of omission were reported, with the majority (13,027 or 70%) not leading to any harm. However, 27 deaths resulted from the omissions. The report clearly highlights the harm that can arise from the delay or omission of critical medicines (included antibiotics, insulin and anticoagulants). Furthermore, the report emphasises that there was no one reason for the delay in administration. Some of the omissions included: a lack of availability of the medicine; loss of IV access; the patient declined to take the medication and/or they were kept nil orally for investigations and/or surgery. One case study described how a patient with a pulmonary embolus had a dose of enoxaparin prescribed but it was not administered and the patient subsequently died (NPSA Report, 2010).

The medicines management process and the nurse's role

1. Nursing assessment

A medication or drug history should be obtained from the patient, or if necessary relatives and friends and/or the GP, as part of the nursing assessment. This assessment should include which drugs are taken, doses, times and any known allergies to medication. The patient should be asked about any side effects from the medication and their understanding of the medication should be assessed. The drug history also needs to include any over the counter medication, recreational drugs and herbal remedies (Greenstein and Gould, 2009). Patients do not always consider herbal remedies as medication but the use of these substances may be related to a current condition and may interact with prescribed medication.

EILEEN

Eileen, a 54-year-old lady with poorly controlled asthma, complains of 'low mood and feeling tired all the time' to the practice nurse during a follow-up appointment at the asthma clinic. During her assessment the practice nurse determines that Eileen has been self-medicating with St John's Wort given to her by a friend. St John's Wort is a herbal remedy that has been used to treat depression for hundreds of years and can be bought from health food shops. It is not classed as a medication and is therefore not regulated and there is no recommended dose (Szegedi et al., 2005). NICE (2009) do not recommend the use of St John's Wort due to concerns which include serious drug interactions, for example it can reduce the effectiveness of theophyllines (a medication sometimes taken by patients with asthma to help open the airways). It was therefore important for the nurse to discover that Eileen was taking this remedy due to its potential interaction with her asthma medication.

(Note: St John's Wort can reduce the effect of theophyllines which may or may not have been the cause of her increasing asthma symptoms.)

2. Knowledge of the individual patient's care plan

Knowledge of an individual's care plan is necessary prior to the administration of medication to determine where the prescribed medication relates to the treatment plan. This is important because a patient's condition may affect the action of the medication, for example, reduced renal function slows the elimination of the medicines. In this example the nurse may need to request a review of the patient by the prescriber as a result of their knowledge of the impaired renal function.

3. Administration of medication

Medicines administration is a key aspect of a registered nurse's role in relation to medicines management. As a student nurse you should never administer medication without supervision by a Registered Nurse (RN). Not least, this is because registered nurses are accountable (i.e. they must account) for their actions in the safe administration of medicines, including the delegation of this task to others. Administration of medication does not occur in isolation. It is one aspect of a collaborative process involving the prescriber, pharmacist and patient. It is complex and requires clear thought to prevent errors and harm to your patient and to promote therapeutic responses.

The Department of Health (2004) recommended the five 'rights' as principles to follow when administering medication:

- The Right Patient.
- The Right Drug.
- The Right Dose.
- The Right Time.
- The Right Route.

The NMC (2007) standards for administration of medication support the five rights and are detailed in Box 4.1.

BOX 4.1   NMC STANDARDS FOR ADMINISTRATION OF MEDICINE

1. Identify the patient – confirm the patient's identity by asking them their name and check the name on the medication/prescription chart matches the patient's identity wristband.
2. Allergy – this should be highlighted on the medication/prescription chart and written in the patient's notes.

(Continued)

(Continued)

3. Knowledge of the drug, the therapeutic dose, its side effects, precautions and contra-indications.
4. Be aware of the patient's care plan.
5. Check that the prescription and/or label on the medicine is clearly written and is unambiguous.
6. Check the expiry date of the medicine.
7. Consider the dose, weight of patient where appropriate, method of administration, route and timing.
8. Administer or withhold the medication according to the patient's condition.
9. Contact the prescriber where contra-indications to the prescribed medication are discovered.
10. Make clear, accurate and immediate records.
11. When medicines are not given the reason for this must be recorded.

It is essential that the patient is identified and that the name on the prescription corresponds with the patient's details. This is because poor checking of the patient's identity can lead to an administration error.

In an inpatient setting, all patients should wear a wristband containing their identification information (NPSA, 2005). This is checked and the patient should be addressed by name or asked to confirm their name to reduce the risk of administering the correct medication to the wrong patient. In some settings an up-to-date photograph may be attached to the prescription to help with identification.

At the point of administration a final check should be made to ensure the patient does not have an allergy to the medication. Some medications, for example penicillin, can produce anaphylaxis, a serious allergic reaction which is potentially life threatening. Any known allergy should be recorded on the prescription chart as well as within the medical and nursing notes. Some hospitals use a red wristband to help alert staff to a patient's allergy status. However, this should not be relied upon and the allergy status must be checked prior to the administration of a drug (Corben, 2009).

The prescription must be legible to avoid any confusion: for example, the drugs *oxybutytnin* (used for urinary frequency) and *oxycontin* (an opiate analgesic) have similar names. Both of these could look similar if the prescriber's handwriting is poor and may lead to very different therapeutic effects. A prescription should be clearly written and contain the following:

- The name of the medicine.
- Dose and route of administration.
- Time.
- Signature of prescriber.
- Start date.
- That the medicine has not already been administered.

Poor documentation is a common factor in drug errors. Therefore you should never accept illegible writing or unofficial abbreviations. You need to feel confident and be able to question a possible mistake made by a prescriber. When in doubt, always seek advice from a pharmacist (Greenstein and Gould, 2009) or the original prescriber.

Whilst tact may be required when approaching the prescriber, basing your enquiry on the individual patient's care plan, their current condition, the reason for the prescription, knowledge of the drug, its dosage, time and route of administration will help.

Once the medication has been administered a clear and immediate record should be made within the relevant documents, and when medication has not been administered the reason for this should be recorded and the relevant person informed of the omission.

ACTIVITY 4.2

Access the case report below which investigated the death of a young patient in Scotland due to an overdose of paracetamol. Available at: www.scotland-judiciary.org.uk/10/0/4/ Fatal-Accident-Inquiries

- How could this patient's death have been avoided?

There are many reasons for an error in administering medication. Two common types are: *procedural error* (e.g. failing to check the patient's identity) and *clinical error* (e.g. administering the wrong drug or dose). Distraction and interruption of the nurse during drug administration have been highlighted as one of the reasons for procedural errors and in some areas specific actions have been taken to try to reduce these. For example, you may have seen the nurse who is undertaking the medicines' round wearing a red tabard or vest during medicine administration. Pope (2002) suggests that this provides a visible symbol to increase awareness among other staff that the nurse is administering medicines and acts as an effective reminder not to interrupt that nurse during drug administration and distract the staff. However, Cloo, Johnson and Manias (2013) found similar numbers of distractions (90%) across two hospital sites despite the use of red tabards. The majority of interruptions were triggered by other staff (including physicians) and patients. Further recommendations suggest that all members of the healthcare team need to be informed and aware of the importance of avoiding the interruption of nurses during medication administration in addition to simply wearing a red tabard.

ACTIVITY 4.3

Next time you are within a clinical setting and medicines are being administered, observe the process and make some observational notes on the following:

- The number of interruptions.
- The people who made them.
- If a red tabard was worn. (If so, did it seem to prevent and reduce interruptions?)
- How the nurse reacted to these interruptions.

The pressures of work related to other aspects of patient care mean that nurses often feel rushed during the administration of medication and under pressure to complete the task (Cloo et al., 2013). This pressure may lead to short-cuts and a reduction in the required checks or a failure to ensure that the NMC (2007) standards for the adminis-tration of medicines are maintained. This in turn may result in medication errors.

Medication devices

A number of devices are available for use when administering medication and as an adult nurse you will need to have sufficient knowledge and skills to ensure the correct and safe use of any such device. These include measuring pots and spoons for oral administration, syringes and needles for parental administration (injections), and oxygen masks and nebulisers for inhalation. The correct use of these devices is important to ensure the accurate dose of medicines is administered, for example oral syringes (coloured purple) must be used for oral liquid medicines and not parental syringes.

Electronic devices such as infusion and syringe pumps may also be used to administer medication and should only be utilised following appropriate training. Prior to their use such devices should always be examined to confirm that they have been maintained appropriately (for example, there is usually a label on the device that indicates when the next service is required). Maintenance of equipment is important because patient harm may result if, for example, medication is administered too quickly (which could lead to serious consequences).

STOP AND THINK

Susan Smith, aged 30 years, has been admitted to hospital with an infected foot after standing on a drawing pin. She has been prescribed co-amoxiclav IV.

What do you need to know and check before administration?

The medication (Drug)	The patient	Aspects of IV administration

---

When considering the Stop and Think activity above, you should have noted the following:

- *The medication:* the dose, type of antibiotic (e.g. does it contain penicillin?) and side effects of the medication. Check that the antibiotic powder is dry, the glass vial is intact, and the expiry date has not passed.
- *The patient:* Susan has consented to the medication administration and her name and date of birth (ensuring this is the correct patient) should be checked against the prescription. Susan's care plan (including any history of taking antibiotics in the past) and any other prescribed medication should also be considered. At the bedside, you should always check again for any known allergies.
- *Aspects of IV administration:* aseptic no touch techniques (ANTT) should be used when checking that an IV cannula is in place and that there is no sign of redness, swelling or pain at the cannula site. Correct reconstitution of the medication,

consideration of which fluid to use, how much and whether this should be given as a bolus dose or an infusion should also be checked carefully.

Monitoring

Once the medication has been administered, the patient should be observed and assessed for any potential benefit and/or adverse effects of the medication. An adult nurse will be involved in this monitoring which will include taking physiological measures such as heart rate, blood pressure, respiratory rate and temperature. Blood glucose levels are carefully monitored prior to and following insulin administration which is administered to regulate blood glucose for patients with diabetes. This is because blood glucose needs to be kept within specific parameters. If they are too high or too low the patient can become drowsy and/or unconscious.

Morphine is an opioid analgesic used in the management of severe pain.
   List the monitoring requirements of a patient following the administration of morphine and the reasons for the observations undertaken.

STOP AND THINK

Adult nurses are expected to have knowledge of the common side effects of the medication they administer so that they are able to observe for potentially serious consequences. The majority of drugs will have some effect that is not related to their therapeutic effect. Morphine for example reduces the respiratory rate. If the dose of morphine administered is too high or the individual patient is sensitive to morphine this can, on rare occasions, lead to respiratory failure. Constipation is a very common side effect of morphine, and it can also induce nausea and vomiting following administration. Anti-emetics and laxatives are usually prescribed alongside morphine to prevent these side effects. A key aspect of the nurse's role is to monitor the patient to ensure that they obtain the pain relief required without these very unpleasant side effects.

Adverse events are serious untoward reactions related to a medication. It is estimated that drug allergies affect up to 10% of the world population and affect 20% of all hospitalised patients, accounting for up to 20% of fatalities due to anaphylaxis. Most commonly this involves antibiotics (e.g. penicillins, cephalosporins and sulphonamides), aspirin and other non-steroidal anti-inflammatory drugs (Panwakar et al., 2011). *Anaphylaxis* is an example of an adverse event, a type of allergic reaction which triggers the immune system to respond to certain substances to which an individual is allergic. In severe cases an anaphylactic reaction can cause airway obstruction, collapse or death. Other symptoms include a rash (urticaria), swelling of the tongue or mouth, wheezing or difficulty breathing, vomiting or diarrhoea, palpitations or a loss of consciousness.

All adverse events or serious untoward reactions to medicines should always be reported. This requires the careful recording of the reaction and symptoms experienced by the patient in the patient's records. These should also be reported to the healthcare team. Within the UK a system of reporting a suspicion of adverse reactions to medicines is known as the yellow card scheme and is available at http://yellowcard. mhra.gov.uk/the-yellow-card-scheme/. Yellow cards are also available in paper form in all British National Formula (BNF). The information gathered from 'Yellow Card

Reports' made by patients and health professionals is continually assessed at the Medicines and Healthcare Products Regulatory Agency (MHRA) by a team of medicine safety experts made up of doctors, pharmacists and scientists who study the benefits and risks of medicines. A patient's reaction to a medication is individual and not predictable and therefore side effects and an adverse event should not be confused with a medication error.

Storage of medicines

Medicines must be stored according to the manufacturer's guidance. The majority of medicines are stored in coloured bottles or in foil strips to avoid exposure to light which may affect the chemical composition of the drug. To maintain their stability some medicines need to be stored at a specific temperature. For example, insulin should be kept in a specifically designated clinical fridge.

Within the hospital setting all medications are stored in locked receptacles, cupboards, fridges, lockers and trolleys. Registered nurses are responsible for their safe storage and keep the medicine keys on their person (Corben, 2009). Traditionally, a medicine trolley containing a stock of commonly used medicines has been used for the administration of medicines. The nurse wheels the trolley to each patient and administers medicines from it. Increasingly though, individual medicine lockers (where each patient has their own stock of medicines at the side of their bed space) are being used. The introduction of individual lockers is intended to reduce medication errors (Lawson and Hennefer, 2010). However, there does not appear to be any evidence that demonstrates a reduction in errors as a result. Therefore, there remains a need for identification checks whether a trolley or a locker is used. It is also essential that the locker is checked after a patient has been discharged or transferred to ensure that their medicines have been removed.

Controlled drugs (CD) (for example morphine) must be stored separate from other medicines in a specifically designed locker or cupboard. This must be secured to a wall that cannot be accessed from outside in line with the *Misuse of Drugs Act* (1971). There is only one key available for an individual ward or unit CDs and it can only be held by a Registered Nurse, usually the senior nurse on duty.

Patient education

Teaching patients and providing explanations about their medication, its indication, dosage, times of administration, route and possible side effects, are important aspects of the adult nurse's role in all settings to increase the likelihood of *concordance* with the course of treatment (Greenstein and Gould, 2009). 'Concordance' is the term used to suggest an equal partnership and negotiation that occurs in the treatment process rather than a patient being compliant or a passive recipient of treatment from a healthcare professional. Good medicines management ensures that the patient (and where appropriate and with the individual's agreement – their carer) has access to advice and information about their medicines, resulting in a shared understanding. By explaining and demonstrating the correct administration of medication, you can help build your patient's knowledge of their medication and at the same time alert them to possible side effects. All opportunities should be used for teaching. When a patient is in hospital this should be incorporated into the act of administrating medicines (Downie et al., 2008). For nurses working in a community setting, the importance of educating patients is an even higher priority because the patients usually self-administer their medication. In order to aid concordance, the patient and/or their relatives need to understand the reasons for the medication and possible consequences of not taking the medication as directed. The patient's ability to open containers and to remember when to take their medication may need to be assessed and monitored. Advice should also be provided about the correct and secure storage of medicines, for example all medicines should be kept out of the reach of children and other vulnerable groups. It is also important to monitor the effects and identify possible side effects or problems experienced by patients in the community.

Prescribing

Traditionally the prescribing of medicines was the remit of medical staff and the nurse's role was limited to the safe and reliable administration of medication. However, as nurses' roles have become more autonomous and advanced (for example nurse-led clinics and services) *nurse prescribing* enables a complete episode of care to be delivered without referral to a medical practitioner. The introduction of nurse prescribing has been a gradual process, and was first introduced following the *Medicinal Products: Prescription by Nurses etc. Act 1992*, allowing District Nurses and Health Visitors to prescribe a limited number of medicines from 1998, following the successful completion of additional education and training (RCN, 2012). However, following robust reviews and evaluations this has been expanded to include all registered nurses. Since 2006 nurse prescribers across the UK have had access to all items in the British Nursing Formulary (BNF). The aim of nurse prescribing is to improve patient care, ensuring that all patients have equal and improved access to their medicines and information about them and to use healthcare professionals' skills more effectively (DH, 2006). To become a Nurse Prescriber you must have been registered for at least three years and have spent the final year within the clinical speciality or field where you will prescribe prior to undertaking an approved course (DH, 2006).

There are two categories of nurse prescribing: *Nurse Independent Prescribing* (NIP) and *Nurse Supplementary Prescribing* (NSP). The number of nurses registered as prescribers with the NMC in 2012 is detailed in Table 4.1.

- An *independent nurse prescriber* can prescribe any medication within the nurse's area of competence for its licensed use (DH, 2006); for example a Clinical Nurse Specialist for Diabetes prescribes insulin to a patient under her care.
- *Supplementary prescribing* occurs in collaboration with the patient and their doctor. A diagnosis is made by a medical practitioner (doctor) and a treatment plan is formulated as a clinical management plan (CMP) which sets out the parameters within which the nurse/healthcare professional can adjust the prescription (for example the dose). This includes any drug (DH, 2006). Supplementary prescribing is frequently used by PAM (Professions Allied to Medicine), for example by physiotherapists and podiatrists.

Table 4.1 The number of nurses registered as prescribers in 2012

[V100] Community Practitioner Nurse Prescriber	33,683
[V150] Community Practitioner Nurse Prescriber	1,369
[V200] Nurse Independent Prescriber	1,460
[V300] Nurse Independent / Supplementary Prescriber	26,347
Total	**62,859**

A Patient Group Directive (PGD) is a specific written direction for the supply or administration of a licensed named medication to a specific group of patients who may not be identified before presenting for treatment (NMC, 2007). As a student nurse you cannot administer medicines under a PGD even if supervised. The registrant using a PGD must be assessed as competent, be identified by name within the document and must not delegate the administration of the specified medicine. An example of a PGD in community is the administration of a vaccine. In secondary care PGD can be used to dispense analgesia (for example, in day case surgery and in A&E departments).

Legal and ethical aspects of medicines management

The *Medicines Act (1968)* regulates the production, testing and marketing of medical products. A licence is required for every medical product to ensure that it is administered appropriately in order to achieve its best possible therapeutic effect. A licence is only granted once the safety and efficacy of the drug have been established, that it is manufactured to the highest standards and has been tested and evaluated. The safety of the patient is always the prime consideration when a licence is granted (Downie et al., 2008).

Categories of medicines

Patients can access medicines from different sources. These are divided into four categories (see the box below for details of the legal categories of medicines in the UK).

LEGAL CATEGORIES FOR MEDICINES

- *General Sales List* (GSL) medications are freely available to buy in many shops (for example, cough medicines, paracetamol and antacids such as Gaviscon).

The advantages of the GSL are convenience and it is a cost effective way of obtaining simple medications without contacting a healthcare professional.

The disadvantages of GSL medication are that these may lead to other health problems. For example, Ibuprofen is a Non-Steroidal Anti-inflammatory Drug (NSAID) that is freely available and can cause gastric ulcers with long-term use. It may also cause renal damage and allergic reactions, including broncho-spasm. NSAIDS can interact with many other medications such as warfarin (an anti-coagulant).

- *Pharmacy* (P) medicines can only be purchased from a pharmacy or chemist's shop where a pharmacist is available. The pharmacist supervises the purchase, will check for potential interactions and other problems and also provide advice about potential side effects. They may also advise an individual to consult with a doctor if they feel this is necessary.
- *Prescription only medicines* (POM) can only be obtained with a written direction or prescription from a registered prescriber, traditionally a doctor but more recently involving other healthcare professionals, including pharmacists, nurses and professionals allied to medicines (physiotherapists, podiatrists etc.).
- *Controlled drugs* (CD) are regulated by the *Misuse of Drugs Act (1971)*. The ordering, dispensing, prescribing, storage and administration of these medicines are strictly monitored and controlled. Many of these medications are opiates (for example morphine).

The *Misuse of Drugs Act (1971)* relates to the licensing of the production, possession and supply of substances that may be misused. A number of changes were introduced following the enquiry into the deaths caused by Dr Harold Shipman (Shipman Inquiry, 2001): these relate to the prescription, record keeping and destruction of CDs, mainly within community settings, and are known as the *Misuse of Drugs Regulations (2001)*.

Ethical aspects of medication management

When medication is prescribed and administered the patient should always be at the centre of the management process. You will need to ensure that your patient's right to self-determination and autonomy is always considered. Patients must be kept informed and given the opportunity to make decisions about their medicines (DH, 2004). To ensure that patients make informed decisions relating to their medication they should be provided with advice and information about both the benefits and any potential side effects of the chosen medicines. In the spirit of concordance patients can chose to decline the prescribed medication and as a nurse you will always need to respect their decision. You can try to persuade your patient by providing further information and explaining the consequences of omitting medication but should not coerce them or administer the medication covertly.

Covert administration of medication or disguising the medication in food or drink has long been an area of debate and is centred around the notion that healthcare professionals can sometimes take on a 'paternalistic' approach when determining what is in a patient's best interest. However, if a patient is able to consent or decline the medication, covert administration should *not* be attempted. If a patient is considered to be unable to understand, or if they have been assessed as lacking capacity (in accordance with the *Mental Capacity Act*, 2005) their best interest needs to be considered prior to the decision to administer medication covertly. This decision will be made only when all other possible methods of administering the medication have been unsuccessful. An individual assessment of the patient is conducted and will often include the views of relatives (or close caregivers) and members of the multidisciplinary team to decide if covert administration is in the patient's best interest. Support should be available to assist with the assessment and decision from local policy and guidelines.

MALCOLM

Malcolm Jones (aged 72) is an inpatient on a medical ward. He takes a number of medicines that have been dispensed by the staff nurse and who has delegated the administration of these to you.

Mr Jones says he is 'fed up with taking all these tablets and doesn't want to take them this morning, thank you'.

- What would you do?
- What factors might you consider?
- Who needs to be involved?
- Where would you record this episode?

When faced with the scenario above perhaps you would initially try to persuade Mr Jones to take his medication by describing why each drug is necessary and highlighting any potential consequences of not taking the medicine. For example, Atenolol is taken to lower blood pressure. If Mr Jones' blood pressure becomes elevated cardiac problems could occur, including a stroke.

You may also consider if there are any specific reasons why Mr Jones might be declining his medication. For example, he might feel sick or be having difficulty swallowing (both of which would warrant further exploration). You would need to respect his decision but you may also need to consider if he has the capacity to make this decision. For example does he appear unusually confused or disorientated? You would also need to inform the nurse in charge of his reluctance to take his medication. The non-administration of his medication would be recorded on Mr Jones' prescription chart/sheet and in his nursing and medical notes according to local policy. Following this, medical staff should also be alerted. Depending upon his reasons for refusal, the pharmacist and doctor could evaluate his prescription and consider an alternative (e.g. see if the medicines could be given at different times rather than all in a morning).

Incident reporting

When or if a medication error occurs it is important to be honest and report the mistake to ensure that action can be taken to minimise any harm that could occur as a result of the error. Failing to act or denying that an error has occurred can not only harm the patient, it would also lead to serious sanctions for the nurse. A number of referrals to the NMC misconduct hearings are related to poor documentation and attempts to change documentation in relation to medication errors. Often the charges made as a result relate to dishonesty rather than a medication error.

Pharmacology: what do adult nurses need to know?

As an adult nurse, you will be responsible and accountable for keeping your own knowledge and skills up to date through continuing professional development and life-long learning. The underpinning knowledge you will require includes the study of drugs or pharmacology and how they are used to treat medical conditions. This section of the chapter aims to provide you with a very basic overview of *pharmacology* and the *pharmacokinetics* and *pharmacodynamics* of medicines, with some examples of commonly used drugs. (To help you to develop your knowledge and understanding, please refer to the suggested Further Reading at the end of this chapter.) You should use evaluation, supervision and appraisal to improve your performance and enhance the safety, quality of care and service delivery (Lawson and Hennefer, 2010). This includes constantly updating your knowledge and skills relating to medicine management because new medicines are constantly being developed.

Pharmacokinetics is concerned with how the body deals with the drug and relates to the absorption, distribution, metabolism and excretion of the drug (Greenstein and Gould, 2009). *Absorption* of a drug depends on the route of administration (Banning, 2007: see Table 4.2 for different routes of administration and the speed of effect). It is important to know how quickly the medication becomes effective when you are monitoring a patient's reaction to it. For example, morphine can be administered intravenously (IV), or by intramuscular (IM) or subcutaneous (SC) injection. It can also be taken orally as a liquid or tablet or in the form of a patch applied to the skin (transdermal). Therefore careful monitoring will need to be within seconds for an IV administration, up to 30 minutes for IM, and two hours for orally.

Table 4.2   Route of administration and time to effect of the medication

Route of administration	Time to effect
Intravenous (IV)	30-60 seconds
Inhalation (inh)	2-3 minutes
Sublingual (SL)	3-5 minutes
Intramuscular (IM)	10-20 minutes
Subcutaneous (SC)	15-30 minutes
Rectal (PR)	5-30 minutes
Ingestion (O)	30 -90 minutes
Transdermal (TD)	Up to 12 hours

The rapid effect of an intravenously (IV) administered drug is because there is direct access of the drug into the blood stream. However, when drugs are administered via other routes they often have to cross cell membranes before they enter the circulation (Downie et al., 2008). The most frequent route of administration is ingestion or oral. Orally administered drugs pass through the gastric or intestinal mucosa to be absorbed by diffusion through the walls of the small intestine and into the blood stream (Banning, 2007). The speed of absorption depends on the form the medication takes, for example liquid medication is absorbed quickly compared to tablets that need to be dissolved. Some tablets have a layer that delays or slows absorption (modified release) or are enteric coated to protect the gastric mucosa. When a patient has difficulties swallowing tablets it is important that these are not crushed because this may affect the absorption and/or alter the action of the drug. Always seek advice and help from a pharmacist when your patient has problems with swallowing tablets as they may be able to dispense an alternative form of the medicine. In older people, delays in absorption may result from changes in gastric emptying, changes in PH and other factors including insufficiency in cardiac output (Banning, 2007).

Metabolism occurs following the absorption of the drug. Following absorption from the small intestine it is transported in the blood to the liver where it is broken down or metabolised. This is known as first pass metabolism. Patients with liver disease may have difficulties in metabolising drugs, resulting in delays in their action. Metabolism ensures that the drug reaches the circulation and can be carried or transported to the site of its action, such as the heart, the brain etc. *Distribution* of a drug in the bloodstream occurs when some of the drug metabolite binds with proteins found in the bloodstream and becomes inactive. Unbound drugs are free to move in the blood and to cross the plasma membranes to the tissues where they exert their effect (Downie et al., 2008). In a poorly nourished individual an increased effect of the drug may occur because of low albumin levels and high levels of unbound drugs. The binding of a drug to proteins can also be affected by poly-pharmacy (multiple drugs) as the drugs compete for the binding sites (Downie et al., 2008). *Excretion* is the removal of the drug from the body. The body's way of dealing with drugs is to try and get them out of the body as soon as possible through further metabolism and excretion (Greenstein and Gould, 2009). The kidneys (specifically the glomeruli in the kidneys) are the most common route for excretion of drugs and their metabolites. Some drugs will be eliminated unchanged without metabolism and others will need to be changed or metabolised to be eliminated (Downie et al., 2008). Factors affecting the excretion of a drug include its fat solubility, the acidity of urine and the health of the kidneys. It is important that a useful level of the drug in the bloodstream is maintained. The speed of metabolism and excretion (or the length of time a drug stays in the body) means that the dose of a drug needs to be repeated at different times to ensure that it has the desired effect (Greenstein and Gould, 2009).

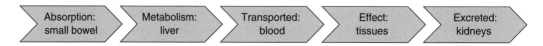

Figure 4.1   The basic life cycle of a drug taken orally

Examine the list of prescribed drugs for three elderly patients under your care.
  Consider what medications have been prescribed and why.

- How many different medications need to be taken and in what form are each of these administered?

Consider any related medical conditions for each patient.

- What is the potential for drug interactions or increased/decreased potency and why?

For example: the non-steroidal anti-inflammatory drug (NSAID) Volterol has a 50% binding capacity at therapeutic levels. In low plasma protein levels (which may be caused by poor nutrition) it displaces Warfarin from its binding sites, allowing more free or unbound Warfarin to exert its biological effect, and increasing the risk of bleeding (Banning, 2007).

Poor nutrition and poly-pharmacy (the concurrent use of multiple medications by one individual) are common in older people. You should be aware that there may be an increase/decrease in drug potency and also potential for drug interactions so you will need to monitor these patients vigilantly. According to Duerden et al. (2013), poly-pharmacy is widespread and increasingly common due to an increasing ageing population and rising numbers of individuals living with a number of long-term chronic conditions. This calls upon the need to have a good level of knowledge and understanding of how drugs work and how to identify and recognise potential interactions as well as the wider demands of effective record keeping and team working.

Pharmacodynamics is the term used to describe the way a drug exerts its effect by producing a physiological response in the body or controlling the changes that result from a disease (Greenstein and Gould, 2009).

Some drugs or medicines act by replacing or substituting a substance such as ferrous sulphate for iron deficiency anaemia. Enzymes are made up of proteins that speed up a chemical reaction and some medications block or inhibit enzymes. An *enzyme inhibitor* drug attaches itself to a particular enzyme to inhibit or stop the reaction. NSAID (e.g. Ibuprofen) is an example of an enzyme inhibitor; it acts by preventing the production of inflammatory chemicals known as prostaglandins, through inhibition of the enzyme cyclo-oxygenase (Downie et al., 2008).

Electrolytes within the body are carefully controlled to maintain homeostasis. Specific *electrolyte channels* are found on cells and tissues and these permit the transportation of certain electrolyte ions into cells (Downie et al., 2008; Lawson and Hennefer, 2010). Muscles have electrolyte channels that allow only calcium to enter causing the muscle to constrict. Some drugs affect the transport process of electrolytes. A calcium channel blocker (e.g. Nifedipine) is used to treat high blood pressure by occupying the calcium channel, preventing the constriction of blood vessels and lowering the blood pressure (Lawson and Hennefer, 2010). One of the ways in which insulin works is to promote the transportation of glucose into cells which results in the lowering of blood glucose (Downie et al., 2008).

Some medications exert their effect by interacting with *receptors*. Receptors are found embedded in the plasma membrane of cell walls to assist in the chemical communication within the cell and they regulate the cell's activity. A receptor *agonist* drug mimics the effects of a neurotransmitter or hormone or alters the physiology of the cell by binding to the receptor (Downie et al., 2008). Morphine is an example of an agonist drug that binds to specific opiate receptors found mainly in the spinal cord and the brain, to produce its analgesic effects. An *antagonist* drug binds with the receptor site and acts by inhibiting or blocking the agonist (Downie et al., 2008). Naloxone is a drug that competes with opiate receptors to block morphine and is used clinically to reverse the effects of opiates.

Synapses are found within the nervous system and these are the gaps between nerve fibres, muscles or glands. A neurotransmitter is released to activate the next nerve fibre or stimulate a muscle or gland into the desired action. Drugs can act as a neurotransmitter or to inhibit the neurotransmitter. Ondansetron inhibits serotonin (a neurotransmitter) in the chemo-trigger zone in the brain to control vomiting (Lawson and Hennefer, 2010).

Chemotherapy drugs act by interfering with cell growth and division to destroy rapidly dividing tumour cells, though unfortunately they also destroy normal cells: an ideal drug would selectively target the cancerous cells (Downie et al., 2008).

In infectious disease *antibiotics* and *antiviral drugs* affect the micro-organisms causing the infection. Penicillin for example inhibits the synthesis of the bacteria cell walls and erythromycin inhibits bacterial protein synthesis. Nystatin acts by increasing the permeability of the invading organism's cell wall (Downie et al., 2008).

STOP AND THINK

Consider carefully what additional information and knowledge you will need to be able to administer medicines safely and effectively. For example:

- How can you ensure that your knowledge of all medicines is kept up to date?
- How will you ensure that you calculate correct drug dosages with confidence and competence?

Note: There is suggested reading material at the end of this chapter.

Chapter summary

This chapter has provided an overview of the role and the skills an adult nurse requires in relation to medicine management and pharmacology. It is not intended to be a substitute for practical experience and adult nurses will participate actively in all aspects of medicine management, especially the administration of drugs in clinical practice.

The administration of medicines is a key element of an adult nurse's role and involves a great deal of their time. Their safe storage, use of medical devices, communication and monitoring of a patient's reaction to medicines are aspects of medicine management that are a nurse's responsibility. As an adult nurse you will need to possess knowledge of the patient, their care plan and the role of the medication in relation to that care plan. You should ensure that you understand the pharmacology of the drugs you administer as well as their possible adverse effects and drug interactions that may occur. Ensuring that legal and ethical aspects of medicine management are adhered to and that the NMC standards and local policy are followed should help to ensure that medication errors are avoided.

Suggested further reading

The *British National Formulary* (BNF) contains all licensed medications available, indications for use and potential side effects as well as sections listing interactions with other drugs.

The National Prescribing Centre is a valuable resource for healthcare professionals (www.nice.org.uk/mpc/index.jsp) and provides evidence for prescribing in addition to BNF access.

Local medicine administration/management policies will provide a practical application for how the information in this chapter is used in everyday practice.

Downie, G., Mackenzie, J., Williams, A. and Hind, C. (2008) *Pharmacology and Medicines Management for Nurses*, 4th edition. Edinburgh: Churchill Livingstone.
Lapham, R. and Agar, H. (2009) *Drug Calculations for Nurses: A Step by Step Approach*, 3rd edition. London: Hodder Arnold.
Lawson, L. and Hennefer, D.L. (2010) *Medicines Management in Adult Nursing*. Exeter: Learning Matters.

References

Audit Commission (2001) *A Spoonful of Sugar: Medicines Management in NHS Hospitals*. Wetherby: Audit Commission Publications.
Baileff, A., Davis, J. and Davey, N. (2012) 'Managing medicines'. In I. Bullock, J. MacLeod-Clark and J. Rycroft-Malone (eds), *Adult Nursing Practice: Using Evidence in Care*. Oxford: Oxford University Press. pp. 378–95.
Banning, M. (2007) *Medication Management in Care of Older People*. Oxford: Blackwell.
Cloo, J., Johnson, L. and Manias, E. (2013) 'Nurses medication administration practices at two Singaporean acute care hospitals', *Nursing and Health Sciences,* 15: 101–8.
Corben, V. (2009) 'Administration of medicines'. In L. Baillie (ed), *Developing Practical Adult Nursing Skills*, 3rd editon. London: Hodder. Chapter 4.
Department of Health (DH) (2001) *The Expert Patient: A New Approach to Chronic Disease Management for the 21st Century*. London: DH.
Department of Health (2004) *Building a Safer NHS for Patients: Improving Medication Safety*. London: DH.
Department of Health (2006) *Improving Patients' Access to Medicines: A Guide to Implementing Nurse and Pharmacist Independent Prescribing within the NHS in England*. London: DH.
Downie, G., Mackenzie, J., Williams, A. and Hind, C. (2008) *Pharmacology and Medicines Management for Nurses,* 4th edition. Edinburgh: Churchill Livingstone.
Duerden, M., Avery, T. and Payne, R. (2013) *Poly-pharmacy and Medicines Optimisation. Making it Safe and Sound*. London: The Kings Fund.
Freedom of Information Act (2000) Available at: www.legislation.gov.uk/ (last accessed 2 June 2014).
Greenstein, B. and Gould, D. (2009) *Trounces Clinical Pharmacology for Nurses*, 18th edition. Edinburgh: Churchill Livingstone.
Lawson, L. and Hennefer, D.L. (2010) *Medicines Management in Adult Nursing*. Exeter: Learning Matters.
Leufer, T. and Cleary-Holdforth, J. (2013) 'Let's do no harm: medication errors in nursing part 1, *Nurse Education in Practice*', 13: 213–16.
The Medicines Act (1968) Available at: www.legislation.gov.uk/ukpga/1968/67 (last accessed 6 March 2015).
Misuse of Drugs Act (1971) Available at: www.legislation.gov.uk/ukpga/1971/38/contents (last accessed 2 June 2014).
Misuse of Drugs Regulations (2001) Available at: www.legislation.gov.uk/uksi/001/3998/ schedule/1/made (last accessed 6 March 2015).
National Coordinating Council for Medication Error Reporting and Prevention (2015) *What is Medication Error?* Available at: www.nccmerp.org/aboutMedErrors.html (last accessed 5 March 2015).
National Institute for Clinical Excellence (2009) *Depression in Adults: NICE Clinical Guidelines*. London: NICE.

National Patient Safety Agency (2005) 'Wristbands for all hospital inpatients improved safety'. Safer Practice Notice 11. London: NPSA.

National Patient Safety Agency (2010) *Rapid Response Report NPSA/2010/ RRR009: Reducing Harm from Omitted and Delayed Medicines in Hospital.* London: NPSA.

NHS Management Executive (1995) *Code of Practice on Openness in the NHS.* London: NHSE.

Nursing and Midwifery Council (2007) *Standards for Medicines Management.* Available at: www.nmc-uk.org/Documents/NMC-Publications/NMC-Standards-for-medicines-management.pdf (last accessed 7 January 2014).

Nursing and Midwifery Council (2010a) *Standards for Pre-registration Nursing Education.* Available at: http://standards.nmc-uk.org (last accessed 19 November 2014).

Nursing and Midwifery Council (2010b) *Standards for Competence for Registered Nurses.* Available at: www.nmc-uk.org/Documents/Standards/Standards%20for%20competence.pdf. (last accessed 19 November 2014).

Panwakar, R., Canonica, G.W., Holgate, S.T. and Lockey, R.F. (2011) *World Allergy Organisation White Book on Allergy 2011–2012: Executive Summary, World Allergy Organisation.* Available at: www.worldallergy.org/publications/wao_white_book.pdf (last accessed 23 September 2014).

Pope, T.M. (2002) 'The effect of nurses' use of focused protocol to reduce distraction during medicine administration' (Dissertation). Houston, TX: Texas Woman's University. (Cited in Cloo, J., Johnson, L. and Manias, E. (2013) 'Nurses medication administration practices at two Singaporean acute care hospitals', *Nursing and Health Sciences,* 15: 101–8).

Royal College of Nursing (2012) *RCN Factsheet: Nurse Prescribing in the UK.* London: Royal College of Nursing.

Szegedi, A., Kohen, R. Dienel, A., et al. (2005) 'Acute treatment of moderate to severe depression with hypericum extract WS 5570 (St John's Wort): randomised controlled double blinded trial', *British Medical Journal,* 5: 330 (7490): 530.

The Mental Capacity Act (2005) Available at: www.legislation.gov.uk/ukpga/2005/9/contents (last accessed 2 June 2014).

Smith, J. (2001) *The Shipman Inquiry, Fourth Report: The Regulation of Controlled Drugs in the Community.* Available at: http://webarchieve.nationalarchives.gov.uk/20090808154959/http:/www.the-shipman-inquiry.org.uk/fourthreport.asp (last accessed 2 June 2014).

Tully, M.P. (2012) 'Prescribing errors in hospital practice', *British Journal of Clinical Pharmacology,* 74(4): 668–75.

5 The NMC Essential Skills Clusters

DEBORAH WARD

The aim of this chapter is to introduce you to the Nursing and Midwifery Council *Essential Skills Clusters* (NMC, 2010a). In doing so, we hope to assist you to reflect upon how you can demonstrate the achievement of these skills in a practice setting, illustrated by the use of activities and case scenarios.

It is important at this point to note that the chapter is not intended to provide specific instruction about how to carry out various clinical skills. There are plenty of excellent resources already available that can help you with this aspect of your development (see the suggested Further Reading at the end of this chapter). Instead, the intention is to outline the basic essential requirements that you will need as a foundation upon which to build your nursing skills in preparation for entry to the register as an adult nurse. (NMC, 2010a) Furthermore, not every ESC statement contained within this chapter will be covered in depth as this would only repeat information which is readily available elsewhere. Instead, we will examine the main statements within each cluster and assist you in identifying how you might go about demonstrating your achievement of these in practice during your pre-registration period.

The chapter will also help to set the scene for Part Two of this book, which will examine specific aspects of nursing and care provision that are commonly encountered within the adult nursing field.

After reading this chapter you should be able to:

- Identify the five NMC Essential Skills Clusters that student nurses are required to achieve prior to registration (NMC, 2010a) and recognise the competency statements within each cluster.
- Discuss the key components within each cluster and identify ways in which competencies may be met and evidenced.
- Explain how each of the clusters can directly impact on patient care.
- Consider the professional and ethical aspects of each cluster.

Background

The Essential Skills Clusters (ESCs) were initially introduced by the NMC in 2007 (NMC, 2007a) for pre-registration nurses in order to ensure such students could demonstrate safe and effective practice in five key areas. They were updated again by the NMC in 2010 (NMC, 2010a) to reflect the move towards an all degree profession.

The ESCs set out the skills that adult nursing students are required to achieve within *five key areas* and at *three transition points*, the final transition being entry to the NMC register as a qualified nurse. However, the ESCs outlined here do not include all the skills required of a registered adult nurse. They are to be achieved in addition to the NMC Adult Nursing competencies (NMC, 2010b) which are outlined at the beginning of this book, and which have been linked to chapters within this book.

The five ESCs are:

1. Care, Compassion and Communication.
2. Organisational Aspects of Care.
3. Infection Prevention and Control.
4. Nutrition and Fluid Management.
5. Medicines Management.

Almost immediately you will perhaps be aware of the areas of overlap, not only with the NMC Competencies for Adult Nursing (NMC, 2010b) but also with the content outlined in this book. In that sense then, we hope that you see this chapter as an opportunity to examine more closely how these all fit together.

Each school and/or department delivering pre-registration nursing programmes may integrate the ESCs in different ways within the curriculum. For example, some may produce a specific document within an overall portfolio of student evidence which requires you as a student to demonstrate the competences required across the three years. Others may integrate the skill requirements into the practice assessment documents linked to each placement. Nevertheless, students, educators and mentors in clinical placement areas should all be left in no doubt as to what evidence needs to be gathered by adult nursing students during their own pre-registration undergraduate programme.

STOP AND THINK

*   How are students at your Higher Education Institution expected to demonstrate achievement of the ESCs? For example:

    o   Are the ESCS outlined within a student portfolio?
    o   Are they cross referenced to your practice placement documents?

*   Find out which skills need to be achieved at each of the NMC's 'progression points' (from year 1 to 2/year 2 to 3, and for entry onto the professional register).

In order to aid your understanding further, each cluster discussion within this chapter will contains a box providing NMC competency statements for that cluster, including in brackets the progression points at which each statement will be assessed, i.e. 1 (Progression from year 1 to 2); 2 (Progression from year 2 to 3); and/or 3 (Progression from year 3 to registered nurse).

NMC Cluster 1: Care, Compassion and Communication

ACTIVITY 5.1

Access the NMC website (www.nmc-uk.org) and carefully review 'The Code' (NMC, 2015).
   Which of the statements within The Code do you think relate to the 'Care, Compassion and Communication' Cluster?
   (It is essential that your practice is underpinned by The Code within this cluster.)
   You will perhaps note that the competency statements from year 1 become more advanced/detailed as students reach the subsequent progression point.

As you will see, this cluster (as with all of the others) contains several competency statements which are shown below.

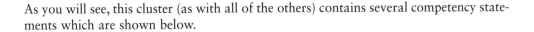

Competence statements for care, compassion and communication

People can trust a newly registered nurse:

- as partners in the care process, to provide collaborative care based on the highest standards, knowledge and competence (1, 2 and 3);
- to engage in person-centred care, empowering people to make choices about how their needs are met when they are unable to meet these themselves (1, 2 and 3);
- to respect them as individuals and strive to help them preserve their dignity at all times (1 and 3);
- to engage with them and their family or carers within their cultural environments in an accepting and anti-discriminatory manner, free from harassment and exploitation (1 and 3);
- to engage with them in a warm, sensitive and compassionate way (1 and 3);
- to engage therapeutically and actively listen to their needs and concerns, responding using skills that are helpful, and providing information that is clear, accurate, meaningful and free from jargon (1, 2 and 3);
- to protect and keep as confidential all information relating to them (1, 2 and 3);
- to gain their consent based on sound understanding and informed choice prior to any intervention, and that their rights in decision making and consent will be respected and upheld (1,2 and 3).

Source: NMC (2010a)

This cluster (as with all of the others) is also broken down further into individual competencies which you are required to meet at the three key progression points. The main foci of this cluster are:

- collaborative care with patients and families;
- working within knowledge and competence limitations;
- projecting professionalism and forming professional relationships;
- effective communication with others;
- learning from experience;
- demonstrating knowledge and skills in the cluster;
- demonstrating self-awareness;
- and ensuring confidentiality and consent and acting as a role model.

The NMC standards (2010a), particularly on *entry to the register* (stage 3), underpin the need to develop and maintain professional relationships and to deliver care without compromise while challenging any personal prejudices, identifying barriers to effective communication and care and developing a greater depth of self-awareness. If we now consider these key issues we should be able to understand more clearly what is required in practice in order to meet this cluster.

In previous chapters we have highlighted the findings of Francis (2013) and the Care Quality Commission (2012), both of which refer to nursing care deficits in terms of care and compassion. Therefore you will be aware of the importance of this cluster in terms of ensuring that adult nurses are able to deliver safe and effective care. Indeed, the requirement of adult nurses to develop and maintain such skills is also outlined within the Department of Health strategy *Compassion in Practice* (DH, 2012), 'the 6 Cs' and the Royal College of Nursing's *Principles of Nursing Practice* (RCN, 2010).

As an adult nurse, you will need to be able to demonstrate that you can collaborate effectively with patients and their relatives/carers, and involve them in decisions about their care, including any problems that you identify and interventions that you decide (under supervision as a student) to implement. Patients need to be considered as partners in their own care. You should be able to demonstrate your ability to provide care which is person-centred and which empowers patients to make their own choices about how their nursing needs are met.

STOP AND THINK

Have a look at the definition of *empowerment* provided in Chapter 8 (see pp. 294–296).

- How might you demonstrate your ability to empower patients in practice? Make a list of all of the examples you can think of.

You can *empower* patients by providing accurate information based upon your knowledge, experience and a sound evidence base so that they are able to give *informed consent* to any care or treatment they are offered. As a new student or member of staff this might mean that you act as a patient's advocate, ensuring that if you are not able to do this yourself, you are able to make sure that your patient can access someone else that can!

When a patient's decisions or choices may have a negative outcome on their care you will need to be able to deal with this, again through imparting your knowledge and ensuring that the patient understands the consequences of their decisions. For example, a patient with an inoperable malignant brain tumour (e.g. a glioma) who has received repeated courses of chemotherapy may decide that they do not wish to have any more treatment. This may be an appropriate decision for your patient, but in your role as an adult nurse you should ensure that they are clear about the consequences of not continuing with treatment.

You will need to communicate effectively with all types of patients in a professional manner, identifying and overcoming barriers to both effective communication and to building an appropriate relationship with a patient and their relatives/carers.

STOP AND THINK

Drawing upon what you have already learnt about effective communication in Chapter 2 consider the barriers to effective communication below – how might you overcome each of these?

- The patient does not speak English.
- The patient is deaf.
- The patient is blind.
- The patient has a severe learning difficulty.
- The patient arrives with chest pain from prison accompanied by two prison officers (you will also need to consider confidentiality here).

Mehrabian (1971) identified three key elements in any face-to-face communication and labelled these the *Three V rule*. These three elements were verbal (e.g. words), vocal (e.g. tone of voice) and visual (e.g. body language and gestures).

Looking beyond the way we verbally communicate and the factors that affect this (e.g. differences in accent or the overuse of acronyms and abbreviations), we need to consider how our gestures, posture and facial expression might be perceived by others. We also need to consider our tone of voice and whether this matches what we are saying. For example, we may stress certain words or use silence to encourage someone to think or speak.

We may also use therapeutic touch (though you will perhaps remember from discussion in Chapter 2 (p.48) that you will need to need to be careful in this area as you may make the patient feel uncomfortable, so take your cues from that individual and remember to maintain professional boundaries). We might also use space so do not sit or stand so close to a patient that they feel uncomfortable. Mehrabian (1971) found that when we decide whether we like someone we consider body language primarily, then tone of voice and finally what the person is saying. Much of our communication is therefore not about what is being said but how it is being conveyed and whether non-verbal messages are positive.

We have already explored the concept of active listening (Chapter 2, pp. 43–7) and have determined that it is a key skill that has several facets to it. However there are several barriers to listening effectively. These include issues such as:

- offering premature advice and reassurance before the patient's main problems have been verbalised;
- explaining away distress as normal;
- attending to physical aspects only;
- changing the subject and trying to 'jolly patients along';
- physical constraints such as time and work pressure.

Hastorf and Isen (1982) also identify less obvious barriers, such as making assumptions which can affect our perception of others and how we categorise and 'pigeonhole' them, errors in interpersonal perception, prejudices and stereotyping. For example, it is often easy to make judgements about patients based on the opinions of other staff members. Yet these views should be approached with caution in order to avoid stereotyping patients.

STOP AND THINK

Consider how you might demonstrate your achievement of the Care, Compassion and Communication ESC in practice. (You might wish to revisit Chapter 2 to assist you with this task.)

Think about a time when you have demonstrated achievement of the Care, Compassion and Communication Skills Cluster within a practice setting.

- What did you do?
- Why did you do it? What informed your actions?

In Chapter 1 (pp. 12–13) we introduced you to the concept of reflection and outlined how you might use this process to inform your professional development by illustrating how Gibb's model of reflection might help in this process. Reflection requires a level of self-awareness which this cluster requires you to increase across your three-year undergraduate programme. Self-awareness is not just recognising and describing an event or what happened, it is also concerned with understanding your own behaviours, personality and motivations (for example, why you became a student nurse, your emotional reactions to patients, staff or situations, your thought processes and how each of these informs not only *what* you do but also *why* you do it). Increased self-awareness can also help us to understand our reactions to other people and situations. Recognising your own feelings and prejudices and ensuring that these do not act as a barrier to providing compassionate care or communicating effectively with your patients, can help you overcome perceptual barriers. Care delivered without compassion becomes task orientated and lacks consideration and empathy.

Organisational aspects of care

The competence statements for this ESC are shown on the following page. Again, many aspects of this cluster are discussed in other chapters (see Chapters 7 and 13) such as *delegation, prioritisation, decision making* and *clinical governance.*

The cluster is mainly concerned with major issues such as the assessment, planning, implementation and evaluation of nursing care, effective team working, risk management (e.g. safeguarding and challenging poor practice), responding to feedback and recording and acting on vital signs and other recordable and observable data. Working within professional boundaries and acknowledging your own limitations are also important as is having knowledge of the theory that underpins practice. This is also stressed for qualified nurses – we should not be undertaking tasks that we are not competent to complete and should work within our current level of competence

Competence statements for organisational aspects of care

People can trust a newly registered graduate nurse to:

- treat them as partners and work with them to make a holistic and accurate assessment of their needs and to develop a personalised plan that is based on mutual understanding and respect for their own individual situation promoting health and well-being, minimising the risk of harm and promoting their safety at all times (1, 2 and 3);
- deliver nursing interventions and evaluate their effectiveness against the agreed assessment and care plan (2 and 3);
- safeguard children and adults from vulnerable situations and support and protect them from harm (1,2 and 3);
- respond to their feedback and a wide range of other sources to learn, develop and improve services (1,2 and 3);
- promote continuity when their care is to be transferred to another service or person (2);
- be an autonomous and confident member of the multidisciplinary or multi-agency team and to inspire confidence in others (1, 2 and 3);
- safely delegate to others and respond appropriately when a task is delegated to them (1 and 3);
- safely lead, co-ordinate and manage care (3);
- work safely under pressure and maintain the safety of service users at all times (1,2 and 3);
- enhance the safety of service users and identify and actively manage risk and uncertainty in relation to people, the environment, self and others (1,2 and 3);
- work to prevent and resolve conflict and maintain a safe environment (1 and 3);
- select and manage medical devices safely (1 and 3).

Source: NMC (2010a)

To illustrate how many aspects of this cluster could be achieved when caring for a single patient, the following patient scenario will be used.

Case Scenario

MRS BIBI

Mrs Bibi is a 58-year-old woman who has been admitted to a general medical ward with an infected leg ulcer and high blood sugar. She has Type 2 diabetes which is controlled by diet and medication. As the student nurse, you are delegated the task of assessing her needs as the first stage of the nursing process.

In this scenario, several of the aspects of the cluster can be demonstrated.

In caring for Mrs Bibi you quickly recognise potential communication difficulties as she is accompanied by her daughter who is acting as her interpreter (she does not speak English). Seeking the support of an independent interpreter you begin to build a therapeutic relationship with Mrs Bibi and provide reassurance to her supporting family, thereby demonstrating kindness and compassion.

Utilising a systematic approach, you begin your nursing assessment by adopting a relevant assessment framework that encourages an holistic approach. You assess the impact of Mrs Bibi's presenting medical conditions on her Activities of Daily Living (Roper et al., 2000) in order to identify which nursing interventions are needed. You also use other assessment tools such as the Waterlow Score (2008) to assess the risk of pressure ulcers, and the National Early Warning Score (NEWS) (Royal College of Physicians, 2012) which could help you with the early detection of any deterioration in her condition.

You undertake vital signs observations which you use to calculate the early warning score and also ascertain information about her current condition. You measure her temperature, pulse, respiratory rate, oxygen saturations and blood sugar. In order to do this you would use various equipment, for example medical devices that you have been trained to use. You would dispose of needles, sharps and/or other devices used as per local policy. You also undertake urinalysis when Mrs Bibi provides you with a urine sample.

You record the results of your observations:

- Temperature 38.5 degrees Centigrade.
- Pulse 98 beats per minute (bpm).
- Respiratory rate 20.
- Oxygen saturations 98% without oxygen.
- Blood sugar reading of 'Hi'.
- Urinalysis showing glucose, blood and protein (indicative of both high blood sugar and a urinary tract infection).

Using your underpinning knowledge of anatomy, physiology and altered pathology you recognise a deviation of vital sign readings (and diagnostic tests) from normal parameters. Working within the limitations of your knowledge and skills and in accordance with local policy (EWS), this triggers you to report the situation to a registered senior nurse. Mrs Bibi is seen by a doctor and assessed medically.

A wound swab is taken from her leg ulcer and a urine sample is sent to the laboratory for testing for culture and sensitivity to ascertain whether she does in fact have an infection. As a previous leg ulcer swab taken recently by her GP demonstrates potential infection, the doctor prescribes antibiotics.

Once medically assessed and immediate nursing actions have been taken to meet priority needs you continue to assess Mrs Bibi's activities of daily living. You find that she has difficulty mobilising due to the leg ulcer and that this is affecting her safety when she tries to mobilise on her own. You undertake a number of other assessments including a Falls Risk Assessment using evidence-based guidelines (NICE, 2013) which leads you to take steps to improve her level of safety while in hospital. You advise her to use the nurse call bell when she wishes to mobilise so that someone can assist her. You also discover that she has not been following her diabetic diet plan.

Following your full assessment you are able to identify Mrs Bibi's nursing problems and produce a plan of care to meet those needs. This plan includes providing health information about appropriate diet, referral to the dietician and physiotherapist and advice from the tissue viability nurse about the appropriate dressing treatment for the leg ulcer.

During Mrs Bibi's stay in hospital you perform evidence-based nursing interventions such as wound dressings, ensure the safe administration of medication supervised appropriately by your mentor, basing your care on both research evidence and your knowledge and previous experience. When the consultant decides that she is fit for discharge home you ensure that a referral is made back to the district nurse for ongoing management of her leg ulcer and to the diabetes nurse specialist in the community to provide continuity of care. However, Mrs Bibi's family are unhappy about her forthcoming discharge as they feel she is not well enough to go home.

- How would you respond to Mrs Bibi's family's concerns?
- What could you do to reassure them?
- Are you aware of local referral criteria and processes?

Find out how to refer to the district nurse and diabetes nurse specialist in your current placement.

STOP AND THINK

The scenario above clearly highlights how you would achieve a number of NMC requirements linked to the *Organisational Aspects of Care* skills cluster, though it is advisable that you access the full skills cluster document on the NMC website to be more fully aware of any additional requirements at the various progression points (e.g. if you are a year 3 student there are issues such as delegating to others, for example healthcare assistants, and demonstrating ward management skills which you would need to demonstrate prior to entry to the professional register).

Two important aspects of this cluster which you might find most difficult to deal with are *conflict resolution* and *challenging poor practice*. Whilst both of these topics are discussed in Chapter 8 (pp. 219 and 227) it would be useful to highlight these here.

In the previous scenario you would need to manage the conflict and respond to her family's concerns with consideration, accepting feedback and providing explanations as needed. This includes giving specific information about the support that she will be provided with at home. For example you would need to consider why conflict has arisen, what has caused this conflict, find out the reason for it and then address the issues appropriately. It is important to try to identify the source of conflict so that this can be more easily addressed.

We can often resolve most issues by communicating effectively with others. Conflict can arise from a number of different sources (Miall, 2011). These may be personal (e.g. related to a clash in personalities and/or values and expectations). This could, for example, be related to past experiences or personal views and opinions. There could also be organisational causes for conflict. As a nursing student for example you will have clinical placements in a variety of different organisations, each with their own rules and ways of working. This can then cause conflict if the policies and procedures in one organisation are different from those of another (for example, conflict related to ways of working, clinical philosophies, the needs of groups of patients and the ways in which groups of staff work).

When in a clinical placement, you might observe practice that you consider to be sub-optimal. This might relate to poor communication or poor clinical care, such as non-compliance with the correct and safe procedures. You may remember that we introduced you to the concept of evidence-based practice and the professional requirements linked to the NMC Code in Chapter 1 (p. 28). All nurses are taught about the importance of evidence-based practice and are therefore called upon to regularly review and consider what best practice is. As research continually strives to inform practice, traditional practice methods can become outdated as evidence suggests a new way of doing things that will bring positive benefits to patients. However, this means that students (and practitioners) can find themselves in a difficult position, caught between the tension of what is considered best practice and the sub-optimal care provision they sometimes witness in practice.

Research has highlighted that there are many barriers to reporting poor practice (Ward, 2010), not least the fear of being viewed negatively by other staff – or in the case of a student – a mentor failing that student's placement because poor practice has been reported. However, challenging poor practice and ensuring that concerns are raised and escalated appropriately are vital for good quality care and positive patient outcomes. Indeed the ability to do so links closely with one of the 6Cs (i.e. *Courage*).

The NMC Code (NMC, 2015) and NMC Guidance on Professional Conduct for Nursing and Midwifery Students (NMC, 2013) require us to *act in the best interests* of our patients, make the care of our patients *our first concern*, and *work to protect and promote their well-being* at all times. Therefore whilst as students and qualified nurses we might be concerned about what happens to us personally if we challenge or report poor practice, we should primarily be more concerned about the consequences for our patients. Each Higher Education Institution and healthcare provider will have their own policies and procedures relating to reporting poor practice. It is important to be aware of the local Raising and Escalating Concerns process so that if you are ever in such a position you are clear about what to do and who you can speak to. (The escalating concerns process is discussed further in Chapter 8, pp. 225–227).

Infection prevention and control

The box below demonstrates the competence statements for this cluster. These require nurses to:

- adhere to standard and other infection prevention and control precautions;
- apply the principles of asepsis for invasive procedures and wound care;
- apply microbiological knowledge to practice and to challenge poor practice in others.

The *Health and Social Care Act 2008* (DH, 2009) stipulates that staff should receive education in infection prevention and control and that policies should be in place which staff should adhere to. In terms of evidence-based practice the precautions which need to be applied are underpinned by relevant guidelines (Loveday et al., 2014) in all settings across the UK (NICE, 2012; DHSSPS, 2013; Health Protection Scotland, 2014; Wigglesworth, 2014).

--------- Competence statements for infection prevention ---------
and control

People can trust the newly registered graduate nurse to:

- identify and take effective measures to prevent and control infection in accordance with local and national policy (1,2 and 3);
- maintain effective standard infection control precautions and apply and adapt these to needs and limitations in all environments (1,2 and 3);
- provide effective nursing interventions when someone has an infectious disease including the use of standard isolation techniques (1, 2 and 3);
- fully comply with hygiene, uniform and dress codes in order to limit, prevent and control infection (1 and 3);
- safely apply the principles of asepsis when performing invasive procedures and be competent in aseptic technique in a variety of settings (2 and 3);
- act in a variety of environments – including the home care setting – to reduce risk when handling waste including sharps, contaminated linen and when dealing with spillages of blood and other body fluids (2 and 3).

Source: NMC (2010a)

Healthcare-associated infection is a problem worldwide. While worldwide prevalence varies, it is estimated at 6.4% in the UK (Health Protection Agency, 2012), with many of these cases being preventable and with a resulting cost of over one billion pounds annually to the NHS (National Audit Office, 2009). In addition, there are costs to the patient in terms of health deficits, time off work and treatment such as antibiotics. It is therefore important that we minimise the risk of infection as far as is possible when we administer care to our patients.

Microbiological knowledge

While standard infection prevention and control precautions should be applied to all patients (including hand hygiene, the use of personal protective equipment, sharps management, decontamination and spillage management), as adult nurses we need to be able to identify when someone has an infection in order to manage it effectively. This involves having some knowledge of microbiology, in particular groups of micro-organisms, routes of transmission of infection, sources of infection and the signs and symptoms of infection. While this knowledge can be gained in a university setting, it needs to be applied in a practice setting.

The starting point is the chain of infection shown in Figure 5.1. In order to prevent infection one of the links needs to be removed from the situation. Some knowledge and appreciation of the links and how these apply to different infections is therefore vital in infection prevention.

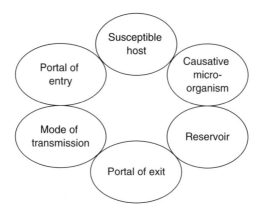

Figure 5.1   The six links within a chain of infection

There are general signs and symptoms of infection which can guide our practice such as pyrexia, redness and swelling, increased pain and pus production. However, there also needs to be an appreciation of specific signs and symptoms for different sites of infection and for symptoms which are not necessarily listed in the usual textbooks – remember that as adult nurses we sometimes need to 'think outside the box'.

STOP AND THINK

Consider the following sites of infection. What might the signs and symptoms of infection be in these sites?

- Eye.
- Chest.
- Surgical wound.
- Urinary tract.

The ability to recognise infection in our patients improves with experience. It is therefore worth asking qualified nurses in practice why they consider something to be infected when they arrive at this conclusion. It may not always be obvious to you initially, but with time the additional symptoms that qualified nurses recognise will become part of your knowledge base. Factors which affect the signs and symptoms of infection also need to be considered. For example, wound dressings can sometimes cause wounds to look infected to the novice and a sound knowledge of wound dressings, their actions and their consequences will help with this.

Understanding the *routes of transmission* of infection is also important in identifying strategies to prevent cross-infection.

There are four main routes of transmission:

- *Airborne* – through aerosol droplets and respiratory secretions (examples of infections transmitted by this route include chicken pox, influenza and pulmonary tuberculosis).
- *Faecal-oral* – hand to mouth transmission (e.g. salmonella enteritidis, campylobacter).
- *Contact* – this can be direct or indirect and is the most common route of transmission in healthcare, usually via staff's hands or the environment (e.g. MRSA).
- *Blood and body fluid* – through vertical transmission (mother to baby) or horizontal transmission (e.g. unprotected sex, sharing needles, bites etc.). This includes the blood- and vector-borne infections such as hepatitis B and C, HIV and malaria.

The route of transmission is one of the links in the chain of infection, thus by interrupting the route of transmission we can therefore remove this link and prevent infection. Application of standard precautions is one way we can interrupt the route of transmission.

Another link identified is the *susceptible host*, namely people at risk of infection. There are many factors which can increase a person's risk of infection and these will need to be minimised in order to reduce that risk. However, we perhaps don't need to point out here that not all risk factors can be negated (e.g. increasing age or some chronic diseases). In healthcare we aim to reduce the risk of infection as far as possible, while working with people who have inherent risks which increase their susceptibility and which we cannot address. Some factors are related to the situation that patients find themselves in when requiring healthcare. This includes the need to take some medications, the presence of invasive devices and surgical intervention. All of these increase the risk of infection but are required both to improve quality of life and save lives. We must therefore accept as nurses that the things that we may do to ultimately help our patients may also increase their risk of infection (e.g. urinary catheterisation) and as a result we must put systems in place to minimise this risk as far as possible. This includes implementing standard precautions.

Standard precautions

All patients (whether known to have an infection or not) should be considered to be a source of infection. The standard precautions previously mentioned should therefore be applied to minimise the risk of both infection and cross-infection. These precautions will often be taught in both the skills laboratory and in practice and they should always be applied in all placement areas.

All of the UK national guidelines (NICE, 2012; Loveday et al., 2014) highlight the importance of hand hygiene in the control of infection. The World Health Organization's (WHO, 2009) 'five moments' campaign highlights when hands should be decontaminated in healthcare.

ACTIVITY 5.2

Access the following website at http://who.int/gpsc/tools/Five_moments/en/. Focus on the WHO's five moments of hand hygiene.

- Identify the 'five moments' of hand hygiene and reflect upon how they align with the evidence base concerning the spread of Hospital Acquired Infections (HAI).

Hand hygiene is a basic but essential aspect of nursing care. In most care situations outside of a theatre environment routine hand hygiene is required. This involves the use of soap and water or an alcohol hand rub. Usually posters above hand basins in clinical areas will demonstrate the steps involved in the technique to ensure that all areas of the hands are cleaned. However, one important aspect that is often neglected is skin care. Using soaps incorrectly and not fully following the correct hand decontamination procedures can result in damaged skin on hands – this then increases the bacterial count on hands and can therefore contribute to infection. It is thus vital that hand hygiene guidelines are followed and that products provided are used correctly. This is particularly the case when using an alcohol hand rub which can cause dry and irritated skin if care is not taken.

Protective clothing such as disposable gloves and aprons, masks and visors should be provided in healthcare settings to protect both you and your patients. Non-sterile items are for the protection of staff. Sterile items such as gloves are worn for both staff and patient protection. You therefore need to understand when sterile and non-sterile items should be used. There are a variety of glove types available, with each one being suitable for different tasks. Being aware of these glove types and what they can be used for is part of your role in protecting both yourself and your patients. These might include polythene (not recommended for use in clinical practice), vinyl, latex, nitrile and neoprene. On each placement it is recommended that you find out what type is available for use. This is particularly important if you have a latex sensitivity. Disposable gloves and aprons are designated as 'single use' items. This demands the need to change them between patients and between different activities on the same patient to avoid contamination. It is worth considering that aprons costs a few pence each whereas a healthcare-associated infection can cost upwards of £4,000 to treat (National Audit Office, 2009).

Other standard precautions include the safe management and disposal of sharps (including needles), the correct management of blood and body fluid, spills and decontamination (Loveday et al., 2014). Perhaps the least simple of these is decontamination – this is really an umbrella term which could mean cleaning, disinfection or sterilisation. It is therefore important that if you are asked to decontaminate a piece of equipment you request further clarification of the correct process required to avoid mistakes. Manufacturers of medical devices are legally obliged to provide information on how their devices should be decontaminated and these instructions should be followed in clinical practice (MHRA, 2014). If decontamination instructions from manufacturers are not appropriate, this should be reported to the MHRA. Instructions might include designating items as single use. This means using the item once and then disposing of it. Some items might be designated as 'single patient use'. This means that it can be used several times on the same patient but not on anyone else.

Compliance with standard precautions

One of the issues that nurses sometimes have to deal with is non-compliance with infection prevention and control precautions. Some understanding of rates of compliance and reasons for non-compliance is therefore useful. The research literature highlights that there is poor compliance worldwide with aspects such as hand hygiene and the use of protective clothing (Gammon et al., 2008). This is the case in both acute and community settings. Many reasons have been identified for this including a lack of or poor facilities, skin problems (related to hand hygiene) and/or a lack of manual dexterity (related to glove use), a lack of time, workload issues, the lack of management support and positive role models, levels of motivation, a lack of risk perception, and/or a lack of knowledge. As a student you need to be aware of the challenges inherent in working in a healthcare setting and should not be willing to accept sub-optimal practice as the norm. Poor practice is not acceptable and puts both patients and staff at risk. Highlighting ways in which we can overcome the barriers to good practice is important, such as education, the provision of better facilities and the correct use of hand decontamination agents to lessen the potential for adverse effects on the skin.

Isolation

In terms of infection prevention and control, there are two main types of isolation: *source isolation* (formerly known as barrier nursing) where patients with a known or suspected infection or infectious disease are isolated to protect other patients; and *protective isolation* (formerly known as reverse barrier nursing) where patients are isolated to protect them from others, such as in bone marrow transplantation. For the purposes of this ESC, we will focus on source isolation. Examples of common infections for which patients may be isolated include pulmonary tuberculosis, norovirus, chicken pox and Clostridium difficile. Different organisations will have different policies and procedures about who is isolated and this may also differ between ward areas in the same organisation in relation to risk. Source isolation generally involves isolating the patient in a single room but in some circumstances might involve what is termed 'cohort nursing'. This means putting patients with the same infection in one room or bay together. Though you need to be aware that this is not appropriate for some infectious diseases, i.e. pulmonary tuberculosis. When in doubt, a member of the organisation's infection prevention and control team should be contacted.

In some situations, a risk assessment and management process has to be utilised to decide which patient should be isolated when there is a lack of single rooms. Cohort nursing is sometimes the answer but in other cases difficult decisions have to be made. Knowledge of different infections and their routes of transmission is important in decision making processes here. Just knowing the name of the infection may not be enough. Consider if there is only one side room available and there are three patients with infections. How do we decide who is placed in isolation? If we take this further and say that one patient has MRSA, one has tuberculosis and one has Clostridium difficile, can a decision be made with that knowledge? The answer should be 'no', as much more information is needed. For example, what part of the body is infected with tuberculosis (it may not be in the lungs), where is the MRSA (is it in a covered wound or in sputum in a patient with a productive cough?) and is the patient with Clostridium difficile symptomatic?

Ensuring that you have full information on each patient combined with knowledge of the routes of transmission will enable you to make an informed decision which minimises the risk to others.

Aseptic non-touch technique (ANTT)

This Essential Skills Cluster requires you to be able to carry out ANTT and apply the principles of asepsis. While it is not within the remit of this chapter to list the stages in an ANTT procedure – these can be found in a clinical skills book such as the *Marsden Manual* (Dougherty and Lister, 2011) – discussing the underpinning principles of asepsis is important so that you understand the rationale for the skills you will use in your placement. Asepsis occurs when the area being managed or treated is kept free from contaminants which may cause disease such as bacteria, viruses, fungi or parasites. This is important when dealing with breaks in the skin or when inserting invasive devices. Surgical asepsis occurs in the operating theatre where hand decontamination involves a surgical scrub, skin is disinfected, sterile instruments are used and air changes reduce airborne organisms. On wards and in the community setting, asepsis will apply to procedures such as wound dressings, the insertion of a urinary catheter and the management of central lines. In addition to the usual standard precautions, an ANTT includes the use of sterile equipment (including gloves) and ensuring that only sterile items come into contact with the key part such as the wound, the catheter and so on. In practice this means using sterile packs. As with other clinical procedures it is recommended that you only carry out ANTT if you have the knowledge and skills to do so.

Uniform policies

In England (DH, 2010) guidance on NHS work-wear has been updated following a review of current research evidence. The review highlights that while there is no direct evidence that uniforms contribute to cross-infection, staff should adhere to good practice guidelines and local policies to reflect professionalism and maintain staff and patient safety. There is a general consensus that to enable better hand hygiene and minimise infection, staff should be bare below the elbows when carrying out patient care activities. This includes jewellery as well as clothing. The current guidance also offers some advice on cultural issues which may arise when asking staff to bare their lower arms and remove jewellery.

ACTIVITY 5.3

Compare the Infection Control Policies in the guidance documents below:

1. **Scotland**: Health Protection Scotland (2014), *National Infection Prevention and Control Manual*, V2.3. Available at www.documents.hps.scot.nhs.uk/hai/infection-control/ic-manual/ipcm-p-v2-3.pdf (last accessed 10 January 2015).
2. **Northern Ireland:** DHSSPS (2013), *The Northern Ireland Regional Infection Prevention and Control Manual*. Belfast: DHSSPS.

3. **Wales:** Wigglesworth, N. (2014) *National Model Policies for Infection Prevention and Control in Wales.*
4. **England**: Department of Health (2010) *Uniforms and Workwear: Guidance on Uniform and Workwear Policies for NHS Employers.* London: DH.

Make a note of the similarities and differences between each of these.

The infection prevention and control team

Each NHS organisation has access to a team of staff who provide a service related to infection prevention and control. The most familiar to nurses is the infection prevention and control nurse.

ACTIVITY 5.4

Find out who is the Infection Control Nurse/Contact for your practice area.
Identify and locate the Infection Prevention and Control policies for your practice area.

Nutrition and fluid management

There are several competence statements related to this cluster as demonstrated in the box below. The majority of these are for achievement at progression points 2 and 3. Each of these have individual competences which you can find in the full ESC document on the NMC website (www.nmc-uk.org).

Competence statements for nutrition and fluid management

People can trust a newly registered graduate nurse to:

- assist them to choose a diet that provides adequate nutritional and fluid intake (2 and 3);
- assess and monitor their fluid and nutritional status and in partnership with them formulate an effective plan of care (2 and 3);
- assist them in creating an environment that is conducive to eating and drinking (1, 2 and 3);
- ensure that those unable to take food by mouth receive adequate fluid and nutrition to meet their needs (2 and 3);
- safely administer fluids when fluids cannot be taken independently (3).

Source: NMC (2010a)

In order to manage a patient's nutritional needs adequately a baseline assessment must first be undertaken and this should then be reviewed regularly . Once a proper assessment has been undertaken problems can be identified and a plan of care developed, implemented and evaluated.

The NICE quality standard for nutrition support in adults recommends that *'people in care settings are screened for the risk of malnutrition using a validated screening tool'* (NICE, 2012a: 7). This suggests that all patients, whether in hospital or in a primary care setting, should be screened. As an adult nurse you will undertake many of these assessments, often as part of the hospital admission process. It is therefore important that you understand the tools you are using in the assessment to ensure an accurate and appropriate outcome for the patient.

One commonly used tool is the Malnutrition Screening Tool or MUST (BAPEN, 2004). This is used in many hospitals across the United Kingdom and is comprised of five simple steps which identify whether a patient is at low, medium or high risk of malnutrition. The overall score is determined by the Body Mass Index which will require you to measure the patient's weight and height; an assessment of unplanned weight loss in the past three to six months; and how acutely ill the patient is in terms of poor nutritional intake for greater than five days. Those individuals identified as *low risk* should have repeat screening – the regularity of this is determined by local protocol and is often influenced by where the patient is being cared for, for example annual screening is recommended for individuals over 75 living in their own homes. Those at *medium risk* should be observed and this involves documentation of their dietary intake for three days with action taken following that. Those at *high risk* should be treated unless this is of no benefit to the patient. This includes referral to a dietician. In a very simple way, the MUST tool identifies level of risk and suggests basic actions to take.

ACTIVITY 5.5

Access a copy of the MUST tool (www.bapen.org.uk/screening-for-malnutrition/must/must-toolkit/the-must-itself) and familiarise yourself with it.

- Do you think this provides an adequate assessment of nutritional status?
- What other tools are available?

It needs to be acknowledged (as with all screening tools) that these are meant to be used as a guide only (in conjunction with your own knowledge and professional judgement). Screening tools are there to support your assessment and clinical decision making regarding nursing interventions and treatment. A sound knowledge base is needed in order to undertake a thorough nutritional assessment. This knowledge should be comprised of an adequate understanding of anatomy and physiology, the normal processes involved in the acquisition and assimilation of nutrients, factors that can influence nutrition and the effects of malnutrition on health and healing for example.

Following on from the assessment, regular monitoring should be undertaken. This may be as a result of the patient being identified as medium risk or on the recommendation of the dietician. This might involve the use of a food diary or fluid balance chart. Some patients will be unable to feed themselves and it is part of the nurse's role to ensure that patients receive adequate nutrition and hydration. This will require assisting patients to eat and drink. Care may need to be taken with some patients due to swallowing difficulties and advice from professionals such as the speech and language therapist about issues such as thickness of fluids will need to be adhered to.

The nurse's role in health promotion and nutrition is vital here. In order to provide advice and support for a patient about their diet, you will need to be knowledgeable yourself. Of course, the dietician can provide additional in-depth information but it is beneficial to have some knowledge and awareness of what a healthy diet is, the impact of nutritional deficiencies and also of some of the diet restrictions involved in conditions such as diabetes mellitus.

Some patients will be unable to take nutrition orally. NICE (2006) provide guidance for these patients in relation to enteral and parenteral nutrition. This ESC requires that students at progression points 2 and 3 are able to ensure that patients who cannot take food orally are adequately fed and hydrated (e.g. due to a swallowing impairment following a stroke or if a patient is unconscious).

In order to gain entry to the register, you will be required to be able to insert naso-gastric tubes and manage them following insertion, in addition to managing the administration of nutrition by other means such as PEGs and intravenous devices.

In order to be able to carry out such procedures safely and effectively, you must ensure that you have the relevant skills and training. Local policies and procedures should be followed and the clinical criteria which permit tube feeding should be adhered to. It is not enough, as a nurse, to be able to undertake the skill of NG tube insertion after watching your mentor or another qualified member of staff carry out the procedure. You will need to understand why the tube is being inserted, what the contraindications are, how the tube works and the problems it may cause to ensure that you are able to provide safe and effective patient care.

NG tubes may be inserted for a number of reasons but of relevance to this cluster is partial or total nutritional support where a patient is unable to meet their own needs orally. The decision should be made following a proper nutritional assessment and a tube should only be inserted if the patient has a functional gastrointestinal tract. NG tubes are usually used to provide short-term nutritional support, sometimes whilst awaiting the insertion of a more long-term feeding tube such as a PEG.

There can also be many negative consequences to inserting an NG tube. The patient should therefore be monitored for potential complications. As a foreign body, the NG tube is a portal of entry for micro-organisms and infection prevention and control procedures should therefore be adhered to. There is also a risk of trauma to the nostrils during insertion and damage from securing the tube to the face. The tube can block during feeding or medicine administration and its position can also change. In order to minimise the risks, care should be taken on insertion and during the administration of feeds and medicines. If complications are suspected, action should be taken by informing the supervising registered nurse.

It is also important that you know when the insertion of an NG tube would not be appropriate. For example, NG tubes should not be used for long-term nutritional support or in patients with a dysfunctional gastrointestinal tract. In some situations more specialist advice may be needed prior to making the decision to insert a tube. This might involve an ENT specialist or radiologist and perhaps the need to carefully consider the risk for patients with oesophageal tumours or varices, skull fractures, those who have had recent head or neck surgery, including a laryngectomy, and patients with maxillo-facial disorders. As a student you should always work under the supervision of a registered nurse. Decisions about whether a tube is appropriate should therefore rest with that nurse.

Documentation (as with other aspects of nursing) is also vital in relation to fluid and nutritional management. Records of the administration of feeds and intravenous fluids should be made so that accurate calculations can be made about progress. This will include keeping accurate records of fluid balance, regularly documenting assessment findings such as the MUST score, recording the patient's body mass index, keeping food diaries and noting any changes and amendments to patient management in the care plan. The NMC (2009) has its own guidance for record keeping which should be adhered to. Correct record keeping, accountability, making continuity of care easier and enabling the early detection of complications are all applicable to nutrition management.

Medicines management

The box below shows the competence statements for this cluster. Chapter 4 on medicines management should be useful to you in terms of the knowledge base for this cluster.

─────────── Competence statements for medicines ───────────
management

People can trust the newly registered graduate nurse to:

- correctly and safely undertake medicines calculations (1 and 3);
- work within legal and ethical frameworks that underpin safe and effective medicines management (2 and 3);
- work as part of a team to offer holistic care and a range of treatment options of which medicines may form a part (2 and 3);
- ensure safe and effective practice in medicines management through a comprehensive knowledge of medicines, their actions, risks and benefits (2 and 3);
- safely order, receive, store and dispose of medicines (including controlled drugs) in any setting (2 and 3);
- administer medicines safely and in a timely manner, including controlled drugs (2 and 3);
- keep and maintain accurate records using information technology where appropriate, within a multidisciplinary framework as a leader and as part of a team and in a variety of settings including at home (2 and 3);
- work in partnership with people receiving medical treatments and their carers (2 and 3);
- use and evaluate up-to-date information on medicines management and work within national and local policy guidelines (2 and 3);
- demonstrate understanding and knowledge to supply and administer via a patient group direction (2 and 3).

Source: NMC (2010a)

Drug calculations

There are many calculations involved in medicines management which may be fairly basic, e.g. calculating the number of pills required to make up the dose, or more complicated, e.g. when administering intravenous drugs which rely on the weight of the patient. Over the course of your pre-registration programme you will be assessed in drugs calculations as this is an NMC requirement (NMC, 2010a, 2010b). It is also becoming increasingly common that a drugs calculation test is included in interviews for registered nurse posts after qualifying. As miscalculation results in drug errors, this is a key aspect of medicines administration.

Legal and ethical frameworks

Such aspects have already been covered in Chapter 4. However it is worth stressing here that it is vital that you are aware of the legal aspects of medicines administration (such as the *Misuse of Drugs Act 1971*, the *Medicines Act 1968* and the *Misuse of Drugs Regulations 2001*). You will also need to be mindful of ethical issues such as being asked to administer medication without consent from the patient or hiding medication in food in order to administer it.

Underpinning knowledge

If you are administering medication, it is important that you have some pharmacological knowledge about the action of the drug, contraindications, side effects and interactions. You will also need to have knowledge of the usual doses for the drugs you administer so that you can avoid drug errors. Knowledge in these areas ensures not only that you fully understand the actions and consequences of the drugs that you are administering, but also that you are able to explain these things to patients and their relatives. It is not expected that you become an expert in every medicine available but you should be aware of the drugs that you are administering. The use of books such as the *British National Formulary* (BNF) is common in practice where the nurse is not fully knowledgeable about a drug being given.

Drug administration

Can you remember the five rights of drug administration outlined in Chapter 4? Write these down and then check your answer below.

STOP AND THINK

You should check that you have the following five things right:

1. *Patient* – by checking their identification band if in hospital.
2. *Drug* – this is particularly important when considering both generic and trade names for drugs.
3. *Dose* – this also includes that the dose prescribed is appropriate.
4. *Route* – i.e. oral, intravenous, intramuscular, subcutaneous and so on.
5. *Time* – though drugs prescribed for 10am are not all administered at exactly 10am, it should be ensured that the drug is being administered at the correct time of day.

Identify at least *10 of the common drugs and medications* used on each of your placements.
   Make a note of the aims of each treatment, drug strengths or concentrations, routes of administration, potential side effects and interactions.
   Keep a record of these in your portfolio, adding to your list each time you undertake a new placement.

When administering medication, it is also important to adhere to other requirements such as infection control and documentation.

Record keeping

As with other aspects of nursing, documentation is vital in medicines management. Correctly completing drug charts after medicines administration is important as is noting allergies and the reasons for medicines being missed/not administered. This includes documentation of intravenous fluids and nutritional support. Again, the NMC (2009) record-keeping guidance should be considered in addition to their standards for medicines management (NMC, 2007b).

Patient Group Directions (PGDs)

According to the Royal College of Nursing (2004), 'a PGD, signed by a doctor and agreed by a pharmacist, can act as a direction to a nurse to supply and/or administer prescription-only medicines (POMs) to patients using their own assessment of patient need, without necessarily referring back to a doctor for an individual prescription'. PGDs should only be used where there is patient benefit as usually patients should be treated as individuals, and in a situation of similarity within the group. Examples might include immunisations, pre-operative drugs for specific procedures where all patients are administered the same drug or drugs or common medications for those with specific chronic diseases. The usefulness of this in areas such as surgery and immunisation clinics can easily be recognised. There are some restrictions on the use of controlled drugs due to some of the consequences of administration and in certain areas only specialist nurses can administer. It is part of the NMC's requirements that as a student you demonstrate the knowledge and understanding of the processes required when administering medications via a PGD. In some universities, for example, this may be measured through the use of an OSCE; an examination using simulation, often in a clinical skills laboratory.

What can help you demonstrate your achievement of NMC Essential Skills Clusters in practice?

Some would argue that the most valuable learning experiences take place in practice. However, Dewey (1933) suggests experience is only the raw material for learning. Therefore it is how you utilise the learning experience from practice and what you do with it that matters. The ability to apply underpinning theories to the care that you provide to your patients in a practice setting is a fundamental part of your learning process. During the first year of your studies it is expected that you will need guidance, help and support to guide your practice. However, as you progress through your programme of study expectations of your abilities in practice will gradually increase as you become more able to use previous experience to plan, assess and prioritise care. At the end of year 3 you will normally be expected to provide co-ordinated care confidently and efficiently.

It is important to take advantage of all the learning opportunities available to you on every placement area, working with your mentor/supervising practitioner regularly. Working with a range of other health and social care professionals can also help you gain additional knowledge of their roles and specialist skills. Similarly, working a range of different shifts (including night duty) will help you get a sense of the differences in 24-hour care provision.

Whilst your achievement of many of the required competencies and skills will be directly observed by your mentor in practice (e.g. focusing upon the communication skills you use to interact with your patients, carers and other team members), the changing nature of the NHS means that most students will not spend *all* of their time with their allocated mentor. This can sometimes present as a challenge to mentors in terms of assessing your ability and achievements at the end of a placement. Therefore, being able to provide your mentor with other examples and evidence from practice which allow you to demonstrate how you have met the required competencies is useful.

This is one of the purposes of the student portfolio we mentioned briefly in Chapter 1 (pp. 11–13). As a student you are expected to gather evidence of your achievements and match these to your learning outcomes, taking a level of responsibility for your own learning. Collecting additional supporting evidence in this way and combining this with your mentor's direct observations of practice will assist your mentor to carry out a more holistic assessment of your achievements.

For example, your supporting evidence may consist of:

- *short briefing papers (*along with your own reflections*)* for your mentor on what has been learned during a spoke placement or brief visit;
- *testimonials* from other practitioners that you have spent time with;
- *reflective accounts* of your experiences with patients or during particular procedures or situations (taking care to ensure the confidentiality of all those involved);
- *written case studies or personalised care plans* (taking care to ensure the confidentiality of all those involved);
- *evidence of reading* certain documents or literature (e.g. policies, protocols and guidelines) and then *discussing* these with your mentor or other healthcare professionals demonstrates your awareness of supporting evidence that can be used to underpin the care you provide to your patients: this is a particularly good way of demonstrating that you have a sufficient theoretical understanding of a particular clinical issue or policy;
- *patient/service user feedback* can often be used to provide a valid and tangible source of evidence of your abilities;
- *verified evidence of attendance at workshops/courses/study days* (though this evidence can be strengthened by the addition of a reflective piece which indicates how you plan to apply your newly acquired knowledge in practice).

Chapter summary

This chapter has served as a brief introduction to the NMC Skills Clusters which adult nursing students have to achieve at three key progression points during their degree programme: the final point being *entry to the register*. We have considered the *Five Core Clusters*, highlighting the overall competencies required.

It is hoped that by briefly explaining how each of the skills clusters can be demonstrated by students in practice, making links to other chapters within this book and providing references to the relevant evidence-based guidelines which underpin practice, we have helped you to understand their relevance to contemporary nursing practice, whatever the clinical setting.

Suggested further reading

Bach, S.A. and Grant, A. (2011) *Communication and Interpersonal Skills in Nursing*, 2nd edition. Exeter: Learning Matters.

Baille, L. (ed.) (2009) *Developing Practical Adult Nursing Skills*, 3rd edition. London: Hodder Arnold.

Best, C. (2008) *Nutrition: A Handbook for Nurses*. Hoboken, NJ: Wiley.

Chambers, C. and Ryder, E. (2009) *Compassion and Caring in Nursing*. Oxford: Radcliffe.

Crouch, S., Chapelhow, C. and Crouch, M.A. (2008) *Medicines Management: A Nursing Perspective*. Harlow: Pearson Education.

Danami, N. (2012) *Manual of Infection Prevention and Control*. Oxford: Oxford University Press.

Docherty, C. and McCallum, J. (eds) (2009) *Foundation Clinical Nursing Skills*. Oxford: Oxford University Press.

Doherty, L. and Lister, S. (2009) *The Royal Marsden Hospital Manual of Clinical Nursing Procedures* (Student Edition). Oxford: Wiley Blackwell.

Endacott, R., Jevon, P. and Cooper, S. (2009) *Clinical Nursing Skills: Core and Advanced*. Oxford: Oxford University Press.

Gibney, M.J., Lantam-New, S.A., Cassidy, A. and Vorster, H.H. (2009) *Introduction to Human Nutrition*. Hoboken, NJ: Wiley.

Gould, D. and Brooker, C. (2008) *Applied Microbiology for Healthcare*, 2nd edition. Basingstoke: Palgrave Macmillan.

Jevon, P., Payne, L., Higgins, D. and Endecott, R. (2010) *Medicines Management: A Guide for Nurses*. Hoboken, NJ: Wiley.

Lapham, R. and Agar, H. (2009) *Drug Calculations for Nurses: A Step by Step Approach*, 3rd edition. London: Hodder.

Lawson, L. and Hennefer, D. (2010) *Medicines Management in Adult Nursing*. London: Sage.

Mayer, B.H., Tucker, S. and Williams, S. (2007) *Nutrition Made Incredibly Easy*. Philadelphia: Lippincott Williams and Wilkins.

Rushforth, H. (2009) *Assessment Made Incredibly Easy*. London: Lippincott Williams and Wilkins.

Smith, B. (2011) *Nursing and Health: Compassion, Caring and Communication*. Harlow: Pearson Education.

Soule, B.M., Memish, Z.A. and Malani, P.N. (2012) *Best Practices in Infection Prevention and Control*, 2nd edition. Illinois: Joint Commission International.

Sully, P. and Dallas, J. (2010) *Essential Communication Skills for Nursing and Midwifery*, 2nd edition. Edinburgh: Mosby.

Weston, D. (2013) *Fundamentals of Infection Prevention and Control: Theory and Practice*, 2nd edition. Oxford: Wiley Blackwell.

World Health Organization (2013) *Meeting the Nutritional Needs of Older Persons*. Geneva: WHO.

Wilkinson, J.M. (2012) *Nursing Process and Critical Thinking*, 5th edition. New Jersey: Pearson.

Zator Estes, M.E. (2014) *Health Assessment and Physical Examination,* 5th edition. New York: Delmar Healthcare.

References

BAPEN Malnutrition Advisory Group (2004) *Malnutrition Universal Screening Tool*. London: BAPEN.

Care Quality Commission (2012) *State of Care Report*. London: CQC.

Department of Health (2004) *Building a Safer NHS: Improving Medication Safety*. London: DH.

Department of Health (2009) *The Health and Social Care Act (2008)*. London: DH.

Department of Health (2010) *Uniforms and Workwear: Guidance on Uniform and Workwear Policies for NHS Employers*. London: DH.

Department of Health (2012) *Compassion in Practice*. London: DH.

Dewey, J. (1933*, How We Think: A Restatement of Reflective Thinking to the Educative Process*. Boston: D.C. Heath.

DHSSPS (2013) *The Northern Ireland Regional Infection Prevention and Control Manual*. Belfast: DHSSPS.

Dougherty, L. and Lister, S. (eds) (2011) *The Royal Marsden Hospital Manual of Clinical Nursing Procedures*, 8th edition. Oxford: Wiley-Blackwell.

Egan, G. (2002) *The Skilled Helper: A Problem Management and Opportunity Approach to Helping*. Pacific Grove, CA: Brooks/Cole.

Francis, R. (2013) *Report of the Mid Staffordshire NHS Foundation Trust Public Inquiry*. London: The Stationery Office.

Gammon, J., Morgan-Samuel, H. and Gould, D. (2008) 'A review of the evidence for sub-optimal compliance of healthcare practitioners to standard/universal infection control precautions', *Journal of Clinical Nursing*, 17(2): 157–67.

Gibbs, G. (1988) *Learning by Doing: A Guide to Teaching and Learning Methods*. London: Oxford Polytechnic.

Hastorf, A.H. and Isen, A.M. (1982) *Cognitive Social Psychology*. New York: Elsevier.

Health Protection Agency (2012) *English National Point Prevalence Surveillance on Healthcare-associated Infections and Antimicrobial Use 2011*. London: HPA.

Health Protection Scotland (2014) *National Infection Prevention and Control Manual*, V2.3. Available at: www.documents.hps.scot.nhs.uk/hai/infection-control/ic-manual/ipcm-p-v2-3.pdf (last accessed 29 September 2014).

Loveday, H., Wilson, J.A., Pratt, R.J., Golsorkhi, M., Tingle, A., Bak, A., Browne, J., Prieto, J. and Wilcox, M. (2014) 'Epic3: national evidence-based guidelines for preventing healthcare-associated infections in NHS Hospitals in England', *Journal of Hospital Infection*, 86(S1): S1–S70.

Miall, H. (2011) *Contemporary Conflict Resolution*. Cambridge: Polity.

MHRA (2014) *Managing Medical Devices*. London: MHRA.

Mehrabian, A. (1971) 'Nonverbal betrayal of feelings', *Journal of Experimental Research in Personality*, 5: 64–73.

Mobley, J. (2005) *An Integrated Essential Approach to Counselling Theory and Practice*. New York: Edwin Wellen.

National Audit Office (2009) *Reducing Healthcare-associated Infections in Hospitals in England*. London: The Stationery Office.

NICE (2006) *Nutrition Support in Adults*. London: NICE.

NICE (2012) *Prevention and Control of Healthcare-associated Infections in Primary and Community Care*. London: NICE.

NICE (2012a) *Quality Standard for Nutrition Support in Adults*. London: NICE.

NICE (2013) *Fall Assessment and the Prevention of Falls in Older People*. Available at: http://pathways.nice.org.uk/pathways/falls-in-older-people (last accessed 23 September 2014).

Nursing and Midwifery Council (2007a) *The Essential Skills Clusters*. London: NMC.

Nursing and Midwifery Council (2007b) *Standards for Medicines Management*. London: NMC.

Nursing and Midwifery Council (2008) *Standards for Medicines Management*. London: NMC.

Nursing and Midwifery Council (2009) *Record Keeping: Guidance for Nurses and Midwives*. London: NMC.

Nursing and Midwifery Council (2010a) *The Essential Skills Clusters*. London: NMC.

Nursing and Midwifery Council (2010b) *Standards for Pre-Registration Nursing Education*. London: NMC.

Nursing and Midwifery Council (2013) *NMC Guidance on Professional Conduct for Nursing and Midwifery Students*. London: NMC.

Nursing and Midwifery Council (2015) *The Code: Professional Standards of Practice and Behaviour for Nurses and Midwives*. London: NMC.

Roper, N., Logan, W.W. and Tierney, A.J. (1980) *The Elements of Nursing*. Edinburgh: Churchill Livingstone.

Royal College of Nursing (2004) *Patient Group Directions: Guidance and Information for Nurses*. London: RCN.

Royal College of Nursing (2010) *Principles of Nursing Practice*. London: RCN.

Royal College of Physicians (2012) *National Early Warning Score (NEWS): Standardising the Assessment of Acute-illness Severity in the NHS*. London: RCP.

Schon, D.A. (1983) *The Reflective Practitioner: How Professionals Think in Action*. San Francisco, CA: Jossey-Bass.

Ward, D. (2010) 'Experiences of infection control in clinical placements: interviews with nursing and midwifery students', *Journal of Advanced Nursing*, 66(7): 1533–42.

Waterlow, J. (2008) *Pressure Ulcer Risk Assessment and Prevention*. Available at: www.judy-waterlow.co.uk/waterlow_score.htm (last accessed 5 March 2015).

Wigglesworth, N. (2014) *National Model Policies for Infection Prevention and Control in Wales*. Available at: www2.nphs.wales.nhs.uk (last accessed 29 September 2014).

World Health Organization (2009) *WHO Guidelines on Hand Hygiene in Healthcare*. Geneva: WHO.

6 Exposure to Other Fields of Nursing

GEORGINA TAYLOR

Adult nursing focuses more on the care of adults and older people than any other client group (NMC, 2010a, 2010b). However, adult nursing students are also required to comply with Article 31 and Annexe V.2 of the European Directive on recognition of professional qualifications (European Union, 2005). This stipulates that adult field students are exposed to other fields of nursing in order to gain an insight into the specific needs of service users across a variety of different client groups, thus enabling them to provide safe and effective basic care to all the individuals they encounter within their nursing role. It also ensures recognition of the professional qualification and freedom of movement within EU member states (NMC, 2010a, 2010b).

This chapter is designed to help you to consider the importance of providing care which meets the essential needs of *pregnant* or *postnatal women* in the context of a co-existing physical condition, and some of the key aspects of caring for *children and young people*, people with *learning disabilities* and people with *mental health issues*. It will also assist you in identifying how you can utilise this knowledge and understanding to support a variety of service users and carers within your placement areas.

After reading this chapter you should be able to:

- Discuss key elements of promoting health during and after pregnancy.
- Discuss key influences on child development.
- Recall the role of the nurse in relation to safeguarding children and adults.
- Discuss key elements of caring for people with learning disabilities.
- Demonstrate an understanding of the importance of promoting mental health.

Related NMC Competencies

All nurses must be able to:

> ... assess and meet the full range of essential physical and mental health needs of people of all ages who come into their care and provide safe and effective immediate care to all people prior to accessing or referring to specialist services irrespective of their field of practice. (NMC, 2010a: 17, 2010b: 6)

————— **To achieve entry to the register as an adult** —————
nurse you should be able to:

- Recognise and respond to the needs of all people who come into your care including *babies, children and young people, pregnant* and *postnatal* women, people with *mental health problems*, people with *physical disabilities*, people with *learning disabilities, older people,* and *people with long-term problems* (such as cognitive impairment), paying special attention to the protection of vulnerable people. Where necessary, you must challenge inequality, discrimination and exclusion from access to care.
- Promote the rights, choices and wishes of adults, children and young people, paying attention to equality, diversity and the needs of an ageing population.
- Work with the midwife and other professionals and agencies to provide basic nursing care to pregnant women and families during pregnancy and after childbirth.
- Understand the normal physiological and psychological processes of pregnancy and childbirth.
- Respond safely and effectively in an emergency to safeguard the health of mother and baby.
- Recognise and interpret signs of normal and deteriorating mental health, responding promptly to maintain or improve the health and comfort of the service-user, acting to keep them and others safe.
- Recognise when a person is at risk and in need of extra support and protection, taking reasonable steps to protect them from abuse.

(Adapted from the NMC Standards of Competence for Adult Nursing, 2010a, 2010b.)

Background

It is important to be aware that individuals with mental health problems and learning disabilities may belong to some of the most vulnerable groups of people in society. Children and pregnant and postnatal women may be in a similar position. For example, it is reported that over three million children live in poverty (Children's Society, 2013) and people with learning disabilities are among the most socially excluded and vulnerable groups in Britain (DH, 2001).

Poorer people have more illness and a shorter life expectancy than richer people. These differences are referred to as *inequalities in health*. The roots of these inequalities lie in the different socio-economic experiences of these groups of people. The Commission on Social Determinants of Health (CSDOH, 2008) was established in order to consider the evidence relating to actions to promote equity in health and a global approach to reducing inequalities in health. Inequalities in health mirror inequalities in wealth. Therefore, poorer people tend to have worse health than richer people. This is the case both between countries and within countries. A range of factors contribute to inequalities in health. These go beyond material factors and are referred to as 'social determinants of health', which are the *'conditions in which people are born, grow, live, work and age ...'* (CSDH, 2008). These include social position, education, occupation, income, gender, ethnicity and race: factors which can have an impact on an individual's material circumstances, social cohesion, psychosocial aspects, behaviours and biological aspects (CSDH, 2008). You can see from the definition of social determinants of health that they cover the lifespan. A poor education can lead to unemployment or insecure employment, possibly in an unfulfilling job, low pay which in turn may cause poor housing, little money for recreational activities and ultimately an inadequate retirement pension (for further discussion see Chapter 9, pp. 251–252). The challenge for governments and for society is to improve the conditions of daily life – i.e. the circumstances in which people are born, grow, live, work and age (CSDH, 2008). In this chapter we will see how vital it is to be aware of social determinants, especially in the early years of life.

Different experiences of the social determinants of health can result in inequalities in health, which in turn result in social injustice. Many government policies concerning health now aim to address this injustice by reducing inequalities in health. But it is important to be aware that the picture of inequalities in health is not a polarised one with a clear difference between the richest and poorest groups in society. Rather there is a social gradient in health – this represents a step-wise gradient in health experience, with people in any social class having a better health experience than those in the class immediately below them. The notion of the step-wise gradient in health experience gains credence from the findings of the Whitehall studies (Marmot, 1996; Bosma et al., 1997; Marmot and Davey Smith, 1997). The Whitehall studies of a large number of civil servants working in government offices in London found that death rates were four times as high among the most junior office support staff as they were among the most senior administrators. Another startling finding was that men in the second from top grade had a higher mortality rate than that for the top grade civil servants, identifying a step-wise gradient relating to the respondents' relative position in the hierarchy (Brunner and Marmot, 1999). The findings of the Whitehall studies have led to explanations emphasising psychosocial factors, giving consideration to the pathways through which the social structure influences health in its widest sense. Syme's (1996) explanation for this phenomenon is that as individuals move down the social hierarchy they have less control over their lives. By less control he means 'less opportunity to influence the events that affect one's life' (1996: 28).

STOP AND THINK

Consider the step-wise gradient in health.

Go to the website of the London Knowledge and Intelligence Team at Public Health England and use the search tool to find the Jubilee line of Health Inequality 2004–2008 (Inequality Tube Map).

This relates to the Jubilee line of the London Underground, which runs from Stanmore to Stratford.

Using data from 2004 to 2008, the London Health Observatory identified differences in male life expectancy within a small area of London – the so-called 'Jubilee line of health inequality' (London Health Observatory, 2010). Travelling from west to east along the Jubilee line from Westminster, every two tube stations represent over one year of life expectancy lost.

Add a few key points here.

As a result of this picture of health across society, universal policies are now in place to improve the health of all people but 'with a scale and intensity that is proportionate to the level of disadvantage. We call this proportionate universalism' (Marmot Review, 2010). These policies for improving the health of people provide the context within which day-to-day nursing practice takes place.

A report on the role of health professionals in relation to reducing inequalities in health (Allen et al., 2013) acknowledges that most of the social and economic factors that contribute to inequalities in health are outside the scope of the NHS, though there are activities that health professionals can engage in to influence these factors, beyond ensuring equity of access and treatment. The report is supported by the RCN (2012) which highlights the key role of nurses in promoting health and minimising the impact of illness, and stresses that all nurses – wherever they practise – should know and understand the health needs of their local populations. Partnership working is also key to addressing the social determinants of health and perhaps you will have noticed that this is a key theme that continues throughout this book. You will see some more examples later in this chapter.

Disadvantaged or vulnerable individuals may also have complex care needs and require services from agencies other than healthcare services. For example, an individual with learning disabilities or mental health problems or a child who is 'in need' or 'at risk' may also be a client of social services. In such cases it is important that health and social care professionals work closely together to ensure that individuals receive the care and treatment they need. It is also necessary to remember that each person is an individual with their own values, beliefs, preferences and needs. Health policies across the UK are pursuing a 'personalisation' agenda, primarily aimed at adults with learning disabilities and mental health issues. Personalisation entails attending to an individual's needs and engaging in shared decision making whilst also ensuring that individuals can exercise both choice and voice:

> Personalisation means recognising people as individuals who have strengths and preferences and putting them at the centre of their own care and support. (SCIE, 2012: 2)

In order to achieve this people need access to information, advocacy and advice to help them make informed decisions about their care and treatment in order to be able to retain control over that care and treatment. During these encounters the individual and the professional will work in partnership: the individual brings their experience of illness, their values and preferences to decision making, whilst the professional brings expertise on the effectiveness of treatments, including their possible benefits and side effects.

Maternity care

We cannot hope to cover all aspects of maternal health and the physiological and psychological processes of pregnancy and childbirth here so we would recommend that you undertake further study by accessing some of the suggested reading material at the end of this chapter to assist you in your studies. However, this section will introduce aspects of maintaining a healthy pregnancy and examples of the help that is available to vulnerable families. It also addresses the importance of recognising potential mental health issues following childbirth. Reading this section and working through the activities will help you work towards meeting the adult nursing NMC competencies related to maternal health needs (NMC, 2010a, 2010b):

─────────── To achieve entry to the register as an ───────────
adult nurse you should be able to:

- Understand and meet the essential needs of pregnant or postnatal women in relation to a co-existing physical condition, mental health problem or learning disability.
- Recognise major risks and act quickly in an emergency to get expert help.

- Have a broad understanding of the physical and psychological effects of pregnancy, childbirth and the postnatal period.
- Have a clear understanding of the role of the midwife and midwifery care, and be able to work in partnership with midwives and other professionals to achieve the best outcomes for pregnant and postnatal women and babies in their care.

A baby's mother needs to be healthy before and during pregnancy and childbirth for the baby to get the best start in life. The evidence here is compelling; the foundations of adult health are laid before birth and during early childhood (Wilkinson and Marmot, 2003). Unfavourable circumstances during pregnancy – for example, poor nutrition, stress, smoking, the misuse of drugs and alcohol – can affect the developing baby and set the scene for health in later life (Wilkinson and Marmot, 2003).

Early experiences have effects on health that last throughout life so ensuring a good start means supporting mothers and young children (Wilkinson and Marmot, 2003). Most families are receptive to help and advice during the perinatal period as most parents will want their children to have the best possible start in life (Hogg, 2013). Therefore healthcare professionals are in a prime position to make use of this opportunity to provide support to families and give advice about a healthy lifestyle during pregnancy.

Nutrition in pregnancy

A healthy diet is key during pregnancy in order to meet the needs of both the mother and the developing foetus (Shepherd, 2008). Epidemiological research led by Barker (1994) concluded that maternal under-nutrition during foetal life or immediately after birth can have lasting consequences on the child and may extend into adulthood. The specific effects of under-nutrition depend on the stage of foetal development at which the under-nutrition occurs. The general advice for nutrition during pregnancy is to find a balance between eating a wide variety of foods, appropriate weight gain and physical exercise (Shepherd, 2008). As an adult nurse you should familiarise yourself with the advice that is offered to expectant mothers concerning their diets.

ACTIVITY 6.1

Nutrition in pregnancy

Locate *The Pregnancy Book* (Department of Health, 2013) at www.publichealth.hscni.net/publications/ by placing the term 'The Pregnancy Book' in the website's search engine.

Read the section 'Your health in pregnancy – advice on nutrition'. You should ensure that you are able to pass on this advice to expectant mothers if required.

The Pregnancy Book aims to provide women with information on many aspects of pregnancy, ranging from advice on planning a pregnancy, enjoying a healthy pregnancy, labour and childbirth and the first weeks with a new baby. As well as the advice you have read about nutrition, the book provides advice on many topics relating to maintaining health during pregnancy, such as smoking and alcohol. It also contains advice on rights and benefits and a list of useful organisations.

Smoking cessation

Smoking is the main cause of preventable illness and premature death across the UK. It is also the main reason for the gap in healthy life expectancy between rich and poor (NICE, 2013a). The effects of smoking on health are well known. Smoking causes many types of cancer, chronic obstructive pulmonary disease and cardio-vascular disease (NICE, 2013a). Stopping smoking at any stage of life has immediate and long-term health benefits (Duaso and Duncan, 2012). In pregnancy, the adverse effects of smoking include the risk of miscarriage, a premature birth, a low birth weight, stillbirth and sudden infant death (Duaso and Duncan, 2012; Percival, 2013). Evidence of an association between smoking during pregnancy and sudden infant death has been established (Wisborg et al., 2000; Anderson et al., 2005). There are also risks attached to exposure to secondhand smoke, for example from a partner smoking. In addition after birth, children who are exposed to passive smoking are at an increased risk of developing pneumonia, bronchitis and asthma. Mothers who are exposed to environmental smoke are more likely to give birth to babies with low birth weights (Duaso and Duncan, 2012).

There is some evidence that people who smoke are receptive to advice on stopping smoking (NICE, 2013a) and smoking cessation interventions have been shown to be effective (Duaso and Duncan, 2012). The NHS Stop Smoking Service is the most effective method for helping people to stop smoking, though not everyone is aware of this service. The service is delivered by professionals who are specially trained to help people stop smoking. As people become addicted to nicotine (and may experience unpleasant withdrawal symptoms) they can find it difficult to give up (Percival, 2013). The NHS Stop Smoking Service includes activities like intensive support through group therapy or one-to-one support. Trying to stop smoking unaided is the least effective method.

Guidelines on quitting smoking in pregnancy and following childbirth (NICE, 2010) state that anyone planning a pregnancy, or is already pregnant or has an infant under 12 months should receive smoking cessation support. Therefore healthcare professionals should assess expectant mothers' exposure to cigarette smoke, inform them of the dangers of smoking, ask smokers if they would like to stop smoking and refer them to NHS Stop Smoking Services appropriately. Many healthcare trusts have a specialist midwife responsible for promoting and supporting women in smoking cessation.

Vulnerable families

Women who experience stress during pregnancy may give birth to babies of low birth weight and as they grow up these children may have emotional and behavioural problems (Wilkinson, 2005). Thus, alongside the mainstream services for pregnant women and young children there are some initiatives that focus on more vulnerable families. Women living in complex social situations (for example, those at risk from substance abuse, recent migrants with language barriers, victims/potential victims of domestic abuse) often avoid antenatal care and so there is a need to reach out to such women. Many healthcare trusts have specialist midwives with a responsibility to target and support vulnerable women.

Sure Start

Sure Start Children's Centres (www.nidirect.gov.uk/sure-start-services) form part of an early intervention programme and provide access to advice and support from pregnancy to primary school as well as a range of services for early childhood. Sure Start Children's Centres are open to all parents, carers and children in England but are primarily aimed at disadvantaged children and families, providing family support services and high quality early years provision to all preschool children. Examples of their services include:

- breastfeeding support;
- high quality childcare and early learning provision;
- advice on issues such as parenting, healthy eating, employment and money management. (Camps and Long, 2012)

Healthy Start

The Healthy Start programme is a UK-wide government scheme to improve the health of low-income pregnant women and families on benefits and tax credits. The programme provides vouchers for healthy food, for example, milk, fresh or frozen fruit and vegetables.

Read more about Healthy Start at www.healthystart.nhs.uk.
    How might you utilise this information to inform your approach in supporting pregnant women and families as an adult nurse?

STOP AND THINK

Family Nurse Partnership Programme

One initiative that aims to help vulnerable young first-time mothers across the UK is the Family Nurse Partnership Programme (FNP) (DH, 2012). This programme aims to:

- improve pregnancy outcomes;
- improve child health and development;
- improve parents' economic self-sufficiency.

All first-time mothers aged 19 and under at conception are eligible and participation in the programme is voluntary. The programme consists of intensive and structured home visiting (provided by specially trained nurses) from early pregnancy until the child is aged two years, when families are transferred to health visiting services so that the remainder of the Healthy Child programme can be completed.

The FNP has a strong evidence base of benefits to families in need in the USA. The original work in the USA found that the FNP resulted in improved outcomes when delivered by highly qualified nurses. The strength of the nursing contribution lies in trust in and respect for the nursing profession as well as the academic preparation in social, life and caring sciences.

There is a strong theoretical base to the programme. Nurses use theory and expertise to engage in behaviour change methods to foster the adoption of healthier lifestyles by the families.

> ### ACTIVITY 6.2
>
> Find out more about how the FNP programme works in your area by undertaking a Google search using the term 'The Family-Nurse-Partnership-Programme' followed by 'Scotland', 'Wales', 'England' or 'Northern Ireland'.

Baby steps

Hogg (2013) describes a collaborative initiative between the NSPCC and Warwick University which developed an evidence-based programme to help vulnerable parents. The programme aims to 'strengthen protective factors such as family relationships, social support and emotional well-being during pregnancy' (Hogg, 2013: 144), and follows the framework set out in the document *Preparation for Birth and Beyond* (DH, 2011a).

The programme focuses on 'hard-to-reach' parents who often have additional needs and chaotic lifestyles. For example, it is sufficiently flexible to allow it to be delivered in a variety of ways to meet the needs of different groups of parents, including groups of parents in prisons and an Urdu language women's group (Hogg, 2013). Parents from black and minority ethnic groups appreciate culturally and linguistically appropriate courses which are based within their communities (DH, 2011a).

These families do not always attend appointments so facilitators will visit them at home. Hogg claims that almost 75% of expectant mothers in low income households do not receive antenatal education, yet the desire to be a good parent has been noted, even in the most troubled situations. The programme adopts a collaborative approach, employing the principles of adult education – for example interactive, group, as well as one-to-one activities (Hogg, 2013). The resources are accessible to a range of parents, for example parents with low literacy skills and learning disabilities (Hogg, 2013). The overall goal of the programme is to foster strong relationships between parents and babies. This goal is supported by promoting good relationships between parents, significant others, encouraging the formation of friendships with other new parents. Hogg argues that evidence suggests that the quality of parental relationships and support networks affects the quality of parenting a child receives.

> ### ACTIVITY 6.3
>
> Find out about the services available in your area that aim to assist pregnant women and support vulnerable families.

Postnatal care and transition to the community

The period of 6–8 weeks after childbirth is referred to as the postnatal period and it is a time of enormous adjustment (Kinge and Gregory, 2011a). NICE (2013b) has developed a quality standard (QS37) for postnatal care, outlining the care and support that every woman should receive during the postnatal period. This care should be individualised to meet the needs of the mother and baby (including partners and family as appropriate). This care and support can be extended beyond the 6–8 week period if necessary. NICE recommends the provision of postnatal education programmes delivered by a multidisciplinary team which provides advice, information and support for new mothers and their families (Kinge and Gregory, 2011a).

Breastfeeding

The NICE Clinical Guidelines (NICE, 2006) describe the postnatal care that every woman and baby should receive in the first 6–8 weeks after birth. The document requires that all maternity care providers should implement an externally evaluated and structured programme that encourages breastfeeding, using the Baby Friendly Initiative (www.unicef.org.uk/babyfriendly).

Breast milk supplies all the nutrients a baby needs for around the first six months of life (NHS, 2010). Policies on breastfeeding across the UK promote feeding babies solely on breast milk for the first six months of life, after which time it is suggested that breastfeeding can continue as long as the mother and baby wish, while gradually introducing a more varied diet (NICE, 2008). Breastfeeding contributes to the health of both mother and baby. It has been found that babies who are not breastfed are more likely to acquire infections such as gastroenteritis during their first year of life (NICE, 2008). Women who are disadvantaged are less likely to breastfeed than their better-off counterparts.

ACTIVITY 6.4

Read about the Baby Friendly Initiative at www.unicef.org.uk/BabyFriendly/About-Baby-Friendly/

Read the following document: NHS (2010) *Off to the Best Start: Important Information about Feeding Your Baby*. Available at www.gov.uk/government/publications/off-to-the-best-start-important-information-about-feeding-your-baby

Now consider patterns of breastfeeding in your local area. Access the Public Health England records statistics on breastfeeding. Go to the following government website at www.gov.uk/government/statistical-data-sets/breastfeeding-statistics-q4-2012-to-2013.

Look at the Excel Spreadsheet for *'Breastfeeding initiation and prevalence at 6–8 weeks 2012/2013 Q4'*. Statistics on breastfeeding are often recorded by local Primary Care Trusts. Look at the figures that are relevant for your locality.

What factors might influence your local breastfeeding rates?

Find out if your local trust has Baby Friendly accreditation and at what level.

Safety in the home

Parents may need advice about how to keep their babies safe. The range of the advice is extensive but can include: the use of car seats and prams; appropriate clothing; sun protection; safety gates; guarding fires; placing hot drinks out of reach; in addition to information about immunisations, signs of illness and first aid.

ACTIVITY 6.5

Read the following document on safety in the home: Department of Health (2013a) *Birth to Five*. Available at www.publichealth.hscni.net/publications/birth-five

    Chapter 7: Protecting your child
    Immunisations
    Common childhood illnesses
    Reducing the risk of accidents
    Safety in the sun.

Now you can consider the situation in your local area.

Have a look at the *'NHS Atlas of Variation in Healthcare for Children and Young People'* (2012) at the following website: www.rightcare.nhs.uk/index.php/atlas/children-and-young-adults/

Look particularly at the chapter on *'Health Promotion and Disease Prevention'* and the maps showing variations in patterns of immunisation in England.

What factors do you think might influence the uptake of immunisations in your local area?

As a nurse, what is your role in influencing patterns of uptake?

Going home

Before being discharged from hospital, mothers will receive a postnatal check by a midwife. This check includes an assessment of the mother's emotional state and her blood loss, ensuring that she has passed urine following delivery (Kinge and Gregory, 2011b). Newborn babies are examined by a paediatrician (Kinge and Gregory, 2011b). Mothers are also advised that they will be visited at home by a community midwife within two days of discharge. They will be offered advice on contraception; they will be advised to make an appointment for a post-natal check up with their GP in six weeks time for themselves and their babies; and they will be advised to register the birth within six weeks at the registration office (Kinge and Gregory, 2011b). A health visitor will also visit the mother and baby at home between 11 and 14 days after the birth and will advise parents where and how often to take the baby for regular checks.

Physical health

The NICE Quality Standard 37 (NICE, 2013b) states that within 24 hours women are informed of the signs and symptoms of conditions that may require urgent treatment, for example signs and symptoms of postpartum haemorrhage, infection, pre-eclampsia/eclampsia and thromboembolism.

Antenatal and postnatal mental health

The NICE clinical guidelines (NICE, 2014) require that at a woman's first contact with services in antenatal and postnatal periods, healthcare professionals should ask questions about past and present severe mental illness, previous treatment by mental health professionals and family history of perinatal mental illness. The aim here is early detection and treatment.

Statement 10 of the NICE Quality Standard for Postnatal Care (NICE, 2013b: 49) states that:

> Women who are still feeling low in mood, anxious, experiencing negative thoughts or lacking interest in their baby at 0–14 days after the birth may be at increased risk of mental health problems. These women should receive an assessment of their mental wellbeing.

It is important to be aware of the mental health problems that can arise in the postnatal period and to be able to differentiate between 'baby blues', postnatal depression, and postpartum (or puerperal) psychosis, by recognising key signs and symptoms. These mental health problems are explained in some detail in the leaflet 'Postpartum Psychosis: severe mental illness after childbirth' (Royal College of Psychiatrists, 2014) – you will find the link in the Further Reading at the end of the chapter.

'Baby blues'

While women may experience many different emotions after having a baby, it is important to be able to differentiate between less serious and mild mood changes associated with 'baby blues' and the more serious signs and symptoms of postnatal depression and postpartum psychosis. 'Baby blues' occurs in over half of new mothers, who may experience irritability, anxiety and become tearful (Royal College of Psychiatrists, 2014). This usually starts three to four days after childbirth and stops by the time the baby is about ten days old (Royal College of Psychiatrists, 2014).

Postnatal depression

Postnatal depression affects 10–15 in every 100 women after childbirth (Royal College of Psychiatrists, 2014). Postnatal depression is 'a depressive disorder that can affect women in the months after childbirth' (Robertson, 2010: 47). It can be difficult to detect because it may present differently in different women. The symptoms of postnatal depression are similar to those for depression at any other stage of life (Royal College of Psychiatrists, 2014). As Robertson points out, the difference is the presence of a baby which is likely to be the focus of the woman's thoughts and difficulties. Also, some of the symptoms of postnatal depression may be similar to the experiences of normal adjustment to life with a baby – for example lack of sleep –which is often experienced in the postnatal period as women wake to feed their babies and change their nappies.

For some women with postnatal depression, anxiety, distress or agitation may be more evident than depression and in some women their mood may vary during the day (Robertson, 2010). The disorder may also be mild or severe. While milder forms might be treated within the primary healthcare team more severe forms will need additional input from psychiatric services. Diagnosing postnatal depression requires the clinical assessment undertaken by GPs or mental health specialists. However nursing and midwifery staff must be alert to the disorder in order to make timely referrals.

Guidance is provided to help healthcare professionals detect signs of postnatal depression and other mental health illnesses (NICE, 2014). The guidelines state that healthcare professionals (including midwives, obstetricians, health visitors and GPs) should ask two questions to identify possible depression at a woman's first contact with primary care, at her booking visit and postnatally:

- During the past month, have you often been bothered by feeling down, depressed or hopeless?
- During the past month, have you often been bothered by having little interest or pleasure in doing things?
- During the past month have you not been able to stop or control worrying?

Healthcare professionals might also consider the use of self-report measures to aid assessment of depression, or for monitoring purposes. You can have a look at these tools in the following Activity.

ACTIVITY 6.6

Access and familiarise yourself with the following assessment tools that might be used in the detection, assessment and monitoring of post natal mental health:
Edinburgh Postnatal Depression Scale (EPDS)
Generalised Anxiety Disorder: Scale-2 (GAD-2) and Scale-7 (GAD-7)
Edinburgh Postnatal Depression Scale (EPDS)
Patient Health Questionnaire-9 (PHQ-9) (NICE, 2014).

Postpartum psychosis

Postpartum (or puerperal) psychosis is a severe episode of mental illness representing a psychiatric emergency, with a sudden onset during the days or weeks following childbirth (Royal College of Psychiatrists, 2014). It is more serious than postnatal depression and can present in different ways. Affected women may have very rapid changes in mood, including symptoms of depression or mania (Royal College of Psychiatrists, 2014). A woman with postpartum psychosis may not be able to care for herself or her baby. The symptoms of postpartum psychosis often begin during the first few days following childbirth, but can present several weeks later (Royal College of Psychiatrists, 2014). Women who have a history of bipolar disorder or schizoaffective disorder and women who have a previous episode of postpartum psychosis are at high risk of developing postpartum psychosis. Women with the signs and symptoms of postpartum psychosis need urgent help (NICE, 2014). An affected mother will need professional help in caring for her baby, and a referral to Children and Families Social Services may be necessary (NICE, 2013b; Royal College of Psychiatrists, 2014).

ACTIVITY 6.7

Have a look at the following patient information leaflet: 'Postpatum Psychosis: severe mental illness after childbirth' (Royal College of Psychiatrists, 2014). Available at: www.rcpsych.ac.uk/healthadvice/problemsdisorders/postpartumpsychosis.aspx
Consider how useful this leaflet might be when educating new mothers about postnatal mental health issues.

This section has introduced some examples of 'proportionate universalism', in terms of universal services that are available to all pregnant women highligthing the need for extra support for the most vulnerable women. This approach also demonstrates how the individual needs of pregnant women can be addressed.

Children and young people

This section focuses on a child-centred approach to care and the promotion of a healthy childhood within the context of the 'Healthy Child Programme'. Focusing upon the universal services that are available to all children, we will explore services that are in place to help children receive a better start in life when and where necessary. You will also need to consider a nurse's role in relation to safeguarding children. Reading this section and working through the activities will help you work towards meeting the Adult NMC requirements related to the needs of children and young people.

--- To achieve entry to the register as an --- adult nurse you should be able to:

- have a broad understanding of the development of children and young people within the family context and how this affects their individual needs, health, behaviour and communication;
- work with children, young people, their families and others to provide family-centred care;
- understand common physical and mental health problems associated with childhood and adolescence, their effects and treatment;
- deliver the basic care required to meet essential needs;
- recognise deterioration and provide safe care to infants, children and young people in an emergency, or act to protect them where there is risk of harm, prior to referral or when accessing specialist services.

(Adapted from the NMC Standards of Competence for Adult Nursing, 2010a, 2010b)

In the early 1900s there was recognition that children had rights and were not simply the property of their parents (Jones, 2000). This period saw a series of laws and developments as part of the emerging welfare state which contributed to policies to protect children. The role of the state in relation to the welfare of children has grown progressively over time.

Can you think of any areas in which the state intervenes in the interests of the welfare of children?

STOP AND THINK

You might have thought of the compulsory use of seatbelts in cars or, more recently, proposals to protect children from passive smoking in cars. In February 2014 MPs voted overwhelmingly in favour of a ban on smoking in cars, making exposing children to smoke in vehicles an offence in England (Mason, 2014). Smoking in cars with children present is outlawed in Australia, Canada and some states of the USA (Mason, 2014). Similar moves across the UK are set to become law in October 2015, although such legislation could be difficult to enforce.

Families

Such state intervention has sometimes been criticised – in these situations the state is sometimes referred to as a 'nanny state' interfering in family life. The family is the place where nurturing takes place and is sometimes described as having the functions of:

- reproduction;
- providing welfare: shelter, food, protection;
- primary socialisation: the process during which children learn about identity, roles, right and wrong and the transmission of culture.

It is important to remember however that there is no 'one' single model of the family. Families may take the 'nuclear' form which refers to adults and dependent children. Extended families include a wider network, e.g. grandparents, aunts, uncles and cousins. However, family structures can be diverse, incorporating co-habiting, lone-parent, same-sex, and reconstituted forms. Therefore ideas about family life and child-rearing may vary according to the family structure and cultural beliefs and values. Nevertheless, current policy retains a child-centred focus, placing the needs of the child foremost. We will see later in the chapter that on occasions there can be a 'dark side' to family life, as the family can also be the place where domestic violence and child abuse occur and inter-generational conflict can arise.

Illness in the family

A child's illness can have an impact on all aspects of family life. Thomas and Price (2012) explored the experiences of seven mothers caring for a child with complex needs. Using semi-structured in-depth interviews they identified the pressures on families of children with complex needs: these included physical burden, isolation and the emotional turmoil of meeting the needs of the sick child and other children. The mothers in this study valued the input from the nursing respite service.

Giving children a healthy start in life

Current policy centres round *Giving All Children a Healthy Start in Life* (DH, 2013b). The background to this initiative is the report *Healthy Lives, Healthy People* (DH, 2010a), which highlights a better health experience of people with higher socio-economic positions in society. This better health experience derives from the enhanced life chances of people in higher socio-economic positions and the opportunities that are available to them to lead fulfilling lives. These influences operate across the life-span.

The *Healthy Lives, Healthy People* strategy for public health is influenced by the Marmot Review's *Fair Society, Healthy Lives* (Marmot, 2010). In terms of children, one policy objective of this review is to 'Give every child the best start in life' and is supported by the following objectives:

- To reduce inequalities in the early development of physical and emotional health, and cognitive, linguistic, and social skills.
- To ensure high quality maternity services, parenting programmes, childcare and early years education to meet needs across the social gradient.
- To build the resilience and well-being of young children across the social gradient (Marmot Review, 2010).

The Annual Report of the Chief Medical Officer for 2012 (DH, 2013c) affirmed the complex interactions of psychosocial events and biological factors, the life course approach and the crucial stages of development during foetal and early life. The report also recognised the need to improve the lives of all but supported the need for 'proportionate universalism', which means that proportionately greater resources should be targeted at the more disadvantaged groups (DH, 2013c).

ACTIVITY 6.8

Locate the Chief Medical Officer's Report on giving children a better start in life, available at: www.gov.uk/government/publications/chief-medical-officers-annual-report-2012-our-children-deserve-better-prevention-pays
Read Chapter 2 'Overview' to get an overview of policy initiatives for children and the challenges faced in improving children's health.
Pay particular attention to:

- Figure 2.8: WHO Commission on the Social Determinants of Health Conceptual Framework for Action (p.13);
- Figure 2.9: Influences and actions along the life course (p.13), and the discussion on p.14;
- Figure 2.10: Key drivers of life change throughout childhood (p.15);
- Box 2.4: Effects of poverty (p.16);
- Figure 2.12: Risk and resilience factors affecting health outcomes (p.19).

Healthy Child Programme

The objectives of *Fair Society, Healthy Lives* (Marmot, 2010) can easily be identified in the related health policy for children, particularly where extra support is available for disadvantaged families. The report also points out that the foundations for almost every aspect of human development are laid in early childhood. The *Healthy Child Programme* (DH, 2009) highlights evidence relating to neurological development that suggests a child's brain develops rapidly in the first two years of life and is influenced by the emotional and physical environment as well as by genetic factors. It is clear then that a child's experiences in these early years are crucial to their development. Therefore, the *Giving All Children a Healthy Start in Life* (DH, 2013b) initiative is also based on the *Healthy Child Programme* (DH, 2009). This programme begins in early pregnancy and ends at adulthood. The importance of pregnancy and the first years of life is stressed in view of the foundations that are laid for future health and well-being.

Universal health and development reviews

Universal health and development reviews are a key feature of the *Healthy Child Programme*. These reviews are carried out by healthcare professionals who have knowledge and understanding of child development, and of the factors that influence health and well-being. These practitioners are usually health visitors. One of the aims of the reviews is to detect any disability and/or developmental delay and to make appropriate referrals if any are identified. It is also important to alert the local education authority if any special educational needs are suspected (DH, 2009).

> ### ACTIVITY 6.9
>
> Locate the following document on developmental stages: Department of Health (2013a) *Birth to Five*. Available at: www.publichealth.hscni.net/publications/birth-five
> Go to Chapter 4: 'How your child will grow'. Read through this chapter in order to acquaint yourself with the key development stages for young children. Pay particular attention to the chart on page 65.

The *Healthy Child Programme* identifies the most appropriate opportunities for development reviews as follows:

- By the 12th week of pregnancy.
- Neonatal examination.
- New baby review (around 14 days old).
- The baby's 6–8 week examination.
- By the time the child is one year old.
- Between 2 and 2½ years old (DH, 2009: 19).

These reviews provide opportunities for screening tests and development surveillance, for assessing growth, for discussing social and emotional development and for referral to early years services as appropriate (DH, 2009).

The rights of children

The care of children is not only guided by government documents. There are also international documents such as the United Nations Convention on the Rights of the Child (1989). While the UN's commitment to the recognition of the inherent dignity and equal and inalienable human rights of all people is well known, it has also decreed that children are entitled to special care and assistance. With this in mind the UN's Convention on the Rights of the Child stresses that the family (as the natural place for nurturing children) should be afforded the necessary protection and assistance to fulfil its responsibilities. The Convention (1989: 3) states that 'children should be brought up in the spirit of peace, dignity, tolerance, freedom, equality and solidarity'. The best interests of the child must always be a primary consideration in all situations concerning children.

There are 54 Articles contained within the Convention, but the following are among those which are most readily applicable to nursing practice:

- Article 19, p. 7: States that are party to the Convention must take legislative, administrative, social and educational measures to protect the child from all forms of violence, negligence and abuse.
- Article 23, p. 8: States that are party to the Convention must ensure that a mentally or physically disabled child should enjoy a 'full and decent life, in conditions which ensure dignity, promote self-reliance and facilitate the child's active participation in the community'.
- Article 24, p. 8: Stresses the right of the child to the enjoyment of the highest attainable standard of health and to facilities for the treatment of illness and rehabilitation of health.
- Article 30, p. 10: Stresses that 'In those States in which ethnic, religious or linguistic minorities or persons of indigenous origin exist, a child belonging to such a minority or who is indigenous shall not be denied the right, in community with other members of his or her group, to enjoy his or her own culture, to profess and practise his or her own religion, or to use his or her own language'. This is clearly very important and relevant in a multicultural country like Britain.

The importance of play

Article 31 (p.10) recognises the right of the child to 'rest and leisure, to engage in play and recreational activities appropriate to the age of the child and to participate freely in cultural life and the arts'.

Protective factors in early childhood, such as secure attachment, consistent parenting, appropriate play and learning opportunities, contribute to children's emotional well-being and chances of reaching their potential (Fearn and Howard, 2012). Play is important for children as it is a pleasurable activity and assists with the development of peer friendships, learning about social dynamics and the rules of engagement (Lester and Russell, 2010). Lester and Russell suggest that without play children's development may be compromised. During play children create imaginary worlds where they have the potential to develop a range of responses to the situations they create and encounter. Thus through play children can develop a range of adaptive capacities and strategies to help them cope with being children.

Lester and Russell (2010: ix) argue that play acts across several adaptive systems to contribute to health, well-being and resilience. These systems include:

- pleasure and enjoyment;
- emotion regulation;
- stress response systems;
- attachments;
- learning and creativity.

Children interact with their environments through play and therefore play can help them adapt to their environments – for example, play can help children to cope with abuse, conflict, displacement and/or poverty (Lester and Russell, 2010). When they are in supportive environments, play can also help children to develop resilience. Fearn and Howard (2012) analysed case studies concerning interventions with children caught up in the bombing in Beirut, children abandoned by their parents to the state system in Romania, and street children in Rio de Janeiro and Cali. They found that play can provide a healing experience for children affected by war and conflict and that it encourages the growth of resilient adaptive systems. Therefore, children can develop the adaptability and flexibility to cope with stress through play (Fearn and Howard, 2012).

ACTIVITY 6.10

Go to the following website regarding the importance of play: www.nhs.uk
    Search for information related to babies and toddlers, the importance of play and play ideas.

Early education

Children's intellectual, social and behavioural development is also enhanced by their pre-school education. Disadvantaged children particularly have been found to benefit from good quality pre-school experiences (Sylva et al., 2004). Children who have attended good pre-schools do better in reading and maths at the age of six years than those who have not. Government policy is to provide universal free entitlement to early education for all children aged three and four years. This education helps the transition to school (Department for Education, 2011a, 2014).

Safeguarding children

All nurses have a responsibility in relation to safeguarding children (NMC, 2015) and UK policy in this area is clearly defined. While your responsibility in this respect is obvious while you are on a placement that deals with children, you might also encounter concerns about the safety of a child while working in an Accident and Emergency Department, in primary care, in any adult care ward or indeed in your personal day-to-day life. Policies to protect children have been in place for a long time but concerns escalated after the death of Victoria Climbié whose high profile case attracted a lot of criticism of the professionals who had contact with her and prompted the strengthening of policy concerning safeguarding children. The Laming Report (DH, 2003) into the death of Victoria Climbié identified poor communication, poor interprofessional working and poor teamwork among the factors that contributed to the professional failure to protect Victoria.

This public Inquiry influenced policy relating to children's services, including the establishment of local Children's Trusts consisting of multidisciplinary teams of professionals from health, education and social services. Other policy developments included the Green Paper *Every Child Matters* (Department for Education and Skills, 2003) and the *Children Act* 2004 which identified the role of new safeguarding boards and duties of agencies working with children to promote health and well-being, as well as protect them from harm (Powell, 2013). The government also produced guidance on inter-agency working to protect children, including a common assessment framework (CAF) (DES, 2007).

Common Assessment Framework

The CAF was introduced as part of a range of policy documents that was published following the death of Victoria Climbié in 2000 (Powell, 2013). The CAF is a tool for early intervention in children's lives, once needs have been detected (Powell, 2013) and where there are issues that might require support from more than one agency. The assessment is based on a *social model of health* and is designed to be shared among relevant professionals in order to avoid repeatedly asking families to provide the same information. Sharing of the assessment also promotes multi-agency working through the formation, implementation and evaluation of a care plan.

However, while policy to protect children was strengthened, abuse of children continues. In 2008 Peter Connelly (originally referred to as Baby P), a 17-month-old toddler, died following non-accidental injuries. A further review of child protection procedures by Lord Laming resulted in the child protection guidance *Working Together to Safeguard Children* (Department for Education, 2010). Lord Laming again noted failures to implement policy, particularly in relation to the use of the CAF.

While guidance was now in place, the Munro Review of Child Protection (Department for Education, 2011b) commented on the culture of compliance with this guidance, targets and rules in relation to child protection which resulted in standardisation and a focus on following procedures and 'doing things right'. The review called for a shift towards more freedom for professionals to use their expertise in helping children and young people, with a focus on 'doing the right thing' and checking whether children and young people were being helped. The review also recommended a better balance between rules and professional judgement, between prescription and the exercise of judgement (Department for Education, 2011b).

In spite of the guidance and reports, there have been further high profile and shocking cases of abuse and neglect. We will consider the case of Daniel Pelka which culminated in his murder at the hands of his mother and her male partner. The case of Daniel was extensively covered in the media and is summarised below. The case was also reported in a Serious Case Review (Coventry Safeguarding Children Board, 2013).

A Serious Case Review (SCR) is commissioned in order to determine what can be learned from a case about the way in which local professionals and organisations worked individually and together to safeguard children.

DANIEL PELKA

Daniel was aged 4 years and 8 months at the time of his death. He had one older and one younger sibling. His family had migrated to the UK from Poland in 2005. Daniel was born in the UK in 2007. His family life was chaotic – his mother had relationships with three different partners while in the UK. All of these relationships involved high alcohol consumption and abuse. The family were known to the police, who were called to the home on many occasions, including 27 reported incidents of domestic abuse. In 2011 Daniel was taken to an A&E department with a spiral fracture to his arm. As the fracture had occurred on the previous day (the mother and step-father had delayed taking Daniel to A&E) and with the knowledge that this type of fracture is associated with non-accidental injury, the hospital referred the case to police. Although a social worker carried out an assessment, professionals accepted the mother's account of what led to the fracture and no continuing need for intervention was identified.

CASE STUDY

In September 2011 Daniel started school and over the ensuing months his attendance was poor. He grew thinner, was constantly hungry, stopped growing and went to school with bruises – his teachers reported seeing facial injuries, black eyes and bruises on his neck and head. Daniel was found scavenging in bins at school for food, but when school staff spoke to his mother about his hunger she told them he had an eating disorder that caused him to feel constantly hungry. She also told them that they should not give him any food.

It is reported that Daniel spoke little English, had few friends, often played in isolation and sometimes displayed ritualistic behaviours. He did, however, have a strong bond with his older sibling. When teachers asked him how he got his injuries, he looked down at the ground and did not answer.

Daniel was murdered by his mother and step-father in March 2012 – they were both sentenced to life imprisonment. He died of a subdural haematoma following a severe blow to the head. The trial and SCR revealed that for a period of at least six months prior to his death Daniel had been starved, assaulted, neglected and abused. Daniel was frequently locked in a 'box room' without a window or heating or toys – the only 'furniture' was a soiled mattress; he was plunged into cold baths; he was beaten and he was denied meals. He was force-fed salt until he vomited. The mother and step-father set out to deliberately harm Daniel and deceive professionals. The SCR claims that it was likely that Daniel existed in a constant state of stress and anguish. His older sibling was primed to explain his injuries as accidental. A post-mortem examination found him to be emaciated, grossly malnourished and dehydrated with bruising over his body – a total of 40 injuries. There was evidence of long-standing neglect.

The professionals who had contact with Daniel and his family included teachers, classroom assistants, school nurses, an education welfare officer, a general practitioner, a community paediatrician, social workers and the police. Three months before he was murdered a learning mentor at the school raised the possibility of completing a Common Assessment Framework from – but it never happened. Teachers variously described Daniel as 'losing weight', 'pale', 'ashen' and 'a bag of bones'. The communication between all professionals was poor, as was their recording of their concerns. This lack of proper reporting and recording meant that child protection issues were not identified. As in previous cases, there were many missed opportunities to protect Daniel. The SCR claims that no professional tried hard enough to engage with him about his eating habits or home life.

The SCR concluded that professionals need to 'think the unthinkable' and believe and act upon what they see before them, rather than accept parents' versions of events unchallenged. The approach of the professionals was not 'child centred' and Daniel was 'invisible' to the authorities.

Not long after the reporting on Daniel's murder, there were reports of another child, 4-year-old Hamzah Khan, being starved to death by his mother (Bradford Safeguarding Children Board, 2013) and of a 2-year-old toddler, Keanu Williams, who was murdered by his mother (Birmingham Safeguarding Children Board, 2013). Again investigators reported many missed opportunities to protect both children. The NSPCC has called for the exercise of 'professional curiosity' on the part of professionals when dealing with cases of suspected abuse.

- Having read the summary of Daniel's case and having had some insight into child development, can you identify any obvious areas where professionals might have used their most basic knowledge to act more appropriately on their concerns?
- From what you have learned so far, what factors, events or observations might initiate your 'professional curiosity'?

Apart from the obvious visible injuries there are several areas that you might have identified. For example, growth is an important indicator of a child's health and well-being and slow growth in childhood has psychosocial causes (Wilkinson, 2005). Daniel's apparent isolation and ritualistic behaviours might have caused alarm. Knowing that attachment is important for child development, you might have considered his relationship with his mother. But in terms of 'professional curiosity', you might have asked the question 'What eating disorder?' in response to his mother's explanation and particularly when Daniel was clearly losing weight and was constantly hungry. Many of the professionals in contact with him did have concerns but they did not act adequately on those concerns and the various professional groups did not communicate with each other.

The revised document *Working Together to Safeguard Children: A Guide to Inter-agency Working to Safeguard and Promote the Welfare of Children* (Her Majesty's Government, 2013) reiterates that safeguarding children is everyone's responsibility – everyone who comes into contact with children and their families has a role to play. The document stresses that a child's needs remain paramount. Failures to protect children are often the result of losing sight of the needs of children or placing the interests of adults ahead of those of children (HMG, 2013). Acknowledging that no single professional can have a full picture of a child's needs and circumstances, the document stresses the need to share information. It is this lack of sharing information that has too often resulted in a failure to protect children.

Nevertheless child protection policy has attracted controversy. In the 1980s child protection policies focused on children as clients of the professionals concerned rather than on the parents. Children were to be listened to and professionals were empowered to act to protect children. However, subsequent debates highlighted the rights of parents and eventually settled on family protection, although in reality the rights of children and the rights of parents may be contradictory. This change of focus had the effect of discouraging professional intervention. The dilemma here is summarised well by Campbell (2013) in the Activity below.

ACTIVITY 6.11

Read the following short article in order to understand the dilemma within child protection policy: Campbell, B. (2013) 'From Jasmine Beckford to Daniel Pelka'. Available at: www.theguardian.com/commentisfree/2013/sep/17/jasmine-beckford-daniel-pelka-history-chaos.

A nurse's role in relation to safeguarding children

There is no shortage of guidance in relation to safeguarding children. The NICE guidance (2009: 4) states that:

> ... child maltreatment includes neglect, physical, sexual and emotional abuse, and fabricated or induced illness.

You need to be aware of the factors that might place a child at risk of maltreatment. The government document *Working Together to Safeguard Children: A Guide to Inter-agency Working to Safeguard and Promote the Welfare of Children* (Her Majesty's Government, 2013: 12) states that professionals should, in particular, be alert to the needs of a child who:

- is disabled and has specific additional needs;
- has special educational needs;
- is a young carer;
- is showing signs of engaging in anti-social or criminal behaviour;
- is in family circumstances presenting challenges for the child, such as substance abuse, adult mental health, domestic violence; and/or
- is showing early signs of abuse and/or neglect.

This document further states that:

> Children are best protected when professionals are clear about what is required of them individually, and how they need to work together. (Her Majesty's Government, 2013: 7)

Guiding principles of child protection include ensuring that:

- the child's needs are paramount;
- all professionals who come into contact with children are alert to their needs;
- all professionals share information in a timely way and can discuss their concerns.

STOP AND THINK

Are you aware of the different types of maltreatment? Are you familiar with the procedures for safeguarding the welfare of children in your area?

Guidance relating to child protection does change from time to time, so you need to be guided by your mandatory training in relation to safeguarding children and alert to policy changes. However, the principles remain the same.

Firstly, you need to ensure you are aware of the following types of maltreatment:

- Physical.
- Emotional.
- Sexual.
- Neglect.

Secondly, you need to ensure that you are familiar with procedures for safeguarding the welfare of children in your area and know who to contact to express any concerns you might have. Every NHS Trust has a named member of staff who takes the lead on concerns relating to safeguarding children. Make a note of the name and contact details of the person in your placement area.

Communicating and recording are crucial in child protection

If you suspect that a child is being maltreated you should report your concerns to a more experienced colleague. He/she may well refer the matter to the named nurse for safeguarding children who could then make a referral to social services. You must record your concerns – exactly what you observed and heard from whom and when. You should also record why this is of concern and what you did about your concerns.

You might want to look at the following document from the Department for Education and Skills (2006), *What to Do if You're Worried a Child is Being Abused*. This is available at www. gov.uk/government/publications/what-to-do-if-youre-worried-a-child-is-being-abused

The focus of this section has been on maintaining health during childhood and protecting children from harm. You will have seen how an assessment of each child's needs can lead to a referral to services that can offer additional support for vulnerable children and their families and how children can be protected from harm.

Caring for people with learning disabilities

This section will enhance your understanding of some of the experiences of people with learning disabilities. You will see how universal services need to be adapted to meet the needs of individuals with learning disabilities. Again each person will have individual needs.

Reading this section, and working through the activities, will help you work towards meeting the Adult nursing NMC requirements related to people with a learning disability.

To achieve entry to the register as an adult nurse you should be able to:

- recognise and respond to the needs of people with learning disabilities who come into their care;
- maintain continuity of care to meet pre-existing intellectual, physical and emotional needs;
- understand the prevention, effects and treatment of common health problems and the links between learning disabilities and physical and mental health;
- ensure that they have access to health and social care networks and specialist services to provide support and protect people who are vulnerable;
- actively listen, provide information and involve people with learning disabilities in decision making, including agreeing reasonable adjustments to minimise disruption to their usual way of life and promote their autonomy, well-being and social inclusion;
- work with families, carers, support networks and, where necessary, specialist advocates to address people's needs;
- use effective communication and active involvement in decision making about treatment options, taking into account the person's wishes, lifestyle and capacity for consent.

(Adapted from the NMC Standards of Competence for Adult Nursing, 2010a, 2010b)

Traditionally services for people with learning disabilities were based around long-stay institutions (Phillips, 2012). However, there has been a move away from institutional care for people with learning disabilities towards practices that promote more ordinary lives (Brown et al., 2010). This shift reflects the move from a medical model to a social model of care (i.e. an approach that considers how disability and dependency are *socially* constructed). This move stems very much from a government White Paper, *Valuing People* (DH, 2001), which emphasises the rights of people with learning disabilities, particularly in relation to exerting choice and control over their lives.

People with learning disabilities may live in a wide range of settings but the majority live in the family home (RCN, 2013a). There is a range of support services available according to the level of ability of the individual. These services may include supported housing provided by social services, the private sector or the voluntary sector.

STOP AND THINK

Spend a few minutes thinking about the term 'learning disability' and jot down all of the thoughts that come into your head.

Then visit the following website: www.mencap.org.uk. Click on the link and then 'About learning disability'. You will see that MENCAP defines learning disability as:

> ... a reduced intellectual ability and difficulty with everyday activities – for example household tasks, socialising or managing money – which affects someone for their whole life.

Phillips (2012) points out that these difficulties mean that an individual with a learning disability needs support in a new environment such as an acute hospital ward. A learning disability can be mild, moderate or severe or profound (RCN, 2013a). Some people experience profound and multiple learning disabilities that include more than one disability, a significant learning disability and complex healthcare needs (Brown et al., 2010). These individuals need full-time care and support with most aspects of daily life. They may also have physical disabilities.

The RCN (2013a) reports that some people prefer to use the term 'learning difficulties', although this term is sometimes used in education to refer to conditions like dyslexia.

What causes learning disabilities?

A learning disability occurs when the brain is still developing. It can happen before birth, for example if a mother has an accident or illness during pregnancy of if the unborn baby develops certain genes. It can happen during birth, for example as a result of oxygen deprivation, or if the baby is born too early. It can also happen soon after birth as a consequence of childhood illness (MENCAP, 2013).

Some people with learning disabilities may also have other conditions, for example:

- *Cerebral palsy*: this is a physical condition that affects movement, posture and co-ordination. The effects on any individual are very varied but some people with cerebral palsy may also have a learning disability.

- *Down's syndrome*: an individual with Down's syndrome will have some degree of learning disability, but again this is very individual. Some of the problems that are associated with Down's syndrome include heart conditions and problems with sight and hearing.

Living with a learning disability

MENCAP is a charity that works in partnership with people with learning disabilities. The website contains a lot of useful information that will help you to gain some insight into the daily lives of people with learning disabilities and also help you to ensure that you are able to provide a good standard of care for people with learning disabilities in your area.

ACTIVITY 6.12

Visit the MENCAP website www.mencap.org.uk. Use the website search engine to find the 'Be Me' series of patient stories. Select and read some of the stories about the day-to-day lives of people with learning disabilities.

Health problems associated with learning disabilities

The Learning Disability Observatory at Public Health England collects a lot of data concerning people with learning disabilities. In the report for 2012 it was estimated that 1.14 million people living in England had learning disabilities: this comprised 236,000 children and 908,000 adults (Emerson et al., 2013: i).

People with learning disabilities experience a greater burden of health problems and premature death than the general population (Thomas and Atkinson, 2011; Phillips, 2012). The median age at death for people with learning disabilities is about 24 years younger than those without learning disabilities (Emerson et al., 2013: i). However, an increasing number of people with a learning disability live into old age and, as a consequence of co-morbidities, can become frequent users of health services (Brown et al., 2010; Phillips, 2012). The governments of the four countries across the United Kingdom promote the provision of mainstream healthcare services for people with learning disabilities, supported by specialist services as appropriate (Gibson, 2009). However, evidence suggests that the needs of people with learning disabilities are often not met sufficiently in general healthcare services (MENCAP, 2007; Brown et al., 2010; Phillips, 2012), resulting in inequalities in healthcare provision (Phillips, 2012).

The health problems that are associated with learning disabilities include the following:

- Respiratory disease – the main cause of death for people with learning disabilities. This may be related to aspiration or gastro-oesophageal reflux, as swallowing problems are more prevalent in people with learning disabilities (Brown et al., 2010; Thomas and Atkinson, 2011; RCN, 2013a).
- Coronary heart disease – the second highest cause of death for people with learning disabilities. People with Down's syndrome experience a higher risk of congenital heart problems (Brown et al., 2010; RCN, 2013a).

- People with learning disabilities have higher levels of gastro-intestinal cancers (RCN, 2013a).
- People with learning disabilities are vulnerable to mental health problems (RCN, 2013a).

The following are also more prevalent in people with learning disabilities:

- Epilepsy.
- Constipation.
- Obesity.
- Dental problems (RCN, 2013a).

Experiences of people with learning disabilities in acute care settings

Phillips' (2012) review of the literature relating to factors influencing general hospital care for people with learning disabilities identified the following themes:

- *Effects of being in hospital*: hospitalisation is stressful for anyone but particularly so for people with learning disabilities.
- *Attitude and knowledge of staff*: staff tend to lack knowledge and experience.
- *Hospital environment*: hospital routines tend to fail to cater for the needs of people with learning disabilities.
- *Role of carers*: most family members choose to stay with their relative in hospital but they are not always valued or supported by hospital staff.
- *Recommendations for improvement*: adjustments are often needed to meet the needs of people with learning disabilities in order to meet the legal requirement of the *Equality Act* 2010.

A worrying phenomenon termed 'diagnostic overshadowing' refers to the practice of attributing possible signs and symptoms of health problems to a person's learning disability. Thus behaviour indicating an underlying health problem may be dismissed (RCN, 2013a).

The report by MENCAP (2007), *Death by Indifference*, relayed the stories of the avoidable deaths of six people with learning disabilities and raised concern about hospital care for people with learning disabilities. The stories include the case of a 43-year-old man (Martin) with a severe learning disability who was admitted to hospital following a stroke. Martin could not speak or swallow so speech and language therapists advised that he should not attempt to eat or drink and alternative feeding methods should be used. Apart from intravenous fluids, no other attempts were made to provide Martin with nutrition and he had no food for the 26 days he spent in hospital prior to his death. His story attracted high profile media coverage.

The inadequacies in care that contributed to these six deaths were attributed to a lack of concern for the individuals' disabilities. A subsequent Ombudsman's report found evidence in some cases of NHS trusts not making *reasonable adjustments* to the organisation and delivery of care in order to accommodate the special needs of these individuals (Parliamentary and Health Service Ombudsman, 2009).

ACTIVITY 6.13

Read some of the case studies in *Death by Indifference* in order to understand some of the difficulties that these individuals faced while in the care of health and social services: MENCAP (2007) *Death by Indifference: Following up the Treat me Right! Report.* London: MENCAP. Available at www.mencap.org.uk/sites/default/files/documents/2008-03/DBIreport.pdf.

The Ombudsman report investigated each of the six cases individually but identified some common areas of concern. These included: communication; partnership working and co-ordination; relationships with families and carers; a failure to follow routine procedures; quality of management; and advocacy.

Policy context

Since the publication of the *Disability Discrimination Act 1995*, there has been a legal requirement for public services to make 'reasonable adjustments' to their services in order to cater for the needs of people with disabilities (Thomas and Atkinson, 2011). This requirement was strengthened by the *Disability Discrimination Act 2005* which requires services to meet the needs of disabled people even if this means the provision of more favourable treatment (Thomas and Atkinson, 2011). The *Equality Act 2010* requires that disabled people are not placed at a substantial disadvantage in service provision. Thus Thomas and Atkinson (2011) argue that a failure to make reasonable adjustments for the needs of people with disabilities may be unlawful.

Following the report by MENCAP a lot of attention was paid to the care and treatment of people with learning disabilities at government and policy levels. An independent Inquiry took place which recommended the establishment of the Learning Disabilities Public Health Observatory, and a confidential inquiry into premature deaths of people with learning disabilities. The Inquiry (Heslop et al., 2013) investigated the sequence of events leading to all known deaths of people with disabilities, aged 4 years and older, over a two-year period (2010–2012) in South West England. The deaths of 247 people with learning disabilities were reviewed. The most common underlying causes of death for these people were heart and circulatory disorders and cancers – a pattern that is similar for the general population. For people with learning disabilities, the final event leading to death was most frequently a respiratory infection (Heslop et al., 2013). Common reasons for deaths being assessed as premature were delays or problems with diagnosis or treatment and problems with identifying needs and providing appropriate care in response to changing needs (Heslop et al., 2013). The Inquiry also noted that established care pathways (for example NICE guidelines) were not always followed, suggesting that the required reasonable adjustments in service provision were not made for people with learning disabilities. The RCN (2013a) provides a helpful summary of recent key reports and inquiries in relation to health and social care for people with learning disabilities.

What are 'reasonable adjustments'?

In the following Case Scenario you will have an opportunity to consider how you might adapt your own practice in order to improve the provision of care to people with learning disabilities.

 SEAN

Sean is 37 years old and has moderate learning disabilities. He lives at home with his parents who are his main carers, although the family has some help from outside agencies. Sean has been admitted to a surgical ward for exploratory surgery to investigate a possible cancer.

From the reading you have done so far, make some suggestions regarding what 'reasonable adjustments' you might make to accommodate Sean's needs.

You will no doubt have started with some reflection on the knowledge you have acquired about people with learning disabilities and the general problems they might encounter on admission to an acute hospital ward. You probably decided that an assessment of Sean's needs would be appropriate in order to apply your general knowledge to his specific and unique situation. It is important to note that according to the Department of Health's (2013d) *Learning Disabilities Good Practice Project* one of the indicators of good practices is a 'capabilities approach'. This entails focusing on people's strengths and what they can do rather than what they cannot.

Thomas and Atkinson (2011: 35) state that *reasonable adjustments* entail:

... providing individualised services that are informed by an empathetic understanding of a service user's unique circumstances.

Making reasonable adjustments to services requires the possession of knowledge of the health vulnerabilities that are specific to people with learning disabilities, coupled with an assessment of the service user's communication abilities, views and preferences (Thomas and Atkinson, 2011). It is also important to involve Sean's family and professional carers.

Thomas and Atkinson (2011: 35) suggest the following reasonable adjustments to services:

- *Health passports*: these documents contain an outline of the individual's health and illness history, health problems, and treatments.
- *Informed decision making*: knowledge and appropriate use of the *Mental Capacity Act 2005* to ensure that an individual makes their own decisions as far as possible, or decisions that are made on the individual's behalf are in that person's best interests.
- *Learning Disability Liaison Nurses*: these professionals use their expertise to co-ordinate care and provide advice.
- *Annual health checks*: in order to monitor health and detect health problems early on.

- Involve families and carers.
- Support families and carers.
- Provide information concerning services and treatments in accessible formats, for example pictures, symbols, DVDs.

The RCN (2013b: 16) also identified the importance of communication in removing barriers to satisfactory use of healthcare services and offer the following advice:

- Use simple language.
- Use pictures, photographs.
- Avoid abstract words or concepts.

ACTIVITY 6.14

Some people with learning disabilities use a signing vocabulary. This system is called Makaton.
  Visit the following website and learn a few useful words: www.makaton.org

---

Informed decision making

The *Mental Capacity Act 2005* provides a framework to empower and protect adults who may lack the capacity to make decisions for themselves. The act aims to provide a balance between an individual's right to make their own decisions and their right to protection from harm if they lack such capacity. Accordingly every adult must be assumed to have capacity unless proved otherwise – you cannot assume someone lacks capacity on the basis of a diagnosis.

The Department for Constitutional Affairs (2007) have produced a Code of Practice for the Mental Capacity Act. Guidance is provided on how to test if someone has mental capacity. In order to assess mental capacity it is necessary to determine if the individual can:

- understand the decision to be made;
- understand the consequences of making or not making the decision;
- understand, retain and use the information necessary to make the decision;
- communicate their decision (Department of Constitutional Affairs, 2007).

The outcome of this test applies to a particular decision. Each time a decision needs to be made the test needs to be applied because sometimes patients can make some decisions but not others.

Safeguarding vulnerable adults

Finally in this section, it is important to raise awareness of a nurse's role in safeguarding vulnerable adults in relation to the care of people with a learning disability. People with learning disabilities are at greater risk of abuse – 20% of the total number of alerts recorded by local authorities during 2011/12 concerned adults with learning disabilities. The most common type of alleged abuse was physical abuse and the most common perpetrator was a member of social care staff (Emerson et al., 2013: vi-vii). We will return to a nurse's responsibilities in relation to safeguarding vulnerable adults later in this chapter.

You will have seen in this section how vulnerable people with learning disabilities might be (especially, though not exclusively, when admitted to hospital for acute treatment). This section has focused on the need to consider each person with a learning disability as an individual with their own needs and preferences. Some suggestions have been made concerning how nursing practice might be adapted to assist personalisation of care and treatment and how individuals might be helped to retain some control over their care and treatment.

Mental health

This section introduces you to the need for the promotion of mental health, particularly in younger people, and also the need to place mental health services on a par with services for people with physical health problems. You will need to consider the stigma that might be attached to mental illness, the vulnerability of some people with mental illness, and the need to safeguard vulnerable people. Reading this section, and working through the activities, will help you work towards meeting the Adult Nursing NMC competencies related to people with mental health needs.

─────────────── **To achieve entry to the register as an** ───────────────
adult nurse you should be able to:

- use basic mental health skills to reduce the distress associated with mental health problems and help promote recovery;
- act promptly to reduce the risk of harm in a crisis and to protect people who are vulnerable;
- have a basic understanding of mental health promotion, the links between physical and mental health problems and the aetiology and treatment of common mental health problems;
- appreciate the impact of mental health problems and distress on a person's cognition, communication, behaviour, lifestyle and relationships;
- be aware of the main provisions of mental health laws, especially those relating to capacity, human rights and safeguarding;
- recognise and address people's essential mental health needs when these exist alongside other primary health needs;
- work and communicate with others to maintain continuity in meeting mental health needs in long-term conditions.

(Adapted from the NMC Standards of Competence for Adult Nursing, 2010a, 2010b)

This is a potentially exciting time for mental health nursing as the government seeks to raise the profile of mental healthcare, treatment and services to put them on a par with services for people with physical health problems. The government strategy for mental health, *No Health Without Mental Health* (DH, 2011b), includes the following aims:

- Mental health to have equal priority with physical health.
- End the discrimination associated with mental health problems.
- Ensure that everyone who needs mental healthcare gets the right support at the right time.

Furthermore, greater priority is being given to preventing mental ill health and promoting mental well-being. At least one in four people will experience a mental health problem at some point in their life (DH, 2011b).

A recent document, *Closing the Gap: Priorities for Essential Change in Mental Health* (DH, 2014), supports the longer-term aims of the mental health strategy but also seeks to speed up the pace of change locally, identifying 25 areas where changes can be made within a shorter timescale. Central to this is the aim of gathering more information about mental health and illness, the needs of clients and the services that are available. One of the aims of enhanced information is to establish waiting time limits for mental health services in order to match the existing standards for access to services for physical health problems (DH, 2014). This is against the background of concerns raised about waiting times for the treatment of anxiety and depression. Another aim is to tackle inequalities in access to mental health services (for example in relation to black and minority ethnic communities and older people) particularly concerning access to psychological therapies, which have been found to help many people manage long-term mental health problems (DH, 2014). Psychological therapies are often referred to as 'talking therapies' (for example cognitive behavioural therapy and counselling).

A further aim of government policy is that of better integration of mental healthcare and physical healthcare. Remember, people whose health problems are primarily physical can develop mental health problems and people whose health problems are primarily psychological can develop physical health problems. There is obviously a clear need for better understanding of the links between mental and physical health.

Mental health – as opposed to mental illness – has many benefits including healthier lifestyles, better physical health, improved recovery from illness and better employment prospects and income (Friedli, 2009). But what is 'mental health'?

> Concepts of mental health include subjective well-being, perceived self-efficacy, autonomy, competence, intergenerational dependence and recognition of the ability to realize one's intellectual and emotional potential. It has also been defined as a state of well-being whereby individuals recognize their abilities, are able to cope with the normal stresses of life, work productively and fruitfully, and make a contribution to their communities. Mental health is about enhancing competencies of individuals and communities and enabling them to achieve their self-determined goals. Mental health should be a concern for all of us, rather than only for those who suffer from a mental disorder. (WHO, 2003: 7)

Mental health is more than a lack of mental illness (WHO, 2003). However, Wrycroft (2009) prefers to view mental health at one end of a continuum with mental illness at the other end.

Mental health ————————————————————— Mental illness

People may move along this continuum at different times in their lives. Mental illness should be understood less in terms of individual pathology and more in terms of the response to adversity (Friedli, 2009).

Culture and mental health

The issue of mental health and illness and ethnicity is a complex and controversial one. The term 'minority ethnic group' encompasses many different groups with different experiences and beliefs about mental health and illness. For example, there is a long history of higher admission rates to psychiatric hospitals for black men than those for the white majority population (Balarajan and Soni Raleigh, 1993; Smaje, 1995). African-Caribbean people are also more likely to be subject to compulsory treatment under the *Mental Health Act* than the UK majority population (DH, 2011b). The boundary between mental health and mental illness is concerned with the question of normality, which is culturally relative (Sashidharan and Commander, 1998; Fernando, 2002). Mental health and illness are socially constructed, both in terms of the person suffering from the 'abnormality' and the person making any judgement on 'abnormality' (Helman, 2000), suggesting that cultural misunderstanding may contribute to some misdiagnosis. Helman notes that, as well having a higher rate of mental illness than the majority population in their adopted countries, immigrants also have higher rates of mental illness than the populations of their countries of origin. This suggests that mental health problems among immigrants may be associated with experiences in host countries. The government acknowledges that progress in tackling inequalities for minority ethnic groups has been disappointing (DH, 2011b).

ACTIVITY 6.15

For further information about culture and mental health, access the following Department of Health report *Race Equality Action Plan: A Five-Year Review* (DH, 2010b). This document reviews the work of the Delivering Race Equality in Mental Healthcare Programme and describes key challenges, successes and learning.

While it has been suggested that some diagnoses may reflect a lack of cultural understanding and be the result of labelling certain behaviours as deviant that might be seen as normal if viewed within its cultural context (Helman, 2000), the role of social disadvantage cannot be ignored. A Manchester-based study (Thomas et al., 1993) exploring compulsory psychiatric admissions found that second-generation (UK born) Afro-Caribbean people had nine times the rate of schizophrenia than white people. However, it is possible that this could be explained by their greater socio-economic disadvantage (i.e. poor inner-city housing and higher rates of unemployment) rather than psychiatric misdiagnosis – socio-economic disadvantage is known to be correlated with schizophrenia (Thomas et al., 1993).

The government strategy (DH, 2011b) also notes that more young people are experiencing behavioural and emotional problems than previously. One in ten children aged 15–16 years have a mental health problem and many continue to have mental health problems into adulthood. Half of those with lifetime mental health problems first experience symptoms by the age of 14 and three-quarters before their mid-twenties (DH, 2011b). The promotion of mental health and well-being in childhood is therefore very important. As well as providing better support for new mothers, schools will be supported to identify mental health problems sooner (DH, 2011b); for example, the government plans to review models of service and practice for health visiting and school nursing.

Labelling and stigma

In a seminal study Rosenhan (1973) described an experiment during which sane people covertly gained admission to psychiatric hospitals in order to explore the experience of being a patient. In order to get themselves admitted, the researchers said that they had been hearing voices. Once they were admitted with a diagnosis of schizophrenia they ceased any pretence of illness – they just carried on recording their observations. While the staff did not recognise that the researchers were not mentally ill, some of the patients did. The researchers were all eventually discharged with a diagnosis of schizophrenia in remission. The label had stuck.

People with mental health problems often suffer social stigma (WHO, 2003). Stigma has connotations of shame and deviations from normal. The process of stigmatising involves making adverse social judgements about a person or a group. People who are stigmatised often experience rejection and exclusion and may be treated as outcasts (Scambler, 2009) so it is not surprising that current policy aims to raise awareness of mental health and illness and to promote positive mental health.

Maladaptive coping strategies

Stressful circumstances can be damaging to health. Ongoing adverse social and psychological circumstances (for example, low pay and difficulties in supporting a family, paying a mortgage or rent, difficult working conditions and/or social isolation) can cause long-term stress, which in turn can have a detrimental effect on physical and mental health (Wilkinson and Marmot, 2003). In such situations some people might turn to health-damaging behaviours as a way of dealing with their problems. Misuse of drugs and alcohol can lead to addiction.

The Centre for Social Justice (2013) reports the following statistics:

- 1.6 million adults (1 in 20) are dependent on alcohol.
- 380,000 people (1 in 100) are addicted to heroin or crack cocaine.
- 335,000 children (1 in 37) live with a parent who is addicted to drugs.
- 1 in 7 children under the age of one live with a substance-abusing parent.

Drug and alcohol abuse has significant effects on individuals, families and communities (WHO, 2003; CSJ, 2013). Such abuse can lead to child poverty, family breakdown, welfare dependency and severe personal debt as well as crime (CSJ, 2013). For example, the WHO (2003: 10) demonstrates how excessive alcohol consumption can result in more money being spent on alcohol, which in turn can lead to financial problems, resulting in less money being available to be spent on food. Living conditions can deteriorate, the individual and family may experience social stigma and the health of the entire family may be affected as a consequence of the stigma and poor nutrition. The impact of drug and alcohol abuse is felt particularly in Britain's most deprived communities (CSJ, 2013). Drinking alcohol at dangerous levels is increasing: and alcohol-related hospital admissions and deaths are rising (CSJ, 2013). Furthermore, coping strategies like smoking are linked to physical health problems (WHO, 2003).

Anxiety

As McGrandles and Duffy (2012) point out, a degree of anxiety is normal and most people will experience anxiety at some point in their lives. Anxiety and stress can initiate protective mechanisms in the body which prepare us for 'fight or flight'. When this happens our heart rate increases, our blood pressure rises and blood is diverted to the muscles to help us respond to the threat, for example by running away. Cortisol is also released into the blood stream, by the adrenal glands, and has the effect of raising blood sugar levels in order to enhance energy. The result of this response is increased vigilance and a preparedness to deal with short-term threats and emergencies (Wilkinson, 2005).

STOP AND THINK

Think about a time when you have experienced anxiety, maybe before an exam or when leaving home to start your nursing course.

• How did you feel?

A traumatic event can cause anxiety which may affect sleep, appetite and the ability to concentrate (McGrandles and Duffy, 2012). Usually anxiety diminishes once the threat has passed but if it persists it may become a mental health problem. Prolonged stress and/or anxiety can also contribute to physical health problems, such as raised blood pressure and reduced functioning of the immune system. Diabetes may result from insulin resistance (Wilkinson, 2005).

Anxiety and hospital admission

Admission to hospital is a major event in many patients' lives and can cause varying levels of anxiety as a consequence of fear of the unknown, fear arising from adverse media reports of poor hospital care and an awareness that hospitals can be dangerous places. In particular, there is potential for anxiety and fear when patients are admitted to hospital for elective surgery (Pritchard, 2011).

Pritchard (2011: 35) defines anxiety as 'an unpleasant state of uneasiness or tension that may be associated with hypertension and tachycardia'. An anxious patient may appear to be aggressive or demanding, require a lot of attention from nurses. High levels of nervousness and apprehension may also hinder the ability to understand or follow simple instructions (Pritchard, 2011).

Pritchard argues that all health professionals should be able to identify patients who are at risk of anxiety or depression and respond appropriately with effective and supportive care. For example, in adult nursing there is a professional responsibility to ensure that patients are adequately prepared for surgery both physically and psychologically. The provision of accurate information about what to expect during the pre- and post-operative periods has been found to contribute to reductions in anxiety (Pritchard, 2011).

Emotional and psychological distress associated with approaching death

Individuals may experience a range of emotions when faced with the prospect of approaching death (see Chapter 13, p. 402). Several authors have attempted to theorise the process of dying. For example, Kubler-Ross (1969) described a series of stages that individuals might go through:

- *Denial* – a reaction to the diagnosis of an incurable illness. Individuals deny the severity of the situation.
- *Anger* – individuals move from denial to being angry at the diagnosis and prognosis. Why me?
- *Bargaining* – individuals make promises that will be fulfilled in exchange for being given more time to live. 'If only ...'
- *Depression* – individuals can no longer deny the progression of the disease.
- *Acceptance* – individuals may come to accept the inevitable if there is sufficient time.

This outline has been criticised as dying is a very individual process and not all patients follow this pattern (certainly not in a linear fashion) and not all individuals achieve acceptance. Nor is the framework prescriptive; patients should not be encouraged to move from one stage to another. Rather, Copp (1998) suggests that patients may oscillate between periods of calm, fear, hope, depression, anger, sadness, and withdrawal.

Law's (2009) exploration of how district nurses meet the emotional needs of dying patients in the community found that patients talked about 'outside' and 'inside' worlds. Outside worlds consisted of hospitals and treatments and the everyday social world where people conduct their daily lives – e.g. shopping and socialising. Inside worlds consisted of the world of disease and illness and the inner emotional world. Law found that district nurses entered the inside world by establishing relationships with their patients and enabling them to express their feelings but she also identified a 'bridging' role whereby district nurses attempted to help patients maintain contact with the outside world. Their approach is consistent with the aim of the hospice movement, 'to help ... to live until you die', expressed by the late Dame Cicely Saunders, a founder of the modern hospice movement.

Patients will vary enormously in their responses to approaching death but most will experience degrees of emotional and psychological distress (see Chapter 13 p.402–3).

Depression

Depression can be a reaction to life events such as physical illness, bereavement, problems with relationships or finances (Hardy, 2013).

What is your understanding of the term 'depression'?

STOP AND THINK

The term 'depression' can be used in common parlance to describe 'a transient low mood state experienced by most people' (Taylor and Ashelsford, 2008: 49) but it is also a clinical syndrome described as a 'medical condition involving changes in mood, appetite, sleep, thoughts and psychomotor activity' (2008: 49). Taylor and Ashelsford point out that depression is not an inevitable consequence of severe illness, but that it is a serious condition and treatable.

It is perhaps important to note that depression in end of life care can be difficult to distinguish from grief and sadness and so it can be hard to differentiate between a severe psychiatric disorder and 'normal' distress (Taylor and Ashelsford, 2008).

Taylor and Ashelsford (2008: 50) describe four domains for the symptoms of depression:

- Mood change (for example low mood).
- Cognitive impairment (for example poor attention).
- Circadian dysregulation (for example changes in sleep pattern).
- Motor deficits (for example restlessness).

Thus as an adult nurse you will need to be alert for signs of depression and engage in accurate assessment as part of a therapeutic relationship with your patients. Taylor and Ashelsford suggest that the involvement of relatives might be helpful in contrasting past mood with current mood in order to detect major changes.

We have already seen that people with learning disabilities are at risk of abuse but they are not the only 'at risk' group. Poor mental health is both a cause and a consequence of the experience of adverse social economic and environmental circumstances (Friedli, 2009). Mental health problems are more common in deprived areas (Friedli, 2009). People with mental health problems can also be vulnerable.

The Department of Health document, *Safeguarding Adults: The Role of Health Service Practitioners,* states that '… safeguarding adults is about the safety and well-being of all patients but providing additional measures for those least able to protect themselves from harm or abuse' (DH, 2011c: 8).

A vulnerable adult is defined as an individual:

who is or may be in need of community care services by reason of mental or other disability, age or illness;

and

who is or may be unable to take care of him or herself,

or

unable to protect him or herself against significant harm or exploitation. (DH, 2011c: 10)

An adult's capacity for self care will be affected by their own personal circumstances such as physical ability, learning disability, mental health, illness and frailty, as well as factors within the local environment, personal strengths, and social contacts and support (DH, 2011c). Harm or abuse may be physical, sexual, psychological, discriminatory, financial or neglectful in nature (DH, 2011c). Nurses are in a key position to identify possible safeguarding concerns, for example when a vulnerable adult is admitted to hospital with unexplained injuries, or when a community nurse makes a home visit and suspects abuse within the family unit. In both cases local protocols and procedures will provide guidance on what action you should take. Whatever the response is, it is likely to involve a range of professionals and agencies. The local authority is the lead agency for safeguarding adults and co-ordinates the local Safeguarding Adults Board. Local Safeguarding Adults services manage responses to safeguarding adult referrals.

ACTIVITY 6.16

Age UK has produced a factsheet providing advice about different types of abuse of older people and what people can do if they suspect abuse. You can read Factsheet 78, 'Safeguarding older people from abuse', on Age UK's website. This is available at www. ageuk.org.uk.

Policy relating to safeguarding adults is shaped by six principles:

- Empowerment.
- Protection.
- Prevention.
- Proportionality.
- Partnerships.
- Accountability.

Read more about these principles in *Safeguarding Adults: The Role of Health Services Practitioners* (DH, 2011c: 12–13). This is available at www.gov.uk/government/publications/safeguarding-adults-the-role-of-health-services.

As with safeguarding children, you will need to ensure that you are familiar with procedures for safeguarding vulnerable adults in your area and also know who to contact to express any concerns you might have. Every NHS Trust has a named member of staff who takes the lead on concerns relating to safeguarding adults. Again, good communication and record keeping are crucial.

If you suspect the abuse of an adult you should report your concerns to a more experienced colleague who can refer the matter to the named nurse for safeguarding adults who in turn can make a referral to social services. You must record your concerns – exactly what you observed and heard from whom and when. You should also record why this is of concern and what you did about your concerns.

This section has focused on the promotion of mental health, providing examples of how adverse socio-economic circumstances can impact on mental health and how individuals may be stigmatised. You will have considered how stressful circumstances can be damaging to health, particularly when individuals resort to health-damaging behaviours. The importance of individual assessment will highlight individual needs and help partnership working to promote resilience and enhance control over care and treatment plans. More vulnerable individuals need to be protected from harm.

Chapter summary

In this chapter we have considered aspects of other fields of nursing – maternity, children, learning disability and mental health. While these fields appear to represent disparate groups of people, we have seen that there some unifying threads in terms of the needs of disadvantaged people within these groups. We have also seen that while the NHS provides comprehensive and universal services on the basis of clinical need, there is sometimes a requirement for additional services to meet the needs of certain groups. For example, we have explored the need for 'reasonable adjustments' to be made for people with learning disabilities who are admitted to hospital for acute care and we have seen the need for initiatives to reach out to disadvantaged expectant mothers and for additional support for young children in low income families. However, whilst we have often referred to groups of people, here it is important to remember that an assessment of each individual will identify their unique needs and preferences. This assessment will assist the identification of a need for additional support for more vulnerable individuals. For all of these groups of people there is a requirement for adult nurses to understand their needs and be alert to safeguarding issues.

Suggested further reading

Bartley, M. (ed.) (2012) 'Life gets under your skin'. Available at: www.ucl/ac.uk/iclspublications/booklets/lguys.pdf. (This document demonstrates the life-course approach to inequalities in health.)

Department of Health (2011) *Preparation for Birth and Beyond: A Resource Pack for Leaders of Community Groups and Activities.* Available at: www.gov.uk/government/publications/preparation-for-birth-and-beyond-a-resource-pack-for-leaders-of-community-groups-and-activities (this document is a useful resource for understanding the importance of early interventions in children's welfare, bonding and empowering parents).

Department of Health (2013d) *Learning Disabilities Good Practice Project.* Available at: www.gov.uk. (This document contains examples of how some service providers have improved the lives of people with learning disabilities.)

Department of Health, Social Services and Public Safety (2011) *Safeguarding Children Supervision Policy for Nurses Regional Policy for Northern Ireland Health and Social Care Trusts.* Belfast: DHSSPS.

Glasper, A. (2013) 'Preventing ill health in childhood', *British Journal of Nursing*, 22(22): 1326–27. (This article summarises the main points of the Chief Medical Officer's Annual Report for 2012, *Our Children Deserve Better: Prevention Pays* (DH, 2013b).)

Hardy, S. (2013) 'Prevention and management of depression in primary care', *Nursing Standard*, 27(26): 51–6.

MENCAP website at: www.mencap.org.uk

You can explore issues related to those highlighted above on the MIND website at www.mind.org

MIND and Mental Health Foundation (2013) *Building Resilient Communities. Making Every Contact Count for Public Mental Health.* London: MIND/Mental Health Foundation. Available at: http://mentalhealth.org/publications/building-resilient-communities.pdf.

NHS Wales (n.d.) *Good Practice Framework for People with a Learning Disability Requiring Planned Secondary Care.* Cardiff: Welsh Government.

NICE (2011) *NICE Pathway: Antenatal and Postnatal Health.* London: NICE. Available at: http://pathways.nice.org.uk/pathways/antenatal-and-postnatal-mental-health (accessed 27 November 2014). (A summary of NICE guidance on antenatal and postnatal mental health.)

NICE (2014): *Antenatal and Postnatal Mental Health: Clinical Management and Service Guidance.* Available at: www.nice.org.uk/guidanceCG192 (these clinical guidelines make recommendations for the prediction, detection and treatment of mental disorders in women during pregnancy and the postnatal period).

NICE's recommendations for local authorities and partner organisations on social and emotional well-being for children and young people, specifically vulnerable children aged under 5 years and all children in primary and secondary education, can be accessed at: https://pathways.nice.org.uk/(search for social and emotional well being for children and young people).

Phillips, L. (2012) 'Improving care for people with learning disabilities in hospital', *Nursing Standard*, 26(23): 42–58.

Royal College of Nursing (2009) Mental Health in Children and Young People: An RCN Toolkit for Nurses Who are Not Mental Health Specialists. Available at: www.rcn.org.uk

Royal College of Nursing (2013a) Meeting the Health Needs of People with Learning Disabilities: *RCN Guidance for Nursing Staff*. London: RCN. Available at: www.rcn.org.uk (This is an excellent resource that is designed to support qualified and student nurses, who are trained in fields other than learning disability, to provide high quality care to people with learning disabilities.)

Royal College of Nursing (2013b) 'Dignity in healthcare for people with learning disabilities'. In *Guidance for Nurses*, 2nd edition. London: RCN. Available at: www.rcn.org.uk

The Royal College of Psychiatrists (n.d.) 'Postpartum psychosis'. Available at: www.rcpsych. ac.uk/healthadvice/problemsdisorders/postpartumpsychosis.aspx (useful informantion on postpartum psychosis for women, partners and friends).

Robertson, K. (2010) 'Understanding the needs of women with postnatal depression', *Nursing Standard*, 24(46): 47–55.

Taylor, V. and Ashford, S. (2008) 'Understanding depression in palliative and end of life care', *Nursing Standard*, 23(12): 48–57.

The Scottish Government (2012) *Strengthening the Commitment*. The report of the UK Modernising Learning Disabilities Nursing Review, Edinburgh, The Scottish Government.

The Scottish Government (2014) *National Guidance for Child Protection in Scotland*. Edinburgh: The Scottish Government.

The Scottish Government (2012) *Mental Health Strategy for Scotland: 2012–2015*. Edinburgh: The Scottish Government.

The Scottish Government (2014) *Adult Support and Protection (Scotland) Act 2007 Code of Practice*. Edinburgh: The Scottish Government.

References

Allen, M., Allen, J., Hogarth, S. with Marmot, M. (2013) *Working for Health Equity: The Role of Health Professionals*. Available at: www.instituteofhealthequity.org/projects/working-for-health-equity-the-role-of-health-professionals (accessed 19 January 2015).

Anderson, M.E., Johnson, D.C. and Batal, H.A. (2005) 'Sudden Infant Death Syndrome and prenatal maternal smoking: rising attributed risk in the *Back to Sleep* era', *BMC Medicine*. Available at www.biomedcentral.com/1741-7015/3/4 (accessed 19 January 2015).

Balarajan, R. and Soni Raleigh, V. (1993) *Ethnicity and Health: A Guide for the NHS*. London: Department of Health.

Barker, D. (1994) cited in M. Wadsworth, Chapter 9: 'Family and education as determinants of health'. In D. Blane, E. Brunner and R. Wilkinson (eds) (1996), *Health and Social Organisation: Towards a Health Policy for the 21st Century*. London: Routledge.

Birmingham Safeguarding Children Board (2013) *Serious Case Review: In Respect of the Death of Keanu Williams*. Available at: www.lscbirmingham.org.uk/images/stories/downloads/executive-summaries/Case_25_Final_Overview_Report_02.10.13.pdf (accessed 19 January 2015).

Boath, E. and Henshaw, C. (2008) 'Women's health: postnatal depression', *British Journal of Healthcare Assistants*, 2(3): 127–31.

Bosma, H., Marmot, M.G., Hemingway, H., Nicholson, S.C., Brunner, E. and Stansfield, S.A. (1997) 'Low job control and risk of coronary heart disease in Whitehall II (prospective cohort) study', *British Medical Journal*, 314: 558–65.

Bradford Safeguarding Children's Board (2013) *A Serious Case Review: Hamzah Khan: The Overview Report*. Available at: www.bradford-scb.org.uk/scr/hamzah_khan_scr/SeriousCaseReviewOverviewReportNovember2013.pdf (accessed 19 January 2015).

Brown, M., MacArthur, J., McKechanie, A., Hayes, M. and Fletcher, J. (2010) 'Equality and access to general healthcare for people with learning disabilities: reality or rhetoric?', *Journal of Research in Nursing*, 15(4): 351–61.

Brunner, E. and Marmot, M. (1999) 'Social organization, stress, and health'. In M. Marmot and R.G. Wilkinson (eds) *Social Determinants of Health*. Oxford: Oxford University Press.

Campbell, B. (2013) 'From Jasmine Beckford to Daniel Pelka: a history of chaos to calumny', *The Guardian*, 17 September. Available at: www.theguardian.com/commentisfree/2013/sep/17/jasmine-beckford-daniel-pelka-history-chaos (accessed 27 November 2014).

Camps, L. and Long, T. (2012) 'Origin, purpose and future of Sure Start children's centres', *Nursing Children and Young People*, 24(1): 26–30.

Centre for Social Justice (2013) *No Quick Fix: Exposing the Depth of Britain's Drug and Alcohol Problem*. London: CSJ. Available at: www.centreforsocialjustice.org.uk/publications/no-quick-fix-exposing-the-depth-of-britain%E2%80%99s-drug-and-alcohol-problem (accessed 17 January 2015)

Children's Society (2013) www.childrenssociety.org.uk/what-we-do (accessed 22 November 2014).

Commission on Social Determinants of Health (2008) *Closing the Gap in a Generation: Health Equity through Action on the Social Determinants of Health*. Geneva: World Health Organization. Available at www.who.int/social_determinants/thecommission/finalreport/en/index.html (accessed 22 November 2014).

Copp, G. (1998) 'A review of current theories of death and dying', *Journal of Advanced Nursing*, 28(2): 382–90 .

Coventry Safeguarding Children Board (2013) *Serious Case Review: Daniel Pelka*. Available at: www.coventrylscb.org.uk/dpelka.html (accessed 27 November 2014).

Department for Constitutional Affairs (2007) *Mental Capacity Act 2005: Code of Practice*. London: The Stationery Office. Available at www.justice.gov.uk/protecting-the-vulnerable/mental-capacity-act (accessed 19 January 2015).

Department for Education (2010) *Working Together to Safeguard Children: A Guide to Inter-agency Working to Safeguard and Promote the Welfare of Children*. London: Department for Education.

Department for Education (2011a) *Supporting Families in the Foundation Years*. Available at: www.gov.uk/government/publications/supporting-families-in-the-foundation-years (accessed 17 January 2015).

Department for Education (2011b) *The Munro Review of Child Protection: Final Report: A Child-centred System*. Available at: www.gov.uk/government/ publications/munro-review-of-child-protection-final-report-a-child-centred-system (accessed 17 January 2015).

Department for Education and Skills (2003) *Every Child Matters*. London: HMSO.

Department for Education and Skills (2006) *What to Do if You're Worried a Child is Being Abused*. Available at: www.gov.uk/government/publications/what-to-do-if-youre-worried-a-child-is-being-abused (accessed 17 January 2015).

Department for Education and Skills (2007) *Common Assessment Framework for Children and Young People: Practitioners Guide*. London: DfES.

Department for Education (2014) *Early Education and Childcare. Statutory Guidance for Local Authorities*. London: DfE.

Department of Health (2001) *Valuing People. A New Strategy for Learning Disability for the 21st Century*. London: Department of Health. Available at: www.gov.uk/government/uploads/system/uploads/attachment_data/file/250877/5086.pdf (accessed 22 November 2014).

Department of Health (2003) *The Victoria Climbié Inquiry: Report of an Inquiry by Lord Laming*. Cm 5730. London: Department of Health.

Department of Health (2009) *Healthy Child Programme: Pregnancy and the First Five Years of Life*. Available at: www.gov.uk/government/uploads/system/uploads/attachment_data/file/167998/Health_Child_Programme.pdf (accessed 19 January 2015) .

Department of Health (2010a) *Healthy Lives, Healthy People: Our Strategy for Public Health in England*. Available at: www.gov.uk/government/uploads/system/uploads/attachment_data/file/216096/dh_127424.pdf (accessed 19 January 2015).

Department of Health (2010b) *Race Equality Action Plan: A Five-Year Review*. Available at: www.hsconsultancy.org.uk/system/resources/1/race-equality-action-plan-a-five-year-review. pdf?1302161027 (accessed 27 November 2014).

Department of Health (2011a) *Preparation for Birth and Beyond: A Resource Pack for Leaders of Community Groups and Activities*. Available at: www.gov.uk/government//publications/ preparation-for-birth-and-beyond-a-resource-pack-for-leaders-of-community-groups-and-activities (accessed 17 January 2015).

Department of Health (2011b) *No Health Without Mental Health: A Cross Government Outcomes Strategy for People of All Ages*. Available at: www.gov.uk/government/uploads/system/uploads/ attachment_data/file/213761/dh_124058.pdf (accessed 19 January 2015).

Department of Health (2011c) *Safeguarding Adults: The Role of Health Service Practitioners*. Available at: www.gov.uk/government/uploads/system/publications/safeguarding-adults-the-role-of-health-services (accessed 17 January 2015).

Department of Health (2012) *Family Nurse Partnership Programme*. Available at: www.gov. uk/government/uploads/system/uploads/attachment_data/file/216864/The-Family-Nurse-Partnership-Programme-Information-leaflet.pdf (accessed 22 November 2014).

Department of Health (2013a) *Birth to Five*. Available at: www.publichealth.hscni.net/publications/ birth-five (accessed 27 November 2014).

Department of Health (2013b) *Giving All Children a Healthy Start in Life*. Available at: www.gov. uk/government/policies/giving-all-children-a-healthy-start-in-life (accessed 19 January 2015).

Department of Health (2013c) *Annual Report of the Chief Medical Officer 2012. Our Children Deserve Better: Prevention Pays*. Available at: www.gov.uk/government/uploads/system/ uploads/attachment_data_file/255237/2901304_CMO_complete_low_res_accessible.pdf (accessed 19 January 2015).

Department of Health (2013d) *Learning Disabilities Good Practice Project*. Available at: www. gov.uk/government/publications/learning-disabilities-good-practice-project-report (accessed 27 November 2014).

Department of Health (2014) *Closing the Gap: Priorities for Essential Change in Mental Health*. Available at: www.gov.uk/government//publications/mental-health-priorities-for-change (accessed 18 January 2015).

Duaso, M.J. and Duncan, D. (2012) 'Health impact of smoking and smoking cessation strategies: current evidence', *British Journal of Community Nursing*, 17(8): 356–63.

Emerson, E., Hatton, C., Robertson, J., Baines, S., Christie, A. and Glover, G. (2013) *People with Learning Disabilities in England 2012*. Cambridge: Improving Health and Lives: Learning Disabilities Observatory. Available at: www.improvinghealthandlives.org.uk (last accessed 20 November 2014).

European Union (2005) Directive 2005/36/EC of the EU Parliament and of the Council on the recognition of professional qualification. Available at: http://ec.europa.eu/internal_market/ qualifications/policy_developments/legislation/index_en.htm (accessed 19 January 2015).

Fearn, M. and Howard, J. (2012) 'Play as a resource for children facing adversity: an exploration of indicative case studies', *Children and Society*, 26: 456–68.

Fernando, S. (2002) *Mental Health, Race and Culture*, 2nd edition. Basingstoke: Palgrave.

Friedli, L. (2009) *Mental Health, Resilience and Inequalities*. Copenhagen: WHO. Available at: www.euro.who.int/__data/assets/pdf_file/0012/100821/E92227.pdf (accessed 19 January 2015).

Gibson, T. (2009) 'Learning disabilities education in the common foundation programme', *Nursing Standard*, 23(46): 35–9.

Hardy, S. (2013) 'Prevention and management of depression in primary care', *Nursing Standard*, 27(26): 51–6.

Helman, C.G. (2000) *Culture, Health and Illness*, 4th edition. Oxford: Butterworth Heinemann.

Her Majesty's Government (2013) 'Working together to safeguard children: a guide to inter-agency working to safeguard and promote the welfare of children'. Available at: www.gov.uk/ government/publications/working-together-to-safeguard-children (accessed 18 January 2015).

Heslop, P., Blair, P., Fleming, P., Hoghton, M., Marriott, A. and Russ, L. (2013) *Confidential Inquiry into Premature Deaths of People with Learning Disabilities* (CIPOLD). Bristol: Norah

Fry Research Centre: University of Bristol. Available at: www.bristol.ac.uk/cipold (last accessed 20 November 2013).

HM Government (2004) *The Children's Act*. Available at: www.legislation.gov.uk/ukpga/2004/31/pdfs/ukpga_20040031_en.pdf (last accessed 7 March 2015).

Hogg, S. (2013) 'Birth and beyond: supporting parents in the antenatal period', *Journal of Health Visiting*, 1(3): 144–7.

Jones, K. (2000) *The Making of Social Policy in Britain: From the Poor Law to New Labour*. London: Athlone.

Kinge, S. and Gregory, I. (2011a) 'Maternity focus: postnatal transition to the community', *British Journal of Healthcare Assistants*, 5(9): 448–50.

Kinge, S. and Gregory, I. (2011b) 'Maternity focus: postnatal classes and effective care', *British Journal of Healthcare Assistants*, 5(8): 399–400.

Kubler-Ross, E. (1969) *On Death and Dying*. New York: Collier.

Law, R. (2009) '"Bridging worlds": meeting the emotional needs of dying patients', *Journal of Advanced Nursing*, 65(12): 2630–41.

Lester, S. and Russell, W. (2010) 'Children's right to play: an examination of the importance of play in the lives of children worldwide'. Working Paper No. 57. The Hague, The Netherlands: Bernard van Leer Foundation. Available at: http://files.eric.ed.gov/fulltextED522537.pdf (last accessed 9 March 2015).

London Health Observatory (2010) *Jubilee Line of Health Inequality*. Available at: www.lho.org.uk/viewResource.aspx?id=15463 (last accessed 22 November 2014).

Marmot, M. (1996) 'The social pattern of health and disease'. In D. Blane, E. Brunner and R. Wilkinson (eds), *Health and Social Organisation: Towards a Health Policy for the Twenty-first Century*. London: Routledge.

Marmot, M. and Davey Smith, G. (1997) 'Socio-economic differentials in health: the contribution of the Whitehall Studies', *Journal of Health Psychology*, 2(3): 283–96.

Marmot Review (2010) *Fair Society, Healthy Lives*. The Marmot Review Executive Summary. Strategic Review of Health Inequalities in England post 2010. London: The Marmot Review. Available at: www.instituteofhealthequity.org/projects/fair-society-healthy-lives-the-marmot-review (last accessed 9 January 2015).

Mason, R. (2014) *Ministers Hope to Ban Smoking in Cars Carrying Children*. Available at: www.theguardian.com/society/2014/feb/11/ministers-hope-ban-smoking-cars-children-election (last accessed 28 November 2014).

MENCAP (2007) *Death by Indifference: Following up the Treat me Right! Report*. London: MENCAP. Available at: www.mencap.org.uk/sites/default/files/documents/2008-03/DBIreport.pdf (last accessed 18 November 2013).

MENCAP (2013) *All about Learning Disability*. Available at: www.mencap.org.uk (last accessed 27 November 2014).

McGrandles, A. and Duffy, T. (2012) 'Assessment and treatment of patients with anxiety', *Nursing Standard*, 26(35): 48–56.

NHS (2010) *Off to the Best Start. Important Information about Feeding your Baby*. Available at: www.gov.uk/government/publications/off-to-the-best-start-important-information-about-feeding-your-baby (accessed 18 January 2015).

NICE (2008) 'Improving the nutrition of pregnant and breastfeeding mothers and children in low-income households'. NICE public health guidance 11. Available at: www.nice.org.uk/guidance/PH011 (last accessed 18 January 2015).

NICE (2009) *When to Suspect Child Maltreatment*. NICE CG 89. Available at: www.nice.org.uk/Guidance/CG89 (last accessed 18 January 2015).

NICE (2010) *NICE Public Health Guidance: PH26 Quitting Smoking in Pregnancy and Following Childbirth*. Available at: www.nice.org.uk/Guidance/PH26 (last accessed 18 January 2015).

NICE (2013a) *Quality Standard 43. Smoking Cessation: Supporting People to Stop Smoking*. Available at: www.nice.org.uk/Guidance/QS43 (last accessed 18 January 2015).

NICE (2013b) *Quality Standard 37. Postnatal Care.* Available at: http://guidance.nice.org.uk/ QS37 (last accessed 22 November 2014).

NICE (2014) *Antenatal and Postnatal Mental Health: Clinical Management and Service Guidance (CG192).* Available at: www.nice.org.uk/guidance/cg192 (last accessed 5 March 2015).

Nursing and Midwifery Council (2010a) *Standards for Pre-registration Nursing Education.* Available at: http://standards.nmc-uk.org (accessed 19 November 2014).

Nursing and Midwifery Council (2010b) *Standards for Competence for Registered Nurses.* Available at: www.nmc-uk.org/Documents/Standards/Standards%20for%20competence.pdf (last accessed 19 November 2014).

Nursing and Midwifery Council (2015) *The Code: Professsional Standards of Practice and Behaviour for Nurses and Midwives.* London: NMC.

Parliamentary and Health Service Ombudsman (2009) *Six Lives: The Provision of Public Services to People with Learning Disabilities.* Available at: www.gov.uk/government/publications/report (last accessed 19 January).

Percival, J. (2013) 'Smoking cessation: reducing harm and improving the health of children', *Journal of Health Visiting,* 1(12): 689–95.

Phillips, L. (2012) 'Improving care for people with learning disabilities in hospital', *Nursing Standard,* 26(23): 42–58.

Powell, J. (2013) 'Use of the Common Assessment Framework in an acute setting', *Nursing Children and Young People,* 25(5): 24–8.

Pritchard, M.J. (2011) 'Using the Hospital Anxiety and Depression Scale in surgical patients', *Nursing Standard,* 25(34): 35–41.

Robertson, K. (2010) 'Understanding the needs of women with postnatal depression', *Nursing Standard,* 24(46): 47–55.

Rosenhan, D.L. (1973) 'On being sane in insane places', *Science,* 179(4070): 250–9.

Royal College of Nursing (2012) Going Upstream: Nursing's Contribution to Public Health. Prevent, Promote and Protect. RCN Guidance for Nurses. London: RCN. Available at: http://www.rcn.org.uk/__data/assets/pdf_file/0007/433699/004203.pdf (last accessed 18 January 2015).

Royal College of Nursing (2013a) *Meeting the Health Needs of People with Learning Disabilities: RCN Guidance for Nursing Staff.* London: RCN. Available at: www.rcn.org.uk/_data/assets/pdf_file/0004/78691/003024.pdf (last accessed 9 March 2015).

Royal College of Nursing (2013b) *Dignity in Healthcare for People with Learning Disabilities: Guidance for Nurses,* 2nd edition. London: RCN. Available at: www.rcn.org.uk/_data/assets/pdf_file/0010/296209/004439.pdf (last accessed 19 January 2015).

Royal College of Psychiatrists (2014) *Postpartum Psychosis: Severe Mental Illness after Childbirth.* Available at: www.rcpsych.ac.uk/healthadvice/problemsdisorders/postpartumpsychosis.aspx (last accessed 27 November 2014).

Sashidharan, S.P. and Commander, M.J. (1998) 'Mental health'. In S. Rawaf and V. Bahl (eds), *Assessing Health Needs of People from Minority Ethnic Groups.* London: Royal College of Physicians.

Scambler, G. (2009) 'Health-related stigma', *Sociology of Health and Illness,* 31(3): 441–55.

Shepherd, A.A. (2008) 'Nutrition through the life-span. Part 1: preconception, pregnancy and infancy', *British Journal of Nursing,* 17(20): 1261–7.

Smaje, C. (1995) *Health, 'Race' and Ethnicity: Making Sense of the Evidence.* London: King's Fund Institute.

Social Care Institute for Excellence (2012) *Personalisation: A Rough Guide.* London: SCIE.

Sylva, K., Melhuish, E., Sammons, P., Siraj-Blatchford, I. and Taggart, B. (2004) *Effective Provision of Pre-school Education (EPPE) Project.* Available at: www.ioe.ac.uk/RB_pre-school_to_end_of_KS1%281%29.pdf (last accessed 19 January 2015).

Syme, L.S. (1996) 'To prevent disease: the need for a new approach'. In D. Blane, E. Brunner and R. Wilkinson (eds), *Health and Social Organisation: Towards a Health Policy for the 21st Century.* London: Routledge.

Taylor, V. and Ashelsford, S. (2008) 'Understanding depression in palliative and end of life care', *Nursing Standard*, 23(12): 48–57.

Thomas, B. and Atkinson, D. (2011) 'Improving health outcomes for people with learning disabilities', *Nursing Standard*, 26(6): 33–6.

Thomas, C.S., Stone, K., Osborn, M. et al. (1993) 'Psychiatric morbidity and compulsory admission among UK-born Europeans, Afro-Caribbeans and Asians in Central Manchester', *British Journal of Psychiatry*, 163: 91–9.

Thomas, S. and Price, M. (2012) 'Respite care in seven families with children with complex care needs', *Nursing Children and Young People*, 24(8): 24–7.

United Nations (1989) *Convention on the Rights of the Child*. Available at: www.unicef.org/crc/ (last accessed 9 March 2015).

Wilkinson, R.G. (2005) *The Impact of Inequality: How to make Sick Societies Healthier*. London: Routledge.

Wilkinson, R. and Marmot, M. (2003) *The Solid Facts*, 2nd edition. Denmark: World Health Organization. Available at: www.euro.who.int/document/e81384.pdf (last accessed 9 March 2015).

Wisborg, K., Kesmodel, U., Henriksen, T.B., Olsen, S.F., and Secher, N.J. (2000) 'A prospective study of smoking during pregnancy and SIDS', *Arch Dis Child*, 83: 203–6.

World Health Organization (2003) *Investing in Mental Health*. Geneva: World Health Organization. Available at: www.who.int/mental_health/media/investing_mnh.pdf (accessed 19 January 2015).

Wrycroft, N. (ed.) (2009) *An Introduction to Mental Health Nursing*. Maidenhead: Open University Press.

7   Clinical Decision Making

MARY COOKE

This chapter will explore the underpinning theories related to clinical judgement and decision-making processes by nurses in healthcare settings. We will focus upon key issues for nurses in managing complexity and will critically review the key determinants that often have an impact on clinical decision-making processes. The chapter will include a critical consideration of higher order intellectual skills associated with clinical (diagnostic) reasoning, empirical (diagnostic) judgements and the outcome for discerning clinical decision making. The aim of this chapter is to help you nurture your ability to critically appraise knowledge (use information) to form a basis for the decisions you make. The chapter also intends to support the development of clinical judgement and decision-making skills for the effective delivery of nursing care.

After reading this chapter you should be able to:

- Determine how the decision-making process can be implemented with compassion, skill and safety, whilst promoting patient dignity, health and well-being.
- Critically review the components of specific theories and discuss the relevance of clinical decision-making theory to practice.
- Identify relevant sources of information and knowledge that can be used to inform the decision-making process.
- Recognise the importance of sharing the decision-making process with service users, carers, families and other professionals.
- Reflect upon and identify key areas for personal development to improve your own decision-making and problem-solving abilities in practice.

Related NMC Competencies

The overarching NMC requirement is that all nurses must:

> ... meet more complex and co-existing needs for people in any setting including hospital, community and at home. All practice should be informed by best available evidence and comply with local and national guidelines. Decision making must be shared with service users, carers and families, and informed by critical analysis of a range of possible interventions including the use of up-to-date technology. (NMC, 2010a, 2010b)

———————— **To achieve entry to the register as an adult** ————————
nurse you should be able to:

- Use up-to-date knowledge and evidence to plan, deliver, assess and evaluate care, communicate findings, influence change, and promote health and best practice.
- Carry out accurate assessments of people of all ages using appropriate diagnostic and decision-making tools.
- Make person-centred, evidence-based judgements and decisions in partnership with others involved in the care process to ensure high quality care.
- Recognise when the complexity of decisions requires specialist knowledge and expertise, and consult or refer accordingly.
- Recognise and address ethical challenges relating to people's choices and decision-making about their care, and act within the law to help them and their families and carers find acceptable solutions.
- Evaluate care to improve clinical decision making, quality and outcomes using a range of methods, amending the plan of care where necessary and communicating changes to others.
- Appreciate the value of evidence in practice, be able to understand and appraise research, apply relevant theory and research findings to their work, and identify areas for further investigation.

(Adapted from NMC Standards of Competence for Adult Nursing, 2010a, 2010b.)

Background

Daily, we face momentous decisions with important consequences: from the time we wake each day; during the process of getting to our clinical workplace, lecture, library or study rooms; to the time we decide that the day's activities are completed or key issues remain for us to face another time. These decisions include what to wear, eat, who to contact, and what is our priority for the achievement of the day – or to leave for our 'to do' list. Fortunately we have never had better access to information and expertise but this data deluge has become a double-edged sword. Which sources of information are credible? How can we separate the 'signal' from the 'noise'? Whose advice do we trust?

We face decisions with important consequences throughout our lives. We become aware of each difficult and challenging issue and problem and we are the person who has sole responsibility for solving them. Some individuals have even measured such things. For example, according to Douglas (2011) we have to make up to 10,000 trivial decisions every day and 227 are just about food (Wansink and Sobal, 2007). Wrong decisions about such issues as whether to have tea or coffee or what type of bread we prefer for the sandwich we eat at midday don't often matter too much – we can always decide to have something different the next time. However decisions about an assignment, our finances, our health options, are frequently faced and wrong choices here can affect our degree, make us poorer or may lose us our job. If those decisions relate to others (e.g. our family, parents, children, the organisation where we work, colleagues or indeed the patients we are assigned to care for) these can irreversibly affect the direction of their lives too, imminently, for days, months and years. So, what is an important personal decision you will be making in the near future?

Consider where you would like to work for your first and second jobs when you qualify.

- Why do you think you should consider two jobs this early in your career?

Decisions can affect us personally, impacting upon our way of life and also our patients, especially if the job we are appointed to is not what we anticipated. The process of decision making is often ignored, misunderstood, or unknown; if many people were asked to describe how they came to a conclusion or decision it may be difficult to untangle the strata of reasons and reasoning. Understanding how we 'see' or understand a problem can assist us to think through a process and gain a solution.

Hertz (2013) describes how our emotions, feelings, moods and memories affect our choices and how these contribute to the way in which we understand our environment – either at work or study – in making key choices at given times. She draws on personalised discussions to develop ways in which the current environment inhibits as well as informs our ability to think smartly and choose solutions wisely.

One of the first activities you may have completed in Chapter 1 was *Why did you become a nurse?* Ask yourself this again and reflect upon the decision you made. Think about what led you to make this decision.

- What factors did you consider?
- What were the alternatives?
- Were there any major factors that led to your final decision?

Write down your answers.

Making decisions often involves choosing an option from a range of alternatives. In this case your decision may have been influenced by:

- a conscious choice;
- rational thinking;
- a discussion with others in your family, or a partner who may be affected by this choice of career;
- your motivation by assuming you would be able to positively affect other people and their lives.

In one study, first-year students undertaking non-medical health professional programmes identified altruism and professional values as rewards which decreased over time (Miers et al., 2007). Alternatively, nurses who had graduated seven years previously stated that their main source of motivation and satisfaction was focused upon 'helping' and the 'people-centredness' aspects of nursing work (Robinson and Bennett, 2007). It seems that most nurses want to nurse because they inherently *care* about others. Perhaps then, the recent reports highlighted in previous chapters of poor workplace practices and disastrous outcomes for patients' health – often through mismanaged processes – offer a backdrop as to the key reasons why we should aim to improve our critical understanding of situations and the people in them.

Clinical decision making

Thompson and Dowding (2002: 1721) define the clinical decision-making process as 'choosing between alternatives'. Standing (2010: 8) goes a little further and suggests that:

> … clinical decision making is a complex process involving observation, information processing, critical thinking, evaluating evidence, applying relevant knowledge, problem-solving skills, reflection and clinical judgement to select the best course of action which optimizes a patient's health and minimizes the potential for harm.

Clearly then the clinical decision-making process is complex and will often involve the use of problem-solving skills. However these two are distinct concepts: problem solving involves working through the details of a problem in order to generate a solution though this usually involves making decisions too. Both clinical decision making and problem solving require the use of higher order cognitive skills such as *critical thinking* and *reasoning* and the ability to *analyse* and *synthesise* information. Therefore, the two concepts are often discussed together and both are integral to a nurse's role.

As nurses we are responsible and accountable for the professional decisions we make (NMC, 2015). The importance of providing good quality, evidence-based nursing care and the growing emphasis on public accountability mean that we have to be able to justify our nursing interventions and approaches, which in turn calls for a good level of understanding of both the supporting evidence and the decision-making processes which inform our actions. Working in partnership with patients, their families/carers and other healthcare professionals demands that we are transparent and are able to provide a good rationale to support the choice of patient-centred care we deliver. Thompson et al. (2013) also suggest that effective clinical decision making by nurses has the potential to assist in the efficient allocation of resources, promote health gains and benefits and prevent patient harm.

So how do nurses make clinical decisions?

One of the original critical nursing decision makers who pursued a notion of nursing care delivery that was not in keeping with the culture of the time was Florence Nightingale. In 1859 Nightingale realised that nurses needed to work with the universal 'Laws of Nature' which expressed 'uniform relations of simultaneity and succession, in which one mode of being is observed to exist to another' (Nightingale, 1970: 73). She recognised that illness caused similar patterns of physiological and sometimes psychological distress or discomfort in all people who had similar symptoms which formed a clinical diagnosis. She acknowledged that a condition or illness had a noticeable process from start to finish in which nurses could intervene or interrupt and potentially improve their patient's chances of survival or reduce their distress and pain.

Nightingale gathered the information related to the disease/condition process and collated it into a logical and structured framework as seen below:

- *Its beginning* – similarities in the presenting symptoms of a condition.
- *Its constitution or nature* – similarities in the condition or the effect of symptoms on the individual.
- *Its history* – adaptations of the individual in their reaction to the condition (e.g. infection or trauma) or the disease to circumstances of specific intervention and the patient's environment of care.

- *Its tendency or future* – the present is a definite preparation or prediction for a definite future. Nightingale indicated that because there were data on several incidences of the disease or condition there was information on the prediction for such outcomes from selected interventions for nursing care. She then considered that 'Nursing has to put the patient in the best condition for nature to act upon him' (Nightingale, 1970: 75).

This early version of nursing practice has developed our understanding of how information about patients (the regular observations and reporting of changes resulting from nursing and medical interventions in a patient's ongoing condition) contributes to the decisions that are discussed with the patient or carer and health team. Henderson (1966: 15) based her thinking about nursing care and decision making on Nightingale's concept of nursing practice to state that:

> ... the unique function of the nurse is to assist the individual, sick or well, in the performance of those activities contributing to health or its recovery ... that he would perform unaided if he had the necessary strength, will or knowledge ...

To summarise, it seems that Nightingale is suggesting that the role of the nurse is to care for patients until they can care for themselves. In order to do this effectively, however, we need to be able to elicit the nursing needs of patients and plan care strategies that aim to support them in achieving their goals. This will require decisions to be made about the plan of care and negotiated agreements that will enable us to carry out such plans. Ideas about how clinical decisions should be made have emerged and changed over time.

Contemporary decision-making theories, models and frameworks

In more recent times, Standing (2010: 8) suggests that there are three main theories used to underpin the decision-making process in nursing:

- *Normative* (systematic-positivistic): rational, logical scientific, evidence-based decisions (risk assessments, etc.), information processing.
- *Descriptive* (intuitive-humanistic): as proposed by Dreyfus and Dreyfus, Benner, Carper, etc.
- *Prescriptive*: the use of frameworks or guidelines which have been designed to assist in the application of principles which lead to enhanced decision tasks (e.g. nursing process, NICE guidelines, etc.). These can be linked to Nightingale's and Henderson's concepts of nursing above.

These theories, models and frameworks help us to think about how we can critically identify and collect appropriate data, consider priorities from key information and predict outcomes from the use of selected material to form a decision. Many of these date back to the 1970s when research into management in health and social sciences was beginning to become important in the USA due to the rise in administration and the costs of their diverse private health systems. Early theorists include Dreyfus (1979), Elstein et al. (1978), Benner (1982), Carnevali et al. (1984) and Phaneuf (2008). Theories based in UK systems also occur in earlier publications from the 1950s, such as Lewin (1951), which have also been adapted for use in healthcare decision making. This chapter will focus upon a number of theories, models and frameworks which have been used by nurses and can therefore be applied to a clinical nursing setting.

Normative theories

Traditionally rationalists take the view that *reason* is the primary path to knowledge and understanding, using deductive or inductive logic. These principles are based upon the following premises:

Deductive logic is a means of reasoning from a set of premises (assumptions) to a conclusion that can be logically inferred from these. An example here is if you see a person has had a surgical operation then they may have a wound of some type and this must be treated aseptically to prevent infection. You may assume that all patients who have been to the operative theatre will have a wound that needs aseptic dressings. With deduction you can provide absolute proof of your conclusions, given that your premises are correct. The premises themselves, however, remain unproven and unprovable: they must be accepted on face value, by faith, or for the purpose of exploration. An example of an idea you could explore related to this concept of assuming facts is 'Do all operations in an operative theatre occur under aseptic conditions?'

Inductive logic is the result of reasoning from specific instances to a general conclusion that is broader than what can logically be inferred from those instances. In the process of induction you begin with some data and then determine what general conclusion(s) can logically be derived from those data. In other words, you determine what theory or theories could explain the data. For example, you may note that the probability of becoming obese is greatly increased if at least one parent is obese and from that you conclude that obesity may be inherited. That is certainly a reasonable hypothesis given the data. However, you might also consider that induction does not prove that the theory is correct. There are often alternative theories that are also supported by the data. For example, the behaviour of the obese parent may cause the child to be obese and not the genes. What is important in induction is that the theory does offer a logical explanation of the data. To conclude that the parents have no effect on the obesity or size or lifestyle of their children is not supportable given the data and would not be a logical conclusion.

STOP AND THINK

Think about your experiences in specialised surgical wards or units:

- Do all patients who attend theatre for an operation have equipment for a venous access in situ when they return?
- Do all operations occur under aseptic conditions?
- Do all patients who have been to theatre for an operation have open wounds?

(Probably your answers to these questions will start with 'Well on some occasions they do' and you can list these, and 'On other occasions they don't' and you can list those also.)

- What does this mean for your deductive skills and therefore your decision making about such patient groups?

(Note: Consider whether your analysis of these patient outcomes – based on your assumptions of the interventions the patient has undergone – are inductive or deductive.)

A second more contemporary theory we will consider here is based historically on work by Elstein et al. (1978) and can be described as an *'information-processing model'* which incorporates an understanding of how doctors undergo their rational decision making based on information processing and clinical reasoning. A nurse called Doris Carnevali, together with Mary Thomas, adapted this way of critical reasoning to form decisions related to nursing interventions (Carnevali and Thomas, 1993). Their theory follows a clear administrative process so that accurate data (information) are used to make a decision and the decision-reasoning process is then recorded for future use. Specific headings are used which develop an audit trail of processes. The diagnostic reasoning process integrates observation and critical thinking to assign meaning in a nursing assessment. Carnevali applied her theory to clinical practice as nurses took on more administrative roles and needed to understand how the process of decision making occurred. Her model or framework attempts to explain the thinking or intellectual processes that underpin effective clinical judgements and clinical decision making. She describes several stages in the decision-making process:

1. The *collection of pre-encounter data about the client/family* would include information gathered by word of mouth, such as the nurse-to-nurse handover either at the bedside or by telephone prior to the patient's admission; the person's health records or notes would also form part of the assessment; and from there assumptions, generalisations and considerations become important in the value judgement about certain clients.

2. Assuming the patient is then introduced to the nurse, in a clinical setting, the next level of decision making is considered: *entry to the assessment situation.* The nurse takes an initial overview and determines the level of priority setting among other patients/clients and the current demand on resources. The nurse considers strategies for further data collection if necessary and the patient's own role in their assessment. This means that the nurse will judge whether and if the patient is mentally or physically fit to participate in the necessary discussion required for such an admission into the system.

3. Following the initial encounter with the patient, a *further collection of data* then takes place. This may entail screening (a pre-determined structure, for example the past medical history is not notified in the medical notes but is important to nurses, such as whether social services and other tertiary services are involved in community support structures for this person) or be problem-oriented (determined by a client's presenting situation, and their immediate and secondary presenting needs, for example whether the patient has family present, whether they require encouragement to mobilise, take note of diet and require dressings or specific treatments). The level of need (to ascertain the resource requirements of the ward or unit because of the admission of this person) becomes nursing's critical judgement. Prioritising is never an exact science. However when making such decisions a nurse should rely on evidence taken from previous similar clinical situations and personal insights – what many nurses would consider to be 'instinct'.

4. *Pivotal cue clusters* are selected according to what is considered to be the greatest urgency or importance (priority) and the subsequent assessment of other cue clusters.

5. *The retrieval of possible diagnostic explanations* allow a nurse to consider moving from general to specific information that underpins their decision. In addition the considerations of competing or alternative diagnostic explanations are included and a secondary assessment, diagnosis from further test results or observations for example will indicate the *diagnostic choices*.

Carnevali defined this model of decision making as a means of understanding the stages in decisions based on clinical systems and in doing so identified the need for sound evidence-based information on which to make a decision.

STOP AND THINK

Return to the example of the assumptions made about what patients will need as they return from an operation:

- How will you know which equipment will be coming back with the patient when they return from an operative procedure?
- How will you decide which equipment to place by the bed area in preparation for the patient returning from their operative procedure?

Four decades ago Elstein analysed how doctors decide the ways in which decisions are made about the interventions patients will have, diagnosis of conditions and plans for care. He based his findings on research with expert physicians who considered their decision making to be based on intuition and derived from years of accumulated knowledge and experience. Other researchers have reviewed and used the model since (for example Tanner et al. (1987)) who found they used a five-stage cognitive strategy – hypothetico-deduction:

1. Cue recognition:

- acts as an alert to the nurse, often in partnership with the patient.

2. Cue acquisition:

- searching for information (initial assessment) – considering sources of information and 'the patient encounter'

3. Hypothesis generation:

- identifying possible problems (initial diagnoses) – from cues identified in first stage
- can be affected by knowledge and experience

4. Cue interpretation:

- gathering more data to accept or reject identified problems (diagnostic reasoning) – allows initial hypotheses to be revisited – assessment as ongoing process

5. Hypothesis evaluation:

- choosing among alternatives (diagnostic reasoning, nursing diagnosis, treatment decisions). How well does data fit with decision alternatives? In partnership with patient? (Nowadays we would expect this to be in collaboration with the patient)

This model can be explained in Figure 7.1 overleaf:

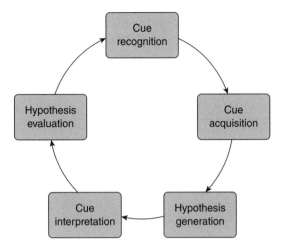

Figure 7.1   A hypothetico-deductive approach to clinical decision making (Tanner et al., 1987)

 NAZIRA

Nazira is a staff nurse in the Accident and Emergency department. She uses a 'triage' system for collating information about patients and is able to make a decision about the priority of individual needs for specific interventions and care or treatment.

By utilising a simplistic triage decision tree based upon a patient's initial observations (an ABDCE approach: **A** – airway, **B** – Breathing, **C** – Circulation and haemorrhage control, **D** – disability and neurological assessment, and **E** – Exposure and environment), she is able to prioritise patients in need of immediate intervention. When the receiving nurse (or triage nurse) continues with the assessment, he/she is able to ascertain the patient's heart rate, blood pressure, temperature, circulating oxygen levels and respiration rate, in addition to the stated reason for the person's visit to the department (e.g. their 'mechanism of injury'). Algorithms (or decision trees) then arise from each decision pathway that is designed to provide standardised interventions adaptable for each individual need. Treatment options and decisions can then be made according to the physiological or psychological state of the patient.

Case Scenario

Early Warning Scores (EWS) (see Chapter 11, pp.322–325) can be used to assist in the detection of deterioration in a patient's physical condition (McGauhey et al., 2007). Vital signs directly demonstrate a patient's current physiological state. The defining characteristics of the patient presentation data are sought in order to compare the current information against previous assessments of the same health problem using the same scoring system in patients with similar symptom patterns. Subtle signs of deterioration can be seen in regular and timely recordings. The appropriate care can then be determined so that morbidity is reduced or death is avoided.

Clinical Decision Making Support Systems (computer software designed to assist in decision-making processes) are based upon this theory and have been used in many clinical areas (e.g. to aid diagnosis, and improve patient outcomes in disease management, prescribing and calculating risk). Information obtained from individual patients is matched to a computerised knowledge base which allows pre-designed software algorithims to generate recommendations based upon specific patient data (Amit et al., 2005). However, frameworks such as these assume that each decision maker's thought processes are systematic and rational and logical (or normative) and that they will measure the same data in the same way. Yet research has clearly demonstrated the inability of healthcare professionals to correctly interpret or act on recorded data – most commonly underestimating the seriousness of the clinical data they have recorded (Thompson et al., 2004, 2005). If data are collected but not interpreted correctly the decisions that are taken are not rational or logical due to the lack of reasoning. Current tragic examples of this misinterpretation of cues and data collected by health professionals are reported in the Francis Report (DH 2013). Here we find the limitations of the inductive theory in practice.

Descriptive theories

The empirical or (sensory) experiential approach takes the view that experience is the primary path to knowledge and seeks to describe the processes used by nurses when making clinical decisions. The *intuitive-humanistic model* outlined by Benner (1982) is based upon the work of Dreyfus and Dreyfus (1986) and raises awareness of differences in the way decisions are made by nurses who have comparable years of experience in clinical practice and decision making. Benner (1982) identifies that nurses use their experiential learning to gain insight into clinical judgement and as

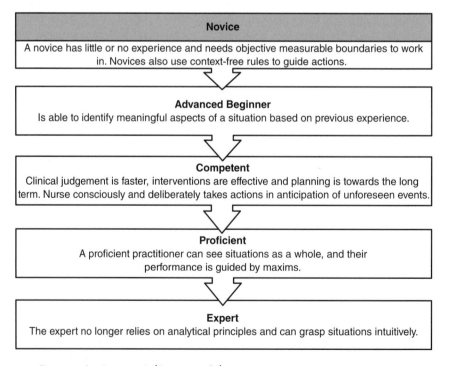

Figure 7.2   From novice to expert. (Benner, 1982)

a result can improve patient outcomes. Phenomenology as a method of defining 'knowing what and knowing how' helps to describe these processes of decision making based on clinical learning through understanding. The various stages of the evolution from novice to expert decision makers (defined by their use of knowledge) are described by Benner in Figure 7.2.

Intuition identified in the realm of expert nursing is often described as a 'gut feeling', 'insight' or 'instinct' (Benner, 1982). However, critics of Benner's thinking and research would suggest that this is merely 'custom and practice', arguing that clinical behaviour that takes place without assessing the differences between patient needs, or current research evidence, or analysing the depth of a complex patient condition, equates to a nurse who is not engaged with their role or the patient's needs.

Think back to a recent shift you completed in the clinical setting.

Consider your interaction/s with a specific patient or their carer/relative where you know you made a difference (e.g. there was a positive change in the patient's response and their condition improved).

Write down the events and describe in detail your responses during that interaction. Now have a short break before you read your description again ...

- What was it that happened?
- How did you make the decisions that caused the difference in the patient or their care/family member?
- Are the thought processes/decision processes you used illustrated by any of the elements identified in Benner's novice to expert continuum (see Figure 7.2)?

STOP AND THINK

Other theorists have considered the ways in which nursing is accomplished and how decision making aids the care process. Phaneuf (2008) describes the decision making process using key factors that form the basis for understanding what is needed to make a decision. Phaneuf considers that *essential knowledge in nursing* and an *ability to apply critical thinking skills* are needed to make judgements. These judgements are made by using a critical assessment of situations, people, systems and rules. This information is gained throughout the years of educational development and training as a student and confirmed by qualification. Clinical experience is then valued externally by judgements made about cause and effect, the impact of nursing interventions and the outcomes of decisions made about care. This means that public acknowledgement of nursing ability is considered and reflected in nursing roles as designated by governments. Policy clearly has an impact on the way nurses are perceived as change makers in healthcare.

Phaneuf goes further in her demonstration of nurse decision making. She suggests that empirical information is used to make decisions (evidence-based nursing care) and that this stems from data perceived by the senses and not necessarily from the literature, publications or theoretical understanding. Experienced nurses are able to pick up non-verbal data and information sub-consciously and use this to assist in making insightful decisions. However, Phaneuf does not consider the length of time a nurse has been in clinical practice and whether this defines their level of ability. She determines a nurse's

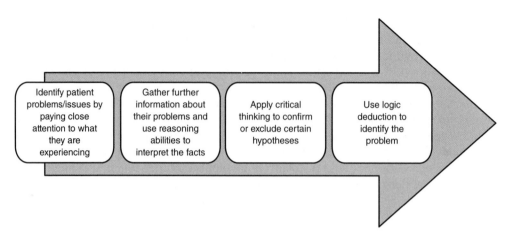

Figure 7.3   Clinical judgement – an essential tool in the nursing profession
Source: Phaneuf (2008)

capacity for intellectual thought as the guiding feature of clinical decision making. Further levels of clinical decision making are dependent upon the nurse's conceptualisation of the problem or solution. The ability to make a decision arises by associating the available empirical data and synthesising the information. Nurses rationally consider the data, the framework of care, the value of the outcome of the range of decisions to be selected and then make a decision arising from critically assembling such information and by responsibly applying the various long- and short-term impact of each part of the decision, analysed in terms of the individual, the unit of care delivery and the organisation.

Returning again to the example above where you 'made a difference' to the care of your patient which resulted in a positive change or improvement, you will have no doubt recognised that in a clinical setting there is often a huge amount of information to process in a short amount of time.

Cioffi (1997) suggests that nurses who are more experienced can prioritise such complex sets of information, re-analyse them and then consider the synthesis of the decision. The use of certain identified and specific cues to ascertain a decision around all the bio-psycho-physiological perspectives of the patient's case has been described as *heuristics* in an attempt to explain intuition. Often referred to as 'rules of thumb', these are used to describe the actions of experienced people who solve complex problems by undercutting or taking 'short cuts' to define the complexity of a situation, analysing the key facts and then determining the preferred outcomes. The nurse requires some years of consistent experience to be able to recall the usual presentation of patterns with particular conditions and compare the presenting patient's condition against any differences between them and other known cases – including the expected and actual progression points of the patient. However, one limitation of this theory is that it assumes that even though the nurse encounters different people, they will all have similar sets of problems which require a simplistic set of solutions. It could also be argued that this is not strictly decision making as decisions require an analysis of the facts which may differ with each encounter. Instead, it reduces individualised decisions towards the nurse's past experience and makes assumptions that patient differences can be factored into 'silos' of solutions. Similarities can be synthesised between this factor-based model and Benner's intuitive model. Therefore by that very fact you may consider that nurses who have many years' experience could either be considered as safe, or perhaps unsafe in their decision making if we were to employ these theoretical analyses. Recent research indicates that patient expectations and priorities are not always the same as those identified by nurses or other professionals. So decisions and their outcomes should be negotiated between all the people involved (Cooke and Thackray 2012).

Alternatively, Carper's (1978) model (see Figure 7.4) illustrates the interconnections between the creative processes and the social/political processes for determining the credibility for each pattern of thinking or decision making about care to be given in clinical practice.

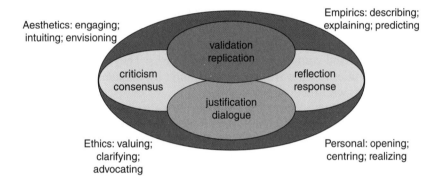

Figure 7.4   Carper's interconnected 'patterns of knowing'

Source: Carper (1978) 'Fundamental patterns of knowing in nursing', *Advanced Nursing Science*, 1 (1): 1113-23.

As processes for forming understanding are engaged, knowledge (as the basis for an assessment of a patient and their care) takes the form of an integrated whole. Each set of processes is distinct for individual nurses' and patients' patterns of knowing, but these draw on and contribute to the processes within the whole patterns of knowing. This framework forms one of the first links between the nurse and patient relationship for assessing and planning care progressions. As each nurse brings their past experiences to each patient encounter, the processes described in this theory/model/phenomenon are always likely to differ a little or a lot. For example, consider one of your earlier exercises where you were asked to think about patients who had been to the operative theatre. One nurse may consider *ethics* (using their moral compass to decide which outcome is preferable) as more important in a specific case or patient care outcome; another may consider *empirics* as more important (the evidence for deciding how to deliver care or the known predictive outcomes of care based on past research). Ask yourself which element or pattern of knowing is more important when deciding how to assist a patient recovering from an operation such as a clinical termination of a pregnancy?

Returning to the earlier discussion about philosophical decisions and the processes and assumptions to be made about patient's needs and what the nurse decides to do:

- Consider a recent time you were in practice and looking after a specific patient. Think about what the patient wanted and how they communicated their desires and needs to you.
- Now consider what your thoughts were about what the patient wanted or needed to happen.

You no doubt considered whether you had been asked to arrange for these needs previously, when you learned how to interpret the patient's needs and understand how best to follow them, and if you had then it would be easier to repeat the process. However, if this was a new experience for you then assumptions or experiential deductions would have to be made. You would be comparing your known experiences with the unknown experiences, reasoning that some things you know about and others are new to you. The patient and their family rely on your duty and commitment to care as well as your compassion, competence and courage to undertake the tasks. They assume that inductively you make opportunities to learn from every encounter by engaging in the ways in which nurses communicate with their responsibilities.

Carper's theory on nurses' 'ways of knowing' helps to unpick these processes and offers the understanding that decisions are complex and often made in complex situations. Carper sets out the sections of knowing, suggesting that decisions and actions depend upon nurses' reflection and responses to common actions in order to respond to patient needs; validity is sought from evidence and the repetition of actions that then form agreed and expected 'professional' decisions that arise from commonly expressed needs. There may have been critical review of the decisions and actions expressed via dialogue and thus justified by agreement; but now there is a consensus of opinion on the action to be taken.

In summary, Benner considers that decisions are made intuitively: the understanding and interpretation of patient needs are honed from experience and knowledge is developed by nurses who are active learners in practice. This aspect of developing decision making over time is not necessarily considered by Carper. However, Carnivali defends the need to record the process of decisions so that each stage is accurately determined by the repetitive collection of data. All of these theories can be seen to have a conceptual contribution to a discussion about decision making.

Over time, professional nurses develop their own intuitive theory about care and/or the responses they can safely make to specific patient needs as they work consistently in a specialism. Often nurses will avoid cases they have had little experience of, knowing it will take time to develop such knowledge. Such selection inevitably reduces the quality of nursing care delivered and limits a nurse in their understanding of the breadth of care required in a diverse population. There is, as a result, little control over professional judgement unless the audit and re-audit of clinical practices and outcomes can determine measures of patient-related outcomes, clinical guidance protocols and local policies that control the clinical setting. Indeed, there is little research or evidence to underpin these 'ways of knowing' other than an implicit understanding of practice. There is also an assumption that all individuals can develop a reflective ability and are then able to clearly articulate their intuitive judgements.

Table 7.1 Theories of decision making in nursing science

Nightingale: Laws of nature: the process of an illness and how nurse interventions are decided	Carnivali: The administration of decisions and recording of the process	Benner: The stages of becoming competent to be a nurse	Phaneuf: The nurse's capacity for intellectual thought as a guiding feature of clinical decision making	Carper: Ways of knowing. Facts underpinning decisions are focused and arise from the nurse's personal moral compass and understanding of her/his professional responsibilities	Cioffi: Heuristics are interpreted as 'rules of thumb' and incorporated into decision making (problem solving) as shortcuts
Its beginning (similarities in symptomology of a condition)	1. The collection of pre-encounter data about client/family	• NOVICE	Empirical information is used to make decisions	Empirics: describing, explaining, predicting	Used in defining processes of problem solving, not decision making; but could be applied in specific understanding or interpretation of facts and needs in a process of moving issues forward (patient, organisation, profession). Assumes few changes or diverse individualistic issues exist when defining problems or solutions
Its constitution or nature (similarities in the condition or symptoms' effect on the individual)	2. Entry to the assessment situation	• ADVANCED BEGINNER	Stems from data perceived by the senses, and not necessarily from literature, publications or theoretical understanding	Personal: opening, centring, realising	
Its history (adaptations of the individual in their reaction to the condition (infection or trauma) or the disease to circumstances of specific intervention and the patient's environment of care)	3. Collection of data	• COMPETENT practitioner	Experienced nurses are able to pick up non-verbal data and information subconsciously and use this to assist in making insightful decisions	Ethics: valuing, clarifying, advocating	
Its tendency or future (the present is a definite preparation or prediction for a definite future)	4. Pivotal cue clusters are selected	• PROFICIENT practitioner		Aesthetics: engaging, envisioning, intuiting	
	5. Retrieval of possible diagnostic explanations	• EXPERT practitioner			
	6. Making diagnostic choices				

Later in the chapter we will consider the above theories in relation to the notion of evidence-based practice. Table 7.1 provides a useful overview of different theories relating to how nurses understand or know what decision to make.

However, it appears that nurses tend not to apply any of these theories or models exclusively. Instead, Hamm (1988) suggests clinicians will often use a combination of approaches. Using the cognitive continuum framework outlined in Figure 7.5 he suggests that the mode of cognition used by a nurse is determined by the task in hand along with the information and time available. Cognition is viewed along a continuum ranging from analytical thinking at one end of the spectrum to intuition at the other end. The framework is further divided into six modes of cognitive practice. Hamm (1988) suggests that most clinicians (including nurses) make decisions around the cognitive modes 5 and 6 (peer-aided or system-aided judgement).

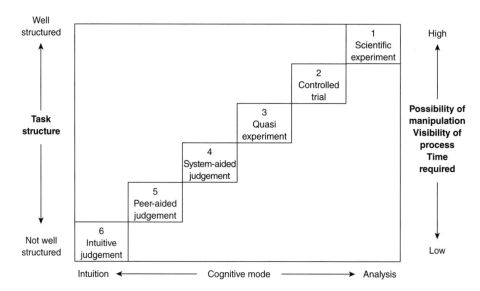

Figure 7.5   The cognitive continuum

Source: Hamm (1988) 'Clinical intuition and clinical analysis: expertise and the cognitive continuum'. In Dowie and Elstein.

Evidence-based nursing and clinical judgement

Evidence-based decision making is a *prescriptive approach* used by nurses to inform clinical decisions and choices. It involves *actively* combining knowledge gained from a variety of sources (e.g. own clinical expertise, patient preference, research evidence, etc.), which is then applied in order to deliver evidence-based care within the context of available resources (Thompson et al., 2004). The ability to carry out this process successfully demands a capacity to locate, retrieve and critically appraise appropriate evidence, then plan care and adapt accordingly to ensure care is individualised and patient-centred (i.e. the clinical judgement process).

Drawing on data from two large UK studies, Thompson et al. (2004) outline the types of clinical decisions made by nurses in acute and primary care settings, highlighting the variety and complexity of decisions required by nurses (see Table 7.2).

Table 7.2   Types of clinical decisions made by nurses in acute and primary care settings

Decision type	Example of clinical choices/decisions
Intervention/effectiveness Decisions that involve choosing between interventions	*Choosing* a mattress for a frail elderly patient
Targeting This is a subcategory of intervention/ effectiveness decisions outlined above. It involves choosing patients who will benefit most from this type of intervention	*Deciding* which patient should get antiembolism stockings
Timing Involves choosing the best time to deploy the intervention	*Choosing* a time to commence asthma education for newly diagnosed patients
Referral Involves choosing a service to which the patient may be referred for ongoing or specialist treatment	*Choosing* to refer a patient with a leg ulcer for medical intervention rather than nursing management
Communication Focuses on choosing ways of delivering information to and from patients, families and other healthcare professionals	*Choosing* how to approach cardiac rehabilitation following acute myocardial infarction for an elderly patient who lives alone with her family nearby
Service organisation, delivery and management Decisions which are related to service configuration or processes of service delivery	*Choosing* how to organise handover so that communication is most effective
Assessment Deciding that an assessment is required and/or choosing what mode of assessment to use	*Deciding* to use the Edinburgh Postnatal Depression screening tool rather than a 'Patient Health Questionnaire-9' (PHQ-9)
Diagnosis Classifying signs and symptoms as a basis for a management or treatment strategy	*Deciding* whether thrush or another cause is the reason for a woman's sore and cracked nipples
Information seeking Choosing to seek (or not to seek) further information before making a further clinical decision	*Deciding* that a guideline for monitoring patients who have had their ACE inhibitor dosage adjusted may be of use, but *choosing* not to use it before asking the advice of a more senior or experienced colleague
Experiential, understanding or hermeneutic This relates to the interpretation of cues in the process of care	Choosing how to reassure a patient who is worrying about a cardiac arrest after having witnessed another patient arresting

(Adapted from Thompson et al., 2004). Available at: www.evidencebasednursing.com

Reflect upon all of the clinical decisions nurses have been involved in on one of your recent shifts (decisions either you or your mentor have made):

- Do they fall into each of the categories outlined above?
- Are there any which do not fall into the above categories? If so, why not?
- Try to identify the cognitive processes involved in each of the decisions that you identified above (you may wish to discuss this with your mentor too).
- What information, knowledge and skills were needed in order to be able to make a decision effectively?
- Were decision processes influenced by patients and/or their family members or other healthcare professionals? If so, how?

Clinical decisions should be based on accurate judgements which are determined after consideration of all of the information cues available. Here we can incorporate the oft-quoted thoughts of Theodore Roosevelt, '... in any moment of decision the best thing you can do is the right thing, the next best thing is the wrong thing, and the worst thing you can do is nothing'.*

From these two considerations we can begin to understand that one of the key qualities of decision making, leadership or management is personal awareness. As student nurses you are expected to participate in structured critical reflection during the three years' education towards qualifying.

Reflective exercises (such as the ones included throughout this book) aim to guide you in identifying and challenging your own assumptions, values and beliefs. This may lead you to alter your rationale or means of making decisions based on your previous assumptions of others, your own strengths and personal development. As you become more successful in analysing your reflections both 'on-practice' and 'in-practice' (Schon, 1991), your reflections and interpretations of learning throughout life become more apparent and your beliefs in self and others are deepened.

In further applying the essence of the key theories or models of decision making we move towards the processes of collection, analysis and organisation of information methodologically in order that it can be tested, compared, assimilated and used in structured planning for decisions. The systematic (either sequential, historical or hierarchical) collection of data or information is important. But so is the knowledge that the information is of a good quality, based on fact, and incorporating all who are involved in making the decision – the 'stakeholders'. Therefore the methodology of facts or data collection is important and defines the quality of the decision eventually made.

Cognitive and practical expertise is the professional understanding that knowledge is generated by an ability to *critically appraise* good quality research and *evaluate* the strength of all the evidence available. You may have come across the Critical Appraisal

*(Above quotes taken from What is decision making? Beginner's Guide, 21st September 2005, para 2: http://beginnersguide.com/executive-coaching/decision-making/what-is-decision-making.php retrieved 20/9/2014).

using Systematic Processes (CASP) when considering literature and its analysis. Indeed, a prime objective of the Department of Health is that research and development becomes integral to healthcare so that clinicians, managers and other staff find it a natural process to rely on research in their day-to-day decision making and in ensuring that the implementation of longer-term strategies of planning service delivery are based upon sound evidence. The rationale behind this policy and its strategic implementation was the critique that strongly held views based on belief rather than sound information have exerted too much influence in healthcare in the past (Department of Health, 1991).

The Centre for Reviews and Dissemination (CRD) and The Cochrane Collaboration are organisations that fund reviews and meta analyses of published research to determine the overview of several results and qualify (as well as quantify) the validity and reliability of the individual results. The view or consensus is that the Randomised Controlled Trial (RCT) is the 'Gold Standard' of research evidence. A well-conducted experiment is considered theoretically the best way of determining the effectiveness of particular interventions for specific conditions. The Centre for Reviews and Dissemination (CRD) also reviews *qualitative* research and funds overviews of published research papers that answer similar questions (systematic reviews).

Many organisations, including professional bodies and agencies such as NICE (the National Institute for Health and Clinical Excellence), SIGN (the Scottish Intercollegiate Guidelines Network) and GAIN (the Guidelines and Audit Implementation Network), issue evidence-based guidelines for practitioners which are usually distillations of research findings focusing on specific treatments and compilations of current best practice as offered by the clinical authors. This 'evidence' of research-based practice is audited in clinical practice to define 'best' or most effective practice by all health professionals.

Outcomes of various national and local audits can be found in the National Audit Office website (www.nao.org.uk). Frameworks for developing research questions to establish evidence for best practice include the PICO technique: **P**atient (or population or problem), **I**ntervention, **C**omparison, **O**utcome (Huang et al., 2006). Additionally, an increasingly important method of interpreting the outcomes of clinical interventions that include nursing interventions reported in research papers is Patient Reported Outcomes Measures (PROM), whereby the results of trials use quality measures designed by patients on whom the trial intervention is tested to understand how useful the outcomes are.

ACTIVITY 7.1

Find out more about the national organisations responsible for publishing evidence-based clinical guidelines by accessing the following websites below:

- NICE (England and Wales): www.nice.org.uk/guidance
- SIGN (Scotland): www.sign.ac.uk/
- GAIN (Northern Ireland): www.gain-ni.org/
- PROM (NHS England): www.england.nhs.uk/statistics/statistical-work-areas/proms

The promotion of evidence-based practice (EBP) in nursing has emerged from 'research-mindedness' in the profession where authors Walsh and Ford (1989) discussed the 'myths, traditions and rituals' of nursing practice. Tensions remain where the Randomised Controlled Trial (RCT) is considered to be the objective and scientific result of outcomes of treatment for a few selected individuals. The critique is that the transfer of this information to the general population, as well as individuals in all their unique complexity, may not identify the diversity of the population and the lack of validity of the original experiment. Conversely, in many cases published currently, holistic treatments applied by nurses are tailored to individual patients, which again loses the impact of approaches drawn from aggregated or meta-data collated in Cochrane or the CRD (Cullum et al., 2008). (Note: At this stage we would advise you to access additional material listed as further suggested reading and supporting websites at the end of the chapter to focus in more detail on research methods and critique.)

As an adult nurse you need to be able to 'understand and appraise research, apply relevant theory and research findings to your work and identify areas for further investigation' (NMC, 2010a: 14, 2010b: 6). Developing a good understanding of the current evidence will also enable you to participate in clinical debates as an equal with other healthcare professionals, knowledgeable patients and carers. The ability to make logical evidence-based arguments and also defend them if challenged will not only help you to justify your clinical decisions, it should also help you to improve your own knowledge and understanding of the evidence base which supports practice, addressing gaps in your personal knowledge and also those of others. Understanding your own beliefs and values through the use of reflection supports the notion that we as professionals will work in partnership with others (including patients) and will carefully, with courage, challenge illogical or unethical beliefs or practices. Indeed, the facilitation of others in developing their own knowledge and skills is another of the NMC competencies for entry to the register (NMC, 2010).

With reference to the illuminating theory of Carper, nurses are also required to become creative in their practice (i.e. 'thinking beyond the box'). This enables us to respond to everyday challenges in the clinical environment, enabling and empowering colleagues as well as individual patients as required. The process of discussion and debate about care often raises issues of complexity in decision making. However, astute nurses who develop an understanding of 'the world view', 'whole picture' or consideration of an issue or series of issues objectively inevitably develop decision-making skills that will enable them to make sound clinical decisions using the resources available. Consideration of these factors will help you to identify and promote new ways of working to address the diverse needs of your patient population.

One of the main foci of nursing judgement is an assessment of the unique situation of the patient/client/service user. This involves the perception of qualitative distinctions in a patient, picking up on differences that are reported by the patients themself. Focusing on the patient has important implications for how decisions regarding treatment are made (Thompson and Dowding, 2002). In fact, nurses who make decisions or organise care packages and pathways without considering the service user and their family or support systems are ignoring 30% of the resources available in the decision-making process. The service user/patient/carer/family/public form one of the major groups associated with patient care and delivery of services, with the other two groups being the managers (policy makers) and the healthcare professionals. The 6Cs (first outlined in Chapter 1 and referred to throughout this book) provide us with a framework which we can use to negotiate positive outcomes with our patients.

Relating the 6Cs to the decision-making process and considering examples from your practice experiences, reflect upon the ways in which you were able to make decisions that made a positive change to a patient and/or their family.

Using short reflective 'bullet points' as outlined below, indicate the process of change that occurred:

- How the person (or you) recognised the problem.
- How the problem had occurred.
- What you or the patient wanted as an outcome.
- How you planned to change or use a nursing intervention to alter the situation.

Consider the resources you used or included to help you make your decision.

- Now identify which of the 6Cs you brought into your decision-making process when deciding what you were going to do and how you did it. Make links to these on the bullet points you produced for the above activity.
- What difference did your decisions make to the overall outcome?

In carrying out this activity you may have considered that *care* can be experienced as a carer or as the person (or other) being cared for. This phenomenon could be considered philosophically and may be used tangibly as a function, a means of management, attentiveness or doing good. Decisions made about care should be based on *compassion* and the *competence* of the carer. Compassion is a personal consideration, often based on leniency or pity for the 'other', and determined by the question 'How would I feel if that was me?', whereas competence is a measurable ability to complete a task or participate in a role. Delegation is included in this, as we should understand the competency of the person we delegate to in order that the standard of care is the same as if we would perform the role ourselves (we will revisit this aspect of care provision again in more detail in Chapter 8, pp. 215–216).

Compassion should drive the considerations of how nurses manage decisions around patient care with and for patients and their carers. Future research and evaluation will indicate the success of nursing compassion and assist in developing new cultural norms of care. *Courage* is not always assumed in a nurse. Most nurses would not consider themselves as courageous or brave – perhaps they may see themselves as performing care under duress, or in favour of the patient against the rules of the organisation – but they would assume they could *communicate* and are committed. 'Whistleblowing' as a decisive action that takes courage comes to mind as in a patient or colleague advocate role. However, many student nurses' reflective analyses are taken from examples of a lack of communication, or misinterpretations, arising from poor understanding of a situation or thought or action. A *commitment* to expressing courage is therefore understood in the context of nursing and caring, to be associated with perseverance, or a personal promise to perform a duty.

It is clear that solving problems using critical analysis of the evidence, as well as ensuring that we involve patients (and other healthcare professions as necessary) in the clinical aking process, calls upon the development of various sophisticated higher order kills needed by nurses to ensure that clinical decisions are evidence based, intellec- ell as factually justifiable, and address the individual needs of patients in their care.

Involving patients in decision-making processes

It is understood that there are three key groups of people who interact in the health systems of the UK. These are health professionals, managers or policy developers, and patients and carers, or service users. Since around 1980 in the UK, government policy has developed the processes by which service users and carers have become involved in managing health services (as members of Trust Boards), by reviewing healthcare (through the complaints services), or by participating in reviews of ser- vice delivery and planning health services, in research, in oversight panels, and in consultations of planned change. Clinical partnerships (patients and health profes- sionals) in decision making about care options have been enacted between patients and their carers, GPs, and senior clinical nurses for several decades.

What can you do to develop your clinical decision-making skills?

Barriers to effective clinical decision-making processes in practice include a heavy work- load, a lack of time, a lack of skills and understanding and a lack of confidence (Mayer, 1992; Thompson et al., 2001; Madjid et al., 2011). However, Gillespie and Paterson (2009) would argue that a useful framework should be adopted to support the develop- ment of decision-making processes by novice nurses that can help overcome at least some of these barriers. They suggest that the *Situated Clinical Decision Making Framework* can be used to guide reflection on decision-making processes in practice and help foster the development of knowledge, skill and confidence in decision-making pro- cesses (see Figure 7.6).

Knowing the Profession: relates to the ability to acknowledge and incorporate rel- evant principles, values and standards of nursing and to use these to inform the decision-making process.

Knowing the Self: highlights the importance of being able to reflect on your own strengths and limitations, skills, experience, competence and learning needs and to be willing to seek help and support if needed.

Knowing the Case: reflects the use of knowledge and understanding of related sci- ences (e.g. patho-physiology and the typical patterns of health, disease and illness, patient responses and predicted outcomes) and the ability to apply this knowledge to the decision-making process.

Knowing the Patient: involves focusing upon the patient's physiological state and being aware of the patient's baseline data and the patterns within their physiological responses to treatment.

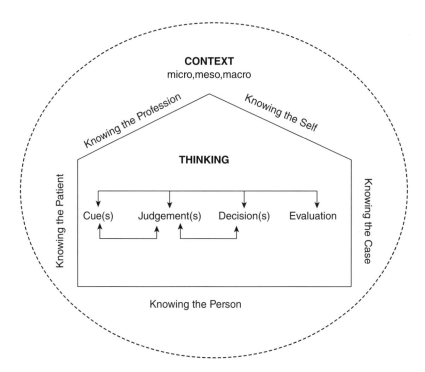

Figure 7.6   Schematic representation of the Situated Clinical Decision Making Framework

Source: Gillespie and Paterson (2009)

Knowing the Person: builds upon the concept of the therapeutic relationship and involves acknowledging that every patient's experience of health and illness is unique, as is their capacity to inform the clinical decision-making process.

Using the above approach may also help you ensure that you utilise the nursing process as it was always intended: as a tool to plan individualised patient care rather than to apply standardised care plans without the critical, analytical approach needed in order to adopt a more person-centred approach (Benner et al., 1996) .

ACTIVITY 7.2

Consider what you need to do in order to enhance your own decision-making abilities and develop the skills you need to make safe and effective clinical decisions.

- How will you ensure that you are able to enhance your critical thinking skills?
- What will this involve?
- What additional help and support might you need?
- How and where can you access this?

Top tips to ensure safe and effective clinical decision making

DO	DON'T
Gather, critically review and collate all relevant information prior to making a decision	Try not to allow decisions to be made to build up and accumulate; make decisions as you go along
Use the available information to the best of your ability	Avoid basing decisions on 'the way things are always done here'
Take time to consider the pros and cons of the issue being dealt with	Make snap decisions, rush, pre-empt or jump to conclusions
Delay or revise a decision as you feel necessary – trust yourself and do not be afraid to do this	Make decisions for the sake of making them; avoid wasting your time making decisions that don't have to be made
Think creatively and 'outside the box'	Feel that there is a right or wrong decision; decisions are choices among alternatives
Remember that any decision you make will have ramifications and consequences which could impact on a wide range of individuals and situations	Procrastinate or be forced or coerced into making a decision
Seek additional help and support from more experienced colleagues if necessary	

Adapted from Peate, I. (2006) *Becoming a Nurse in the 21st Century*.

Summary

This chapter has focused upon some of the various theories, frameworks and models which seek to explain how nurses act and react when deciding how to manage complexity in clinical settings. We have examined key determinants that will often impact on clinical decision-making processes and have explored ways in which the 'art' of nursing knowledge implementation can be addressed. We have also outlined the higher order intellectual skills associated with a critical appraisal of knowledge (using information), clinical (diagnostic) reasoning, empirical (diagnostic) judgements, and provided some examples of how you can develop these in order to ensure that you are able to make effective clinical decisions in practice.

Suggested further reading

You can find more information on Critical Appraisal using Systematic Approaches (CASP) at www.casp.uk.net

Department of Health (www.evidence,nhs.uk) – an index of index of authoritative, evidence-based information from trustworthy and accredited sources.

Standing, M. (2011) *Clinical Judgement and Decision Making for Nursing Students*, 2nd edition. London: Sage.

Thompson, C. and Dowding, D. (2002) *Clinical Decision-Making and Judgement in Nursing*. Edinburgh: Churchill Livingstone.

References

Amit, X., Garg, A.X., Adhikari, N.K.J., McDonald, H., Rosas-Arellano, M.P., Devereaux, P.J., MD; Beyene, J., Sam, J. and Haynes, R.B. (2005) 'Effects of computerised support systems on practitioner performance and patient outcomes: a systematic review', *Journal of American Medical Association*, 293 (10): 1223–38.

Benner, P. (1982) 'From novice to expert', *American Journal of Nursing*, 82: 402–7.

Benner, P., Tanner, C.A. and Chelsa, C.A. (1996) *Expertise in Nursing Practice: Caring, Clinical Judgement and Ethics*. New York: Springer.

Beginner's Guide (21 September 2005) 'What is decision making?'. Available at: http://beginnersguide.com/executivecoaching/decision-making/what-is-decision-making.php (last accessed 23 September 2014).

Carnevali, D.I., Mitchell, P.H., Woods, N.F. and Tanner, C.A. (1984) *Diagnostic Reasoning in Nursing*. Philadelphia: Lippincott.

Carper, B.A. (1978) 'Fundamental patterns of knowing in nursing', *Adv Nursing Sci*, 1(1): 13–23.

Cioffi, J. (1997) 'Heuristics, servants to intuition, in clinical decision making', *Journal of Advanced Nursing*, 26: 203–208.

Cooke, M. and Thackray, S. (2012) 'Differences between community professional and patient perceptions of COPD treatment outcomes: a qualitative study', *Journal of Clinical Nursing*, 21(11–12): 1524–1533.

Cullum, N., Ciliska, D. et al. (eds) (2008) *Evidence-based Nursing: An Introduction*. Oxford: Blackwell and BMJ and RCN Publishing.

Department of Health (1991) *Research for Health: A Research and Development Strategy for the NHS*. London: HMSO.

Department of Health (2013) *Report of the Mid Staffordshire NHS Foundation Trust Public Inquiry*. London: HMSO. Available at: www.midstaffspublicinquiry.com (last accessed 26 March 2015).

Doris, L., and Carnevali, M. and Thomas, D. (eds) (1993) *Diagnostic Reasoning and Treatment Decision Making in Nursing*. London: Lippincott Williams and Wilkins.

Douglas, K. (2011) 'Decision time: how subtle forces shape your choices', *New Scientist*, 14 November: 38–41. Available at: www.newscientist.com/article/mg21228381.800-decision-time-how-subtle-forces-shape-your-choices.html (last accessed 17 March 2015).

Dreyfus, H.L. (1979) *What Computers Can't Do: The Limits of Artificial Intelligence*. Rev. edition. New York: Harper & Row.

Dreyfus, H.L. and Dreyfus, S.E. (1986) *Mind over Machine: The Power of Human Intuition and Expertise in the Age of the Computer*. Oxford: Basil Blackwell.

Elstein, A.S., Shulman, L.S. and Sprafka, S.A. (1978) *Medical Problem-solving: An Analysis of Clinical Reasoning*. Cambridge, MA: Harvard University Press.

Gillespie, M. and Paterson, B.L. (2009) 'Helping novice nurses make effective clinical decisions: the situated clinical decision-making framework', *Nursing Education Perspectives*, May/June, 9 (3): 165–70.

Hamm, R.M. (1988) 'Clinical intuition and clinical analysis: expertise and the cognitive contiuum'. In J. Dowie and A. Elstein (eds), *Professional Judgement: A Reader in Clinical Decision Making*. Cambridge: Cambridge University Press.

Henderson, V. (1966) *The Nature of Nursing*. New York: The Macmillan Company.

Hertz, N. (2013) *Eyes Wide Open: How to Make Decisions in a Confusing World*. London: Harper-Collins.

Huang, X., Lin, J. and Demner-Fushman D. (2006) Evaluation of PICO as a knowledge representation for clinical questions, *AMIA Annual Symposium Proceedings 2006*: 359–3.

Lewin (1950) *Field Theory and Social Science Selected Theoretical Papers*. Edited by Dorwin Cartwright. New York: Harper.

Mayer, R.E. (1992) *Thinking, Problem Solving, Cognition*, 2nd edition. New York: W.H. Freeman and Company.

Majid, S., Foo, S., Luyt, B., Zhang, X., Theng, Y., Chang, Y. and Mokhtar, I.A. (2011) 'Adopting evidence-based practice in clinical decision making: nurses' perceptions, knowledge, and barriers', *Journal of the Medical Library Association*, 99(33): 229–236.

McGauhey, J., Alderdice, F., Fowler, R., Kapila, A., Mayhew, A. and Moutray, M. (2007) 'Outreach and early warning systems (EWS) for the prevention of intensive care admission and death of critically ill adult patients on general wards', *Cochrane Database of Systematic Reviews 2007*, 3, Art. No.: CD005529. doi: 10.1002/14651858.CD005529.pub2.

Miers, M.E., Rickerby, C.E., et al. (2007) 'Career choices in healthcare: is nursing a special case? A content analysis of survey data', *International Journal of Nursing Studies*, 44 (7): 1196–209.

New Oxford Dictionary of English (2001) *New Oxford Dictionary of English*. New York: Oxford University Press.

Nightingale, F. (1859) *Notes on Nursing: What it is and What it is not*, p.75. (Reprinted 1970.)

NMC (2010a) *Standards for Pre-Registration Nursing Education*. Available at: http://standards.nmc-uk.org (last accessed 19 November 2010).

NMC (2010b) *Standards for Competence for Registered Nurses*. Available at: www.nmc-uk.org/Documents/Standards/Standards%20for%20competence.pdf. (last accessed 19 November 2010).

NMC (2015) *The Code: Professional Standards of Practice and Behaviour for Nurses and Midwives*.

Peate, I. (2006) *Becoming a Nurse in the 21st Century*. Chichester: Wiley.

Phaneuf, M. (2008) 'Changes in our profession: an upgrading or downgrading of our role'. In M. Phaneuf (ed.), *Extrait des Aphorismes sur la Sagesse dans la Vie*. Toronto: Sage.

Robinson, S. and Bennett, J. (2007) *Career Choices and Constraints: Influences on Direction and Retention in Nursing*. London: King's College, Nursing Research Unit.

Schon, D. (1991) *The Reflective Practitioner: How Professionals Think and Act*. Aldershot: Avebury.

Standing, M. (2010) (ed.) *Clinical Judgement and Decision Making in Nursing and Interprofessional Practice*. Berkshire: OUP.

Tanner, C., Padrick, K., Westfall, U. and Putzier, D. (1987) 'Diagnostic reasoning: strategies for nurses and nursing students', *Nursing Research*, 36: 358–63.

Thompson, C., Aitken, L., Doran, D. and Dowding, D. (2013) 'An agenda for clinical decision making and judgement in nursing research and education', *International Journal of Nursing Studies*, 50: 1720–6.

Thompson, C., Cullum, N., McCaughan, D., Sheldon, T. and Raynor, P. (2004) 'Nurses, information use, and clinical decision making: the real world potential for evidence-based decisions in nursing', *EBN Notebook*. Available at: www.ebn.bmj.com (last accessed 23 September 2014).

Thompson, C. and Dowding, D. (2002) *Clinical Decision-making and Judgement in Nursing*. Edinburgh: Churchill Livingstone.

Thompson, C., McCaughan, D., Cullum, N., Sheldon, T. and Raynor, P. (2005) 'Barriers to evidence-based in primary care nursing – why viewing decision-making as context is helpful', *Journal of Advanced Nursing*, 52 (4): 432–44.

Thompson, C., McCaughan, D., Cullum, N., Sheldon, T., Thompson, D. and Mulhall, A. (2001) *Nurses' Use of Research Information In Clinical Decision Making: A Descriptive and Analytical Study, Final Report*. London: NCC/SDO.

Traynor, M. (2013) *Nursing in Context: Policy, Politics, Profession*. Basingstoke: Palgrave Macmillan.

Walsh, M. and Ford, P. (1989) *Nursing Rituals, Research and Rational Actions*. Oxford: Heinemann.

Wansink, B. and Sobal, J. (2007) 'Mindless eating: the 200 daily food decisions we overlook', *Environment and Behavior*, 39 (1): 106–23.

8   Leadership and Management

DIANNE BURNS

So far in this book we have focused upon the knowledge, understanding and skills required by an adult nurse in order to effectively assess the needs of patients and deliver evidence-based care in a variety of settings. Yet this is not enough; being able to manage the delivery of care, co-ordinate team activities, delegate care tasks and supervise the work of others is an essential part of every qualified nurse's role (NMC, 2015), and there is an increasing expectation and further opportunities for nurses to take on more leadership roles in the future.

The aim of this chapter is to introduce you to a selection of leadership and management theories, models, styles and approaches that can be applied within any contemporary healthcare setting. The activities in this chapter are designed to help you reflect upon the importance of key leadership and management skills, recognising areas for personal development in order to help you successfully lead healthcare teams in the future.

After reading this chapter you should be able to:

- Identify theories, models, styles and approaches to leadership and management in nursing and consider how these can be applied in any healthcare setting.
- Reflect upon your own leadership and management philosophy, style, skills and qualities and the extent to which these can be developed to make a positive impact on multi-professional care delivery to service users.
- Explore contemporary change management theories and their application to healthcare practice, identifying effective strategies for managing change and overcoming potential barriers.
- Explore effective strategies for risk assessment and management in relation to providing a safe environment for patients, visitors and staff.
- Appraise the concept of quality, focusing upon quality assurance frameworks and methods of monitoring and improving the quality of care for quality management and service provision.

Related NMC competencies

The overarching NMC requirement is that all nurses must:

> ... take the lead in coordinating, delegating and supervising care safely, managing risk and remaining accountable for the care given. They must act as change agents and provide leadership through quality improvement and service development to enhance people's well-being and experiences of healthcare. (NMC, 2010a: 20, 2010b: 6)

To achieve entry to the register as an adult nurse you should be able to:

- Use clinical governance processes to maintain and improve nursing practice and standards of healthcare.
- Create and maximise opportunities to improve services.
- Provide leadership in managing adult nursing care and understand and co-ordinate interprofessional care when needed, liaising with specialist teams as appropriate.
- Systematically evaluate care and ensure that you and others use these findings to help improve people's experience and care outcomes and in order to shape future services.
- Identify priorities, managing time and resources effectively to ensure the quality of care is maintained or enhanced.
- Take the lead in responding to the needs of people of all ages in a variety of circumstances, including situations where immediate or urgent care is needed.
- Recognise your leadership role in risk and disaster management, major incidents and public emergencies and respond appropriately according to your level of competence.
- Respond autonomously and confidently to planned and uncertain situations, managing yourself and others effectively.
- Know when to consult a third party and how to make referrals for advocacy, mediation or arbitration.
- Demonstrate the potential to develop further management and leadership skills during the period of preceptorship and beyond.
- Facilitate nursing students and others to develop their own competence using a range of professional and personal development skills.
- They must aim to improve their performance and enhance the safety and quality of care through evaluation, supervision and appraisal.

(Adapted from the NMC Standards of Competence for Adult Nursing, 2010a, 2010b.)

Background

The main purpose of leadership and management in healthcare settings is to maintain and improve patient care. This can be challenging when healthcare provision is constantly changing and there are a wide variety of competing factors to consider. An ageing and increasingly culturally diverse population; continuous pharmacological, technological and surgical advances coupled with demands to meet government quality targets whilst also coping with rapid patient turnover; maintaining patient safety, managing risk and containing rising costs in current financial climates – all of these are very complex challenges. Added to this is evidence of serious deficiencies in care which have undermined public confidence and where leadership deficits have been clearly highlighted (Kennedy, 2001; Francis, 2010; Care Quality Commission, 2012). There are now increasing calls for stronger leadership which promotes a caring and compassionate culture and also positively influences the quality of patient care (Cummings and Bennett, 2012; Onyett, 2012). It seems clear that healthcare organisations will need strong successful leaders and managers who have the ability to inspire and motivate others to achieve desired goals (DH, 2010a, 2010b; Cummings and Bennett, 2012; NHS Leadership Academy, 2014a).

So what exactly are we talking about when we refer to 'management' and 'leadership' and what part, if any, do 'followers' play?

What do the terms 'leadership' and 'management' mean to you?

Often leadership and management are viewed as being the same thing. However some would argue that they are in fact distinct entities, albeit with some area of overlap. Most would agree though that nurse managers *and* leaders are equally important and necessary to ensure that desired goals are successfully accomplished – although the focus of each of these roles may be different.

Management is mostly about *processes*. Huber (2010: 5) defines management as 'the co-ordination of resources through planning, organising, co-ordinating, directing and controlling to accomplish specific institutional goals and objectives'. Put simply, managers focus on *systems* and *structure*. A manager's role is based on authority and influence. Managers are usually formally appointed to a designated position, although you could argue of course that the role of any qualified nurse involves some aspect of management, particularly when directing the work of support staff or co-ordinating the delivery of patient care. Good management relies heavily on maintaining effective systems and involves ensuring that employees meet organisational goals and objectives; in essence managers *maintain stability* (Huber, 2010). More specifically a nurse manager's role 'combines responsibility for the daily delivery of care and the physical environment in which care is delivered with managerial responsibility of those who deliver the care (the nursing team) and a responsibility for those who receive that care' (RCN, 2009: 4). This role often involves:

- implementing new organisational policies and directives;
- managing human resources such as recruitment, off-duty rotas, sickness and absence management and disciplinary procedures;
- meeting government and organisational targets;
- ensuring quality and maintaining patient safety – setting standards for care, data collection, audit and service improvement;
- undertaking budgetary and resource management and control.

Furthermore, nurse managers are legally and professionally accountable for the decisions they make. They have a duty of care to ensure the safety of patients, visitors and other staff within their sphere of influence. This involves making sure that there are adequate resources available (including safe staffing levels) to deliver patient care and that these are used effectively 'according to the approved standards of care' (Dimond, 2005: 64). However, this does not detract from the fact that each registered nurse is also personally accountable for the actions and omissions of their own practice.

Leadership on the other hand is mostly about *behaviour*. Leadership is often an informal role rather than an officially designated position and as such, can occur spontaneously in any group. In order to influence others, leaders will often rely on their personal character and attitude to develop good interpersonal relationships. Described by Huber (2010: 4) as 'a complex and multi dimensional process of influencing people to accomplish goals' – leaders focus primarily on people (Bennis, 1994). Leadership is considered an interactive event based on human relationships (Kouzes and Posner, 2007), and can best be described as the ability to inspire confidence and encourage followers to follow; collaborating effectively in order to enthuse and motivate others to create and innovate. Moreover, leadership is necessary at all clinical levels and is not an activity reserved for those in positions of authority (The Kings Fund, 2011).

Leadership and followership behaviours are closely related as each of these affects the other. Being a follower is as important as being a leader because without followers a leader would have no-one to lead. *Followership* is also just as complex and multifaceted. Carsten et al. (2010) suggest that a follower's behaviour can be passive (i.e. obediently following direction with reduced responsibility taking), active (i.e. speaking up and making suggestions or verbalising ideas) or proactive (challenging the status quo for the good of the organisation). Chaleff (2009) suggests that the most effective followers are the ones who have initiative and can think for themselves. Therefore competent and committed followers are a valuable asset to be nurtured, developed and valued by every aspiring leader. A leader should always have an understanding of the interests, ideas, attitudes and motivation of potential followers and an ability and desire for their followers to release their potential.

In management, leadership and followership behaviours, *power* is also closely linked. According to Bass (1990) power is the underlying force for all social exchange. This falls into two broad categories; personal power or positional power (French and Raven, 1960), which can be utilised in order to influence others. Some managers may rely heavily on positional power while most leaders will rely primarily on personal power.

Table 8.1 Leaders, managers and followers

Leaders	Managers	Followers
Informal role	Formally designated role.	A member of an informal group or formal team.
Personal power (Expert/Referent) based on ability to influence	Positional (Legitimate/Reward/Coercive) power based on assigned position.	Information/Connection power based on ability and choice of whether to cooperate and collaborate effectively with leaders/managers.
Focus on people	Focus on processes, systems and structure (achieving organisational objectives by planning, organising, supervising, negotiating, evaluating and integrating services).	Support managers, leaders and other team members. Contribute to creating a comfortable and safe working environment.
Influence, motivate, inspire and energise followers	Direct and control followers, ensuring adherence to policies and procedures.	Follow the directions of managers Cooperate and collaborate with leaders and managers
Focus on the future. Visionary – they identify future goals and show the way forward. Innovate and create.	Focus on the here and now. Responsible for maintaining quality and managing resources. Maximise output and productivity.	Focus on agreed tasks.
An achieved position.	An assigned position.	A chosen position.
Do the right thing.	Do things right.	Carry out agreed tasks.
Do not need to be a good manager to be a good leader.	Need to be a good leader to be a good manager.	Good followers can be leaders, managers or neither!

Source: Adapted from Barr and Dowding (2012)

The personal power of followers is based upon being effective communicators, sharing relevant information and sustaining strong relationships with others.

Although managers, leaders and followers all have different power bases, they may use similar strategies, skills and attributes to achieve their goals. Indeed a leader, follower and manager may also be one and the same person playing different roles at different times. Whichever role you adopt in any given circumstance, it is clear that managers, leaders and followers need to work together to improve the quality of patient care and the working environment. However, each of us will have preferred management, leadership or followership behaviours and styles and you may need to reflect upon the type of leader or manager you want to be. Gaining a deeper understanding of your own preferences should help you identify areas for development in order to become a more effective manager, leader and follower in the future.

The activities suggested below should help you identify your own preferences. It is a good idea to try to be honest with yourself rather than focusing on what you think is the right or wrong answer.

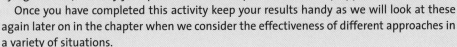

ACTIVITY 8.1

Using one of the Leadership Assessment Instruments (accessible via links on our accompanying website), identify your preferred leadership and followership approaches.

Once you have completed this activity keep your results handy as we will look at these again later on in the chapter when we consider the effectiveness of different approaches in a variety of situations.

What are management theories?

Management theories first arose during the nineteenth century at the time of the Industrial Revolution when the focus was upon looking at ways to improve productivity, efficiency and the relationship between managers and employees (Fayol, 1916). Theorists attempt to describe the role and function of managers and how they engage with employees in order to achieve organisational goals. It is thought that by developing a greater understanding of how to efficiently manage situations and people we can achieve better outcomes whilst simultaneously maintaining or improving levels of productivity. There are many different management theories and it is beyond the realms of this chapter to discuss all of these in any depth. What follows is a very brief summary of management theory development:

Human Relations Theory – promotes the idea that people want personal fulfilment, good social relationships and to be an accepted member of a group (Mayo, 1949). The main principle of this theory is the belief that individuals cannot be coerced and forced to do things that they consider unreasonable – willing participants are needed.

Theory X and Theory Y – McGregor (1960) explored the motivation of workers and their attitude to work, suggesting that by understanding these two aspects managers can develop a better understanding of how their own viewpoints of human behaviour influence their chosen management approach (i.e. Theory X people dislike work and need to be directed and controlled as they want security rather than responsibility, and Theory Y people like work, are self motivated and accept or seek responsibility).

Contingency Theory – some suggest that a manager's or leader's effectiveness is dependent upon the match between leader/manager style and the setting or situation (Fiedler, 1967) and describe styles that are task or relationship motivated (Northouse, 2012).

Situational Theory – focuses upon the idea that the effectiveness of a leader's/manager's style will be influenced by the situation itself and that as a basic principle managers/leaders will need to consider the situation alongside the competence and commitment of staff when making a decision. This approach has both directive and supportive dimensions and each of these will need to be applied according to what is required in any given situation. The essence of this approach suggests that leaders need to match their approach to follower readiness (Blanchard et al., 1993).

Systems Theory – supports the idea that to be effective organisations need to consider a complex network of numerous factors and the interplay between structure, people, technology and the environment (e.g. the provision of excellent patient care is dependent upon the effective integration of effort across departments and disciplines). It is argued that changing one part of the system will affect the whole system as each system is a set of inter-related parts designed to achieve common goals (Senge, 1990). It is worth noting that systems theory has been seen by some as a way of understanding management needs within the NHS (Iles and Sutherland, 2001).

Chaos Theory – draws upon the emerging science of complexity in an attempt to explain the unpredictable nature of organisations like the NHS and the limitations associated with trying to organise a complex system into a 'manageable' state using rule-based frameworks (NHS Alliance, 2003). For a more in-depth analysis of these various theories Further Reading is recommended at the end of this chapter.

What are leadership theories?

Leadership theories attempt to enhance our understanding of the desired characteristics and specific qualities, skills and approaches that are considered helpful in distinguishing a successful leader from a follower. By developing a greater appreciation of successful leadership approaches we can use our influence as leaders to improve not only patient care but also the working environment for ourselves and others.

In general, leadership theories will vary according to

- the emphasis placed on the personal characteristics of a leader;
- the effect of a leader on organisational functioning and culture;
- the emphasis placed on the leader and group behaviour (social interaction processes).

'*Great Man*' or *Trait theories* are based on the belief that leaders possess exceptional qualities that influence the way a person leads (Bass, 1990). Over the years numerous research studies have attempted to identify key traits – although there is still no complete agreement on the desired characteristics. Critics also argue that this fails to take into account the influence of organisational culture and negates the part that social class, gender and race inequalities play in the opportunity for leadership development. *Behavioural theories* focus upon the actions of effective leaders and how they behave (Hersey and Blanchard, 1988; Yukl et al., 2002; Marquis and Huston, 2006). The current NHS Leadership Quality Framework (NHS Leadership Academy, 2014b) identifies what it believes to be the desired behaviours and attributes of leaders in healthcare – suggesting that both trait and behavioural theories still influence current thinking. For example, these are often reflected within desired attributes contained within some person specifications and job descriptions. *Situational theories* attempt to explain how leaders use task behaviours and relationship behaviours in an organisational setting (Blake and Mouton, 1964). Theorists suggest that different situations demand different kinds of leadership and that leaders adjust their leadership styles in accordance with the readiness of their followers (Hersey and Blanchard, 1988). *Contingency theories* focus upon the match between leader style and situational variables – Fiedler (1967) for example concluded that no one particular style met the needs of every situation. *Functional theories* suggest that leadership effectiveness is dependent upon the relationship between leader and group (Kouzes and Posner, 2007; Adair, 2009). These theorists focus on how leadership supports the function of the organisation to carry out work and relates to a leader's source of power and influence over others (i.e. how various roles relate to the organisational functions to meet the needs of the organisation): task needs, needs of the team, needs of the individual and effects on group behaviours.

Leadership and management styles

Leadership and management styles can be described as 'different combinations of tasks and relationship behaviours which are used to influence others to accomplish goals' (Huber, 2010: 6). Looking closely at the literature around leadership and management styles it is possible to identify the similarities and how they overlap. A number of commonly observed leadership and managements styles are outlined in Table 8.2.

Healthcare organisations are often very complex and the varied nature of the work involved along with the diverse nature of the workforce have led some to argue that alternative approaches to traditional top-down (autocratic) methods are required. A model of 'shared/distributed' leadership is now considered much more appropriate. The NHS Leadership Academy (2014b) suggest that effective leaders need to be able to work through others – supporting, motivating and encouraging followers to achieve objectives and empowering them to use their skills effectively, recognising their achievements and thereby creating an engaged workforce. The demand for more openness within organisations is also growing. The 'ethical leadership' framework encourages leaders/managers to take account of key ethical principles when making decisions and to use their authority or influence for the common good. Ciulla (2003) for example recommends that a leader's focus should always be to do the right thing, in the right way for the right reason. *Servant* (Greenleaf, 1977) and *spiritual* leadership models emphasise the 'caring' principle (Northouse, 2012) where leaders demonstrate care and compassion and are sensitive to the needs of others.

There has been considerable debate as to whether leadership abilities are traits we are born with or if they are skills which can be taught. Some would argue that leadership

Table 8.2   Leadership and management styles

Leadership Style	Advantages/Strengths	Disadvantages/Weaknesses
Laissez-faire Leaders exert minimal influence and take a 'hands-off' approach (e.g. try to please everyone and therefore takes a non-directive or inactive approach – leaving the followers to decide upon the actions needed themselves).	Groups of fully autonomous and independent care providers working together can feel empowered to make decisions.	Can often result in a lack of direction (chaotic, frustrating, disheartening and unproductive), particularly where there is disharmony or a clash of work ethic values amongst team members.
Autocratic/Authoritarian/ Transactional Top-down approach (controlling, directing, goal/target setting). Use of recognition and reward incentives to influence motivation. Transactional leaders focus more on tasks (e.g. dominate and make all decisions without allowing for the views of others to be considered).	Can be very efficient in certain situations (i.e. emergencies). Focuses upon the ability of leader/manager to monitor and correct subordinates.	Stifles creativity, fosters dependence, submissiveness and loss of individuality. Very little/limited collaboration and delegation. Shared values are not communicated. This can create discontent, hostility and even aggression amongst group members or followers.
Democratic Leaders work with and guide rather than direct followers. *Transformational* Based on the idea that leaders motivate others to perform by encouraging a shared vision and changing their perception of reality (e.g. shares the decision-making and planning processes as well as responsibility for their implementation).	Increased job satisfaction for followers (feel more motivated to get involved, empowered).	Takes more time and effort to execute effectively.

skills can be developed (Large et al., 2005; Kouzes and Posner, 2007; Adair, 2009) and this is now exemplified by the introduction of nationally recognised NHS Nurse Leadership programmes (NHS Leadership Academy, 2014c) which set out a consistent standardised approach to developing excellent leadership.

The new evidence-based Healthcare Leadership Model (NHS Leadership Academy, 2015) provides an outline of nine 'leadership dimensions', calling upon future healthcare leaders to consider these when seeking to identify personal strengths and areas for development:

- Inspiring a shared purpose.
- Leading with care.
- Evaluating information.
- Connecting the service.
- Sharing the vision.
- Engaging the team.
- Holding to account.
- Developing capability.
- Influencing for results.

It is clear that there are many different styles of leadership. The most effective leaders are likely to be those who are able to recognise that one leadership style is not necessarily better than another. In order to achieve optimum patient outcomes, enhance nurse satisfaction and maintain healthy work environments, as a leader you will need to be able to recognise various factors that will influence your chosen leadership style – adapting and adopting a range of leadership styles where possible – depending upon the demands of the situation. Leaders who perform well tend to be highly visible and thrive on collaboration and network building – which in turn encourages distributed leadership (Lucas and Buckley, 2009; Hardacre et al., 2011; The Kings Fund, 2012).

STOP AND THINK

- As a leader or manager what kind of difference do you want to make?
- Reflecting upon your current abilities as a manager, leader and follower, and reviewing your answers to the previous activities, do you have any areas for development?

For example, what additional areas/skills/attributes do you think you need to develop in order to make yourself a better leader/manager/follower in the following scenarios:

- An emergency situation (e.g. dealing with a patient who has suddenly collapsed).
- Implementing a new way of working (e.g. introducing bedside handovers).

You might want to consider creating a personal skills self-development plan based on these findings.

Table 8.3 contains some useful tips for enhancing your leadership behaviours.

Table 8.3   Enhancing your leadership behaviour (Northouse, 2012)

Trait/Behaviour	Suggested Activity
Intelligence	Keep well informed, read widely about topical issues.
Confidence	Develop a clear understanding of what is required. This will help you feel more confident when identifying and using future opportunities to take on leadership roles (e.g. leading a student discussion or speaking out in group work activities, volunteering, serving on committees and interest groups). Getting involved in all of the above activities can help to boost your confidence.
Charisma	You may or may not be a naturally charismatic or outgoing person. Nevertheless, by demonstrating that you are competent and can clearly articulate your goals, that you have strong values and high expectations; that you can encourage and show confidence in the ability of others – inspiring and exciting others with your ideas – will motivate others to follow.
Determination	Know where you are going and how you intend to get there. Show initiative, be persistent, proactive and persevere; give direction to others if needed.
Sociability	Make an effort to establish pleasant, social relationships. Try to be friendly and outgoing, courteous, tactful and diplomatic, kind, thoughtful and supportive to others in the group (i.e. make others feel included).
Integrity	Be open with others. Always act honestly and be loyal and dependable.

Similarly the six pillars of character in Table 8.4 outline how you might exhibit these in practice (Northouse, 2012).

Table 8.4   The six pillars of character (Northouse, 2012)

Ethical Principles	Six Pillars of Character
Veracity & Fidelity	**Trustworthiness:** being open and honest, representing reality as fully and completely as possible. Keep promises. This element also links to professional **integrity** (e.g. adhering to high moral values and professional standards) and **confidentiality** (in relation to personal or private matters).
Justice	Try to be non-judgemental, treat everyone **equally** and **fairly, respecting** and valuing their views and ensuring that you do not use followers as a means of meeting your objectives rather than their own. Encourage informed decision making processes of the group based on a sound knowledge and understanding of issues. Involves using morally appropriate actions to achieve goals. Give credit to others when deserved.
Autonomy	**Responsibility** and freedom of choice (e.g. accept responsibility for the actions you take as a leader).
Non-maleficence	**Care** for others to avoid harm. Caring leadership behaviour links to the notion of **servant** leadership outlined by Greenleaf (1977) and highlights the requirement to be attentive to the needs of others (e.g. establish goals that all parties can mutually agree to and assist others to develop emotional resilience).
Beneficence	**Develop good citizenship** by making decisions which promote the common good of 'doing the right thing'. Develop collegiality and share goals. Leaders as **servants** focus upon the followers' needs in order to help them become more autonomous and knowledgeable (Barr and Dowding, 2012), mentoring/teaching, team building, empowering others. Demonstrating compassion involves listening deeply to others in order to try to understand things from their perspective (Greenleaf, 1977).

The Five Dimensions of Courageous Followership (Chaleff, 2009) outlined in Table 8.5 below also provide a useful framework when considering areas for developing your followership skills.

Table 8.5   Five Dimensions of Courageous Followership (Chaleff, 2009)

The courage to assume responsibility	Know what you are expected to do and how you will achieve it. Take personal responsibility for completing (or not) the agreed tasks. Utilise effective communication skills to keep the leader and other team members fully informed.
The courage to serve	Followers do not serve leaders. Rather, followers and leaders each serve a common purpose by supporting agreed decisions and shared values – creating a relationship of trust and support. Offer encouragement to the leader when necessary and help to communicate the leader's vision to others throughout the organisation. Cooperate and work energetically with others to achieve the agreed common goal. Provide timely and accurate feedback to the leader and other members of the group.

The courage to participate in transformation	Make time and effort to consider what skills and attributes you will need to develop in order to transform the leader-follower relationship.
The courage to challenge	This does not equate to being argumentative and unreceptive. However good followers should not be afraid to constructively challenge the leader when necessary. Be courageous and voice your opinion when it really matters to challenge current thinking or leadership decisions that you believe are misguided or unethical. Providing accurate feedback on plans will help to ensure that the leader has the necessary information to make critical decisions.
The courage to take moral action	Be honest and trustworthy. Demonstrate a 'courageous conscience'. You should always seek to carry yourself with integrity and self-respect. If you do not morally agree with a leader's approach or agenda then this is the time to stand up for what you believe is the right thing to do. Leaving the group/team or even *whistle-blowing* is one option that may need to be exercised rarely.

Leading and managing people

Every qualified nurse needs to be able to co-ordinate work activities and delegate care to co-workers and other members of the team (NMC, 2010). This requires a variety of skills such as the ability to communicate clearly and directly and being able to provide support, guidance and feedback. Delegating to others will allow more time for leadership activities and will also help you develop the skills and abilities of other members of the team. The most effective leaders and/or managers are those who are able to build a culture where all the members feel valued and will flourish irrespective of their role. However, to ensure that the quality of patient care is not compromised you should only delegate those tasks that you know others can manage. As a qualified nurse you will remain legally and professionally accountable for the decision to delegate care and for the overall management for care delivery. Therefore delegation should always take into account the context of the situation rather than just focusing upon the task alone (RCN, 2011).

When delegating care to others you should always consider:

- the stability of the person being cared for;
- the complexity of the task being delegated;
- the expected outcome of the delegated task;
- the availability of the resources to meet those needs (NMC, 2010).

You will also need to ensure that you only delegate to someone who has had 'appropriate training' and has been deemed competent to carry out the task. On occasions this might be difficult to ascertain, particularly if you are working in unfamiliar surroundings or with unfamiliar people. Therefore you should check that this person fully understands what is required and expected of them. You will also need to provide clear instruction and direction. Once the task has been completed you will also have to check that it has been carried out satisfactorily and offer appropriate feedback (NMC, 2010). Offering coaching, support and guidance in this way will help you foster team work and collaboration (Huber, 2010). However delegating work to others can sometimes be difficult, particularly when staffing levels are low, when the delegated task is considered unpleasant or due to a fear of causing conflict (Hasson et al., 2013).

STOP AND THINK

- What tasks might you consider delegating to other members of staff in what situations?
- What might influence your ability to delegate effectively?
- What strategies or skills could help you further develop your delegating abilities?

Improving your own delegating abilities

Obviously the potential range of tasks you could delegate to someone else is considerable. However, the use of a recognised framework such as the *Five Rights of Delegation* (National Council of State Boards of Nursing, 1997) can help you to decide whether delegation is appropriate or not:

- Right task.
- Right circumstance.
- Right person.
- Right direction/communication.
- Right supervision and evaluation.

You may also want to reflect upon other factors which might impact on your delegating ability. For example, is your ability hampered by:

- a lack of confidence in either in your own abilities or in the abilities of others?
- a fear of losing your authority or control?
- wanting to avoid risk?
- merely a lack of ability to provide clear direction to others?

The following checklist (adapted from Huber, 2010: 246) provides key pointers that may help you to further develop your abilities:

- Developing a good attitude.
- Deciding on what you want to delegate.
- Selecting the right person (e.g. qualified or unqualified practitioner?).
- Communicating responsibilities clearly.
- Granting the authority to act.
- Providing adequate support.
- Monitoring the delegated task.
- Evaluating the outcome.

Developing a healthy work environment

The NMC (2010) requires you to be able to work co-operatively with other members of staff, sharing your skills and experience and respecting their own contribution to the efforts of the team. As a manager or leader, part of your role will involve maintaining a healthy work environment. However this might not be as easy as it sounds.

The population of the UK is changing and along with it the workforce is becoming more diverse in terms of educational background, roles, professionalisation (e.g. different value systems), ethnicity, gender and age (Hutchinson et al., 2012). All of these factors can influence how people act and communicate with each other (for example expectations of behaviour and conformance or differing styles of communication). A nurse leader will need to have an understanding of how these differences can be harnessed in order to build and maintain a healthy workplace (Stanley, 2010).

Furthermore, changes in healthcare during the past decade have led many to question whether the organisational culture within many healthcare settings is *toxic* (i.e. controlling and repressive, where nurses are often afraid to speak out due to a worry of reprisal) rather than facilitative (Francis, 2010; Cummings and Bennett, 2012). A healthy work environment correlates to job satisfaction which in turn positively influences recruitment and healthier patients (International Council of Nurses, 2007; Cowden et al., 2011). Equally, a poor work environment adversely affects health: employees spiral into burnout, leading to frequent absences and recurrent sickness and impacting negatively on professional attitudes and behaviours (RCN, 2013). Therefore the workplace culture has a huge influence on how employees carry out their work and this in turn will ultimately influence patient care. There is a growing call for nurse leaders and managers to embrace the core principles of nursing (for example caring and compassion), and translate these into the type of nurse management and leadership needed in today's contemporary healthcare settings (Sieloff and Wallace Raph, 2011; Onyett, 2012). Cummings and Bennett (2012: 11) suggest that 'leaders at every level have a responsibility to shape and lead a caring culture'. Indeed, an effective leader needs to be able to deconstruct a work culture if that becomes necessary (Sherwood, 2003). Hewison and Griffiths (2004) agree, arguing that without paying attention to the wider need of transforming a 'sick' organisational culture all of the effort placed in developing future leaders could be wasted.

LUCY

Lucy's first post as a qualified nurse was on a 30-bedded female rehabilitation ward. She was happy to be joining a well-established team and was looking forward to her new role. The ward appeared well organised and well resourced, serving mainly elderly females recovering from elective orthopaedic surgery or falls at home. The ward manager was a forthright, well-organised individual who believed that 'you sometimes had to be cruel to be kind' in a bid to ensure that the rehabilitation process (particularly the re-mobilisation of patients) facilitated their return home as quickly as possible. However, after the first few weeks Lucy quickly realised that all was not as it seemed. Long-serving Healthcare Assistants were often seen to apply the 'mantra' of the ward manager inflexibly and sometimes a little too literally when attempting to encourage patients to mobilise, using behaviour and language that she felt often lacked compassion and which she perceived as 'bullying'. Protests from patients were either ignored or resulted in some staff labelling them as 'uncooperative' or 'lazy'. Lucy raised her concerns with other qualified members of staff. Some agreed with the approach favoured by the ward manager, others appeared a little more uncomfortable but admitted they had done nothing about it due to a fear of retaliation if they 'stepped out of line'. Lucy quickly established that anyone who had challenged this approach was quickly put in their place by key staff (supported by the manager) or had simply left. Members of staff who complained were either ignored or ridiculed, labelled as 'soft' and/or 'unhelpful'.

- Do you consider the culture of the ward above to be toxic or facilitative? Give your reasons.
- What are the key influencing factors?

Case Scenario

According to the International Council for Nurses (2007) positive practice environments are characterised by the following:

- Occupational health, safety and wellness policies that address workplace hazards, discrimination, physical and psychological violence and issues pertaining to personal security.
- Fair, manageable workloads and job demands.
- An organisational climate reflective of effective management and leadership practices, good peer support, worker participation in decision making and shared values.
- Work schedules and workloads that permit a healthy work–life balance.
- Equal opportunity and treatment.
- Opportunities for professional development and career advancement.
- Professional identity, autonomy and control over practice.
- Job security, decent pay and benefits.
- Safe staffing levels.
- Support, supervision and mentorship.
- Open communication and transparency.
- Recognition programmes.
- Access to adequate equipment, supplies and support staff.

STOP AND THINK

In relation to your current practice and the points characterised above, reflect upon whether there is anything that you can do to ensure that your current workplace is a healthy one.

Managing difficult situations

Managing the delivery of health and social care in the UK involves collaborating with a variety of complex organisations and professionals within a diverse workforce. Nowadays, healthcare staff are constantly under pressure to improve services often when resources are stretched. In certain circumstances this can result in a communication breakdown or poor provision of care which leads to frustration, particularly when this involves patients and relatives who may be anxious and upset, distressed or angry. Therefore it is somewhat inevitable that you will encounter difficult situations at some stage in your career.

Conflict is defined as 'a serious disagreement or argument'; 'a state of mind in which a person experiences a clash of opposing feelings or needs' and 'a serious incompatibility between two or more opinions, principles, or interests' (*Oxford English Dictionary*, 2014) and can potentially arise in any situation but particularly where changes have taken place due to restructuring, team working is poor or where there are differing management styles, individual personalities or behaviours. However, whilst dealing with 'difficult' people or situations can be very uncomfortable and stressful, if ignored or handled inadequately, conflict can have a negative impact upon individuals, organisations and patient care, resulting in poor job satisfaction, sickness and poor staff retention (Brinkert, 2010). Yet conflict is not always unhealthy. A degree of conflict can sometimes increase understanding and problem solving, leading to higher levels of creativity, and can enhance team motivation if handled appropriately (Almost, 2006). To be able to do this effectively you will need to have an appreciation of all of the contributing factors and an understanding of ways in which conflict can be resolved successfully.

Sources of conflict can be *intra*-personal (e.g. a poor work–life balance or role conflict), *inter*-personal (e.g. a personality clash or differences in beliefs, values, objectives and priorities), or organisational (e.g. competing for resources). Perhaps not surprisingly a common source of inter-personal conflict involves other nurse colleagues (Duddle and Boughton, 2007; Leiter et al., 2010), often resulting in incivility, verbal abuse or bullying. Other sources of inter-personal conflict include other healthcare professionals (i.e. nurse–doctor conflict) and patients or their families – usually as a result of poor communication or perceived shortcomings in provision of care (Brinkert, 2010).

ACTIVITY 8.2

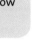

- Identify and list the potential sources of conflict within your current workplace. What are the aggravating or mitigating factors?
- Use the Thomas and Kilman (1974) Conflict Mode Instrument available via the supporting rescources website to help identify how you would normally respond to conflict situations. Your score will help to reveal the repertoire of conflict handling skills which you currently use and also help you identify areas for development and reflect upon how you might do this.

In stressful circumstances each of us will adopt certain strategies or styles in an attempt to manage the situation (Almost et al., 2010). Furthermore there are recognised gender differences in the way men and women handle conflict. Women commonly use avoidance or accommodating tactics (Duddle and Boughton, 2007) whilst men tend to use power (Almost, 2006).

Thomas and Kilman (1974) suggest that there are five common approaches to managing conflict:

- *Avoiding* (e.g. ignoring or withdrawing from the situation).
- *Competing* (e.g. dominating as a way of controlling a situation, using whatever power is at your disposal to achieve your goal).
- *Compromising* (e.g. respecting and accepting the needs of others which involves seeking common ground to find a mutually acceptable solution that partially satisfies both parties).
- *Accommodating* (e.g. neglecting your own concerns to satisfy the other person, i.e. yielding to another person's point of view).
- *Collaborating* (e.g. working with the other person to find some solution which fully satisfies both parties – this involves a full exploration of underlying concerns from all points of view in order to understand the needs of others to find a creative solution).

As with other leadership and management styles no one approach is applicable in every situation. However, Friedman et al. (2000) claim that people who use accommodating, compromising and collaborating styles tend to experience lower levels of conflict and stress. Northouse (2012) also suggests that problem-solving skills (i.e. being able to identify problems and potential solutions and developing effective strategies to deal with conflict) are very useful. At the very least, taking time to actively identify, explore and discuss differences in a non-threatening environment should help to resolve some difficult situations and reduce workplace stress.

In order to be able to do this effectively many would argue that you need to be able to understand your own emotions and those of others and then apply this knowledge and understanding when choosing strategies to deal with difficult situations as they arise. The five integrated domains of EI asserted by Goleman (1995) have already been highlighted in previous chapters (pp. 18 and 41–42). However, Huber (2010: 4) interprets these further in relation to the concept of team working as the following:

- *Self-awareness* (e.g. an ability to read your own emotional state and be aware of your own mood and how this might affect relationships).
- *Self-management* (e.g. the ability to take corrective action so as not to transfer your own negative moods onto staff relationships).
- *Social awareness* (e.g. intuitive skill of empathy and expressiveness: being sensitive and aware of the emotions and moods of others).
- *Relationship management* (e.g. using effective communication with others to disarm conflict and an ability to develop the emotional maturity of other team members).

STOP AND THINK

Make a list of the qualities, skills and abilities that you think may be important when dealing effectively with conflict.

- What could you do to help develop your emotional intelligence (EI)?
- What measures could be taken to help minimise the sources of conflict in your workplace?

Being open-minded and listening carefully and empathetically to someone else's point of view will help you to demonstrate fairness, respect and emotional maturity. Well-developed communication skills should also assist you to negotiate and collaborate with others in order to attempt to resolve issues and disputes.

Unfortunately however, workplace bullying does exist and can be a major contributing factor to unhealthy and toxic environments (Francis, 2010; Care Quality Commission, 2014). Bullying has been identified as a factor that not only affects patient outcomes but also increases occupational stress, decreases job satisfaction and adversely affects staff retention (Carter et al., 2013). Bullying can manifest itself physically (e.g. hitting or pushing), verbally (e.g. name calling or arguing) or psychologically (e.g. being ignored, excluded or undermined).

Dealing with negative behaviour (whether you are personally on the receiving end or not) can obviously be very challenging. However, Bennett and Sawatzky (2013) argue that individuals with greater EI are not only more able to recognise early signs of negative behaviour but are also more able to deal with it more effectively.

Steps you can take to help minimise sources of conflict include:

- setting out and clearly verbalising behavioural expectations to other members of staff – linking these expectations of local policies (e.g. bullying and maintaining dignity in the workplace) will help to identify negative behaviours;

- improving reporting mechanisms by facilitating a supportive, non-blame and responsive culture to encourage 'victims' to come forward;
- treating complaints seriously, enforcing expectations where necessary by reiterating these in line with identified policies and clearly outlining these to all parties.

The skill though will be dealing with conflict in a way that does not add to the stress of the situation within the workplace. It is worth remembering also that there are other sources of help that individuals can turn to if necessary (e.g. your mentor, line manager, university tutor or the Royal College of Nursing or other Trade Union representative).

Managing quality

It is imperative that healthcare systems across the UK are able to deliver high quality patient care. Good quality care is defined by the National Quality Board (2013: 4) as 'care that is effective, safe and provides as positive an experience as possible'. In light of recent failures highlighted by Francis (2010), monitoring and improving the quality of care we deliver to our patients has never been higher on the political or professional agenda. However it is also a complex and demanding task. Having a working knowledge of the relevant frameworks, policies, tools and techniques, alongside an ability to enable and facilitate others is central to leading improvement in the NHS, particularly when dealing with more complex issues (Hardacre et al., 2011).

Table 8.6   NHS Outcomes Framework Five Domains for Improvement

Domain 1	*Preventing people from dying prematurely;*
Domain 2	*Enhancing quality of life for people with long-term conditions;*
Domain 3	*Helping people to recover from episodes of ill health or following injury;*
Domain 4	*Ensuring that people have a positive experience of care;*
Domain 5	*Treating and caring for people in a safe environment and protecting them from avoidable harm.*

Source: Department of Health (2012a) *The NHS Outcomes Framework.* London: DH

In England, the recent *Health and Social Care Act* (2012) has placed new duties on the Secretary of State for Health, the NHS Commissioning Board and clinical commissioning groups to act with a view to ensuring continuous improvement in the quality of NHS services across all care providers. The NHS Outcomes Framework 2013/14 (DH, 2012a) sets out the national goals that NHS England should be aiming to improve within five key domains.

Aligned with two other key frameworks – the Public Health Outcomes Framework (DH, 2012b) and the Adult Social Care Outcomes Framework (DH, 2013) – the aim is to abolish centrally driven targets and create local accountability, with an emphasis on outcome-focused measures that have a more holistic drive towards quality improvement. Similar quality improvement strategies have been implemented in Scotland, Northern Ireland and Wales.

Clinical governance is defined as:

a framework through which NHS organisations are accountable for continuously improving the quality of their services. (DH, 1998)

In England this encompasses a whole range of quality improvement activities falling within three main strands: *clinical effectiveness*, *safety* and *patient experience* (National Quality Board, 2013). As a qualified nurse you will be accountable for the standard of nursing care, dignity and well-being of your patients so you will have a vital role to play in putting these into practice (NMC, 2015). As a nurse manager you will also have the responsibility of promoting awareness of essential standards of quality and safety, monitoring the standard of care delivered and taking action where necessary in the interests of patients. This will involve ensuring that the workplace culture is one in which quality improvement activities flourish and where frontline staff are able to grasp opportunities to make a positive contribution not only by enhancing their own professional development but also by engaging collaboratively with service users to improve and enhance care delivery.

Clinical effectiveness

> Quality care is care which is delivered according to the best evidence as to what is clinically effective in improving an individual's health outcomes. (National Quality Board, 2013: 13)

The provision of good quality patient care is of great interest to providers and purchasers of care alike. In recent years, the emphasis for care providers has focused upon evidence-based practice. Indeed the NMC Code (2015) demands that you deliver care based on the best available evidence. This requires you to keep your knowledge and skills up to date, ensuring that you have a good understanding of the current evidence base and an ability to apply this to your day-to-day practice. Additionally, purchasers are keen to ensure that healthcare provision is cost effective and provides value for money. However, concerns about the quality of care within some healthcare settings have continued to attract national publicity and often focus upon the failure of organisations to provide services that deliver high standards of care. For example, in 2011/2012 the Care Quality Commission reported that only 85% of NHS hospitals met the required standard of ensuring that patients had access to the right food, drink and help that they needed (Care Quality Commission, 2012).

STOP AND THINK

Consider how you might go about improving patient care and experience in your current practice setting? What would you need to know?

Clinical effectiveness is about improving patient care and experience by critically reviewing what you/your team do by considering the following:

- What should be happening? (Identifying evidence of best practice)
- What is happening? (Reviewing current practice)
- How can we do it better? (Comparing your practice with good practice and implementing change)
- Evaluating change (Using clinical audit and other measures, i.e. Patient Reported Outcome Measures – PROMs – to demonstrate improvement).

Measuring quality

It is more than thirty years ago since the concept of quality improvement in healthcare settings was introduced by Donabedian (2005) amongst others who suggested that by observing *structure* (the setting in which care is delivered – e.g. nurse-patient ratio, staffing levels), *focus* (the process or means by which the end point is achieved – e.g. patient care pathway) and *outcomes* (end point – e.g. readmission rates, number of reported falls or hospital acquired infection rates) we can measure the quality of healthcare. More recently the introduction of agreed standards of care has allowed us to measure the care we deliver against a set standard (e.g. benchmarking). As a bare minimum, current requirements dictate that we should meet essential standards for quality and safety set out by the Care Quality Commission (2010). We should also be aiming to meet standards set by the National Institute for Health and Care Excellence (NICE) – for example recognised care pathways (http://pathways.nice.org.uk/) and Department of Health National Service Frameworks (http://nhs.uk/nhsengland/NSF/) – which focus upon the care of patients with a particular condition and set out what high quality care looks like for a particular patient group.

Regularly participating in activities that continuously measure and monitor the quality of care delivered in your current workplace is essential. However, to do this effectively requires the use of robust systems and processes designed to monitor performance. *Quality Indicators* (QI), also referred to as *Clinical Quality Indicators* (CQI), are reliable and valid measures which can be used to assess health processes and outcomes (Maintz, 2003). Additionally, *clinical audit* is a cyclical staged process that seeks to improve patient care and outcomes through a systematic review of care measured against explicit criteria (e.g. quality indicators), a course of action taken to improve services and followed by continued monitoring to sustain improvement. Similarly, data collated from *Patient Reported Outcome Measures* (PROMs) can be used to evaluate the effectiveness of current service provision, recognise deficits and assist in the development of new evidence-based services. However, in order to be successful healthcare professionals need to fully understand the importance of collecting data and also the value of collating data as the success of such strategies is almost entirely dependent on the values and behaviours of staff working within the system. For example, some nurses may be somewhat sceptical about the benefits of time-consuming 'number crunching' and do not always understand the importance of data collection and how information can be used to benefit patient care.

Managing risk and patient safety

> Quality care is care which is delivered so as to avoid all avoidable harm and risks to an individual's safety. (NQB, 2013: 13)

Earlier in this chapter we explored the notion that that the work environment is influenced not least by the quality of leadership provided within the placement and organisation. Equally, effective leadership plays a pivotal role in maintaining patient safety by creating and maintaining safe working environments and practices (Squires et al., 2010). Critical incidents commonly occur as a result of poor organisational systems – for example a failure to follow good practice, poor communication, poor record keeping or as the result of equipment failure (RCN, 2003). As a qualified nurse, ensuring that you have sufficient knowledge and critical understanding of the input and resources needed to manage risk effectively will be crucial to help maintain patient, public and staff safety. Risk can be predictable or unpredictable, environmental (e.g. linked to levels of cleanliness, light, temperature and/or adequacy of space) or human related (e.g. working practices or impaired functioning).

Risk assessment is defined as 'a careful examination of what, in your work, could cause harm to people, so that you can weigh up whether you have taken enough precautions or should do more to prevent harm' (Health and Safety Works NI, 2014: 1).

ACTIVITY 8.3

Reflecting upon your experience so far:

- Closely examine your current workplace or placement area. Make a list of the common risks and adverse incidents that can occur within this setting.
- Consider the role that effective leadership might have in creating safe working environments.

Common incidents in healthcare settings (HSE, 2013) are outlined below:

- Trips and falls.
- Exposure to materials or substances at work (e.g. soaps, disinfecting agents or latex).
- Spillages and/or chemical injuries.
- Needlestick injuries.
- Moving and handling incidents.
- Equipment failure.
- Procedural failure (e.g. resulting in the development of pressure ulcers, incorrect surgery and drug errors or hospital acquired infections).
- Workplace violence.

Indeed a survey (National NHS Staff Survey Co-ordination Centre, 2013) revealed that 29% of all staff and 33% of those working in acute hospital trusts said they had witnessed potentially harmful errors, near misses or incidents during a one month period.

The term 'risk management' refers to the process of identifying, assessing/evaluating and reporting risks in order to maintain the safety of patients, relatives and staff as well as improve the quality of patient care (RCN, 2003). Risk management is about practising safely and ensuring that the occurrence of harmful or adverse events is reduced by:

- anticipating and preventing potential problems;
- learning from incidents, near misses, patient complaints and litigation;
- introducing systems to help clinical staff reflect on and develop their practice.

The HSE (2014) have outlined a five-step process to risk assessment: (1) Identify the hazards; (2) Decide who might be harmed and how; (3) Evaluate the risks and decide on precautions; (4) Record findings and implement them; (5) Review assessment and update if necessary.

Nurses will need to ensure that risk assessment and management strategies are utilised and applied to both the clinical area and current work practices.

Critical Incident Reporting is a system which was introduced with the aim of improving patient safety. By thoroughly investigating an 'incident' the intention is for practitioners to learn from the event and put additional measures or solutions in place to ensure the situation is improved. However, fear of reprisals and sometimes a lack of understanding of how these should be reported can sometimes deter individuals from reporting incidents. Nevertheless, all nurses have a statutory duty to report concerns when they believe there is a potential danger to patients. You have a legal responsibility to ensure that no-one is harmed as a result of an act or omission on your part. Indeed it is important to remember that you can still be pursued for compensation as an individual even if what you are doing is part of your contractual duties and can be prosecuted for criminal damage or negligence. The NMC Code (2015: 11) demands that you 'make the care and safety of your patients your main concern and that you share information to identify and reduce risk and act immediately to put right the situation if someone has suffered actual harm for any reason'. This will involve documenting any concerns carefully as soon as possible, making sure that records are clearly signed, dated and timed and asking for additional help where necessary (e.g. from more senior staff and/or risk managers). Therefore familiarising yourself with local/national risk management policies and the role/functions of numerous patient safety agencies (outlined in Table 8.7) as well as required reporting systems is essential.

Table 8.7   Risk management agencies

National Patient Safety Agency (key functions and expertise for patient safety transferred to the NHS Commissioning Board Special Health Authority in 2012)	Lead and contribute to improved, safe patient care by *informing, supporting* and *influencing* organisations and people working in the health sector. Aim to identify and reduce risks to patients receiving NHS care and lead on national initiatives to improve patient safety.
NHS Litigation Authority	A not-for-profit part of the NHS that manages negligence and other claims against the NHS in England.
Care Quality Commission (CQC)	Statutory independent regulator of health and social care in England responsible for registering and monitoring services and regulating care provided by healthcare providers.
Medicines and Healthcare products Regulatory Agency (MHRA)	Regulates a wide range of materials from medicines and medical devices to blood and therapeutic products/ services that are derived from tissue engineering.
Health and Safety Executive	Enforces health and safety law in industrial workplaces.

When incidents occur it is important to ensure that lessons are learned to prevent the same incident occurring again or elsewhere. A *root cause analysis* framework can be helpful when trying to identify exactly what has happened and more importantly why. Getting to the root of the problem and understanding why something has happened will help to ensure that the real cause of the incident will be uncovered rather than just the details of the incident itself. You should then be able to focus on identifying and implementing solutions to improve the situation and ensure that the risk of it happening again is minimal. The National Patient Safety Agency (www.nrls.npsa.nhs.uk/rca/) and the

NHS Institute for Innovation and Improvement (www.institute.nhs.uk/quality_and_service_improvement_tools/) both provide an array of tools and templates that can be used to assist this process. The 'five whys' approach used in the example below is one of the simplest approaches as it is considered one of the easiest to learn and apply (NHS Institute of Innovation and Improvement, 2013a).

———— Root Cause Analysis using the five 'whys' approach ————
(NHS Institute, 2013a)

Step 1: Write down the details of the specific problem. This helps you formalise the problem and describe it accurately. It will also help the team focus on the same problem.

Step 2: Brainstorm to ask why the problem occurs and then write the answer down.

Step 3: If this answer doesn't identify the source of the problem, ask 'why?' again and write that answer down.

Step 4: Loop back to Step 3 until the team agrees that they have identified the problem's root cause. Again, this may take fewer or more than five 'whys?'

Case Scenario

 ### SABRINA

Practice nurse Sabrina is covering for a colleague who is ill. There is a busy nurse-led travel vaccination clinic taking place and several waiting patients have already complained due to the delays in their appointments as a result of staff shortages. As Sabrina is a little unfamiliar with the clinic processes – and in order to try to save time – a receptionist has offered to assist with the necessary paperwork (completing forms and checklists before sending the patients through to the treatment room). Sabrina rapidly calls the first patient into the treatment room and quickly checks the paperwork before administering the required injections. However, immediately after doing so she quickly realises that she has given the patient the wrong set of injections. The paperwork she looked at belonged to a different patient and had been mixed up in the process.
  Using the 'five whys' approach outlined above consider the following:

- What is the probable cause of the accident/incident?
- What are the underlying causes – if any?
- What immediate action should be taken?
- How could the incident have been prevented?
- Are there any other issues that need to be considered or addressed?

It is clear that several factors contributed to the incident above, for example staff shortages, escalating waiting times leading to patient complaints, unfamiliar processes, poor delegation and/or a lack of acknowledgement on Sabrina's part of her limitations. Obviously the most immediate action would be ensure that the patient had not come to any harm as a result of the mistake. It is also clear that measures could have been taken to prevent this (e.g. informing patients of staff shortages, rearranging appointments, ensuring the availability of appropriately experienced staff or even cancelling the clinic if necessary). Staff education, training and support are also issues that should be considered.

Tackling poor performance

All organisations should have internal mechanisms for investigating and dealing effectively with patient complaints or concerns (e.g. robust policies and procedures). Healthcare professionals also have a duty to report any concerns they may have about the quality of care in their organisation or indeed any other organisation with which they have contact (NMC, 2010). Raising and escalating concerns or 'whistleblowing' defines the act of bringing an important issue to the attention of someone in authority (Bach and Ellis, 2011). Normally in the first instance this would involve informing senior staff or clinical leaders. If unresolved, additional external mechanisms – e.g. reporting concerns to the Care Quality Commission – may also be implemented, although if this is necessary it is advisable to follow your organisation's published whistle-blowing procedures (NQB, 2013). In all instances where practice or procedures are brought into question, clear and comprehensive records will be crucial in determining what has happened. Good record keeping, as well as being a duty of professional practice (NMC, 2015), will also protect staff too.

In your role as a clinical leader you will be responsible for supporting junior staff to fulfil their own professional obligations. Occasionally you may also need to investigate concerns about the behaviour or clinical practice of others in your team. However, fear and mistrust could lead to staff keeping quiet and not reporting concerns. Therefore as a nurse leader one of your key aims should be to build an effective organisational culture in which there is trust and accountability amongst members of your team, fostering a culture of openness and transparency in order to build an atmosphere where all staff are encouraged to identify and report unsafe conditions within a 'non-blame' culture (Francis, 2015).

STOP AND THINK

The Royal College of Nursing's Principles of Nursing Practice (RCN, 2010) set out what patients, colleagues, families and carers can expect from nurses.

- What factors could contribute to situations where nurses might fail to meet such expectations?
- Are you confident about the quality of care that you and your colleagues deliver?
- If so, what evidence do you have that this is the case?
- If not, what can you do about it?

Patient experience

> Quality care is care which looks to give the individual as positive an experience of receiving and recovering from the care as possible, including being treated according to what that individual wants or needs with compassion, dignity and respect. (NQB, 2013: 13)

Patients and service users are being encouraged to take more control of their own care (Department of Health, 2009) and they have an important part to play in determining how services are designed, implemented and evaluated (The Kings Fund, 2012). By collaborating closely with service users and responding appropriately to their feedback, nurses can deliver more appropriate care and ensure that any concerns raised are dealt with quickly and appropriately (Coulter, 2012). This will usually involve collecting and using information provided by patients (e.g. patient satisfaction surveys or focus groups) in order to deliver the kind of services that patients want. Whichever approach is used, the key aim is to find out what patients really think about the services we provide and provide supporting evidence of this.

Ultimately it is very rewarding when you receive compliments from patients about their care. However, unfortunately from time to time complaints will also feature and when they arise it is important to ensure that they are not ignored.

STOP AND THINK

Think of some examples currently used in your practice setting to elicit patient feedback:

- How effective are these methods?
- How is the feedback used?

In summary the following list of factors are critical in assuring the quality of patients' experience of care (Luxford et al., 2011):

- Strong and committed senior leadership.
- Communication of the strategic vision.
- Engagement of patients and families.
- A sustained focus on employee satisfaction.
- Regular measurement and feedback reporting.
- Adequate resourcing for care delivery design.
- Building staff capacity to support patient-centred care.
- Accountability and an incentives culture – strongly supportive of change and learning.

Leading and managing change and service improvement

In order for us to be able to deliver safe and effective person-centred healthcare in a timely and efficient manner we need to continually improve the way we work.

However it sometimes seems that healthcare provision in the UK is constantly changing and this can be unsettling for everyone. Yet change is an integral part of service improvement and being able to live with and manage change is an essential skill. Moreover, as a nurse you have a professional responsibility to make a positive contribution towards shaping a healthcare environment that promotes excellent care and patient satisfaction (NMC, 2015).

Local – small scale:	Medium scale:	Large organisational scale:
e.g. protected patient meal or rest times	e.g. The Productive Ward Programme (NHS Institute for Innovation and Improvement)	e.g. Health and Social Care Bill and Reconfiguration of the NHS

Figure 8.1　Scales of leadership

Improving the quality of nursing care and services involves 'the combined and unceasing efforts of everyone to make the changes that will lead to better patient outcomes (health), better system performance (care) and better professional development (learning)' (Batalden and Davidoff, 2007: 2).

Service or quality improvement projects can vary from local small-scale schemes to the complete redesign of an organisation (Figure 8.1). As a nurse you will be in an ideal position to identify opportunities to make a positive difference to patient care or the working environment, perhaps getting involved in numerous service improvement initiatives or even taking the lead on change management projects.

Whilst the reasons for change in healthcare settings are numerous, the focus should always be on improving services for patients. This will often include the introduction of new policies and guidelines (in line with an emerging evidence base), new technology and equipment, changes to the workforce/team and effective resource management. Whatever the circumstances, being able to 'think differently' about care delivery options is considered a crucial skill for future healthcare leaders (Bevan, 2013).

ACTIVITY 8.4

Closely observing the care that is delivered to patients within a chosen healthcare setting:

- Record the care processes (from a patient perspective) that are encountered throughout the day (e.g. waiting times, provision of patient information, contact with other healthcare professionals, investigations and procedures performed).
- Now identify those aspects of care which could be improved.

When attempting to make improvements you should try to ensure that your goals are SMART (Blanchard and Johnson, 1982):

- Specific-focused – specific objectives are much easier to manage and execute.
- Measureable – you must be able to measure the extent to which your objective has been achieved.
- Attainable – goals within reach but challenging enough to motivate.
- Relevant – goals aligned to professional or organisational goals.
- Timely – goals have target dates which monitor and maintain progression.

Change management and service improvement are complex and demanding processes and it is worth remembering that seeking to change or improve services will always have an impact on someone. Having a critical understanding of the key issues, influencing factors and potential barriers is crucial if you are going to succeed in managing change and improving services within healthcare settings.

Moreover, there are many various change management approaches suggested in the literature and these can often appear contradictory or confusing. For example, some advocate a *planned* (proactive) approach which involves moving from one stage to another in a pre-planned and deliberate manner (see for example Lewin, 1951; Bullock and Batten, 1985). Others argue that change can also be *unplanned* (emergent/reactive) or ad hoc – particularly in rapidly changing environments or when triggered by organisational crisis – and that change will always contain complex emergent elements (Olson and Eoyang, 2001) especially in large-scale projects. Approaches can also be top down (from management downwards) or bottom up (generated by frontline staff upwards). Pearson et al. (2008) suggest that both can be successful in disseminating nursing interventions depending upon the requirements and circumstances.

The *Plan, Do, Study, Act* (PDSA) *cycle* (Langley et al., 2009) is advocated for use by the NHS Institute for Innovation and Improvement when attempting to test new change ideas on a small scale by temporarily trialling a change and assessing the impact. For example:

- Trying out a new way to make appointments for one consultant or clinic.
- Trying out a new patient information sheet with a selected group of patients before introducing the change to all clinics or patient groups.

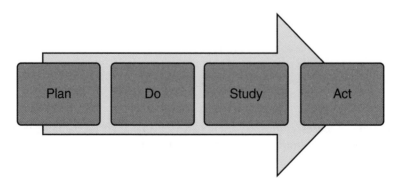

Figure 8.2   Plan, Do, Study, Act Cycle

Source: Langley et al. (2009)

By building on the learning from these test cycles in a structured way, new ideas can be put in place with a greater chance of success.

Another useful approach is the 'Six-stage Framework for Service Improvement' (see Table 8.8) (NHS Institute for Innovation and Improvement, 2013c).

Resistance to change

Service improvement and change management would be relatively easy if everyone involved readily accepted the need for change and supported the development. However it is never that simple – not everyone will be willing or interested. Changing entrenched clinical styles can be a difficult and lengthy process. Defensive reactions from colleagues, a lack of awareness, incentives or training, time pressures and a fear of losing power can all act as barriers (Coulter, 2012). The organisational culture, changes in roles and responsibilities, and policy shifts, can also affect the outcome of improvement work.

Table 8.8   Six-stage Framework for Service Improvement

Phase	Aim
1. Start out	To establish a rationale for any improvement work and obtain support from stakeholders.
2. Define and scope	To ensure the project starts in the right areas and develop a project structure to provide a solid foundation.
3. Measure and understand	To measure the current situation and understand the level of change required to achieve the defined aims and objectives.
4. Design and plan	To design and plan the activities required to achieve the objectives that have been established.
5. Pilot and implement	To test proposed changes via pilots before changes are implemented fully.
6. Sustain and share	To ensure changes that have been implemented are sustained and shared to aid learning.

According to Silber (1993), the degree of resistance for each individual will often depend upon four factors:

- Their flexibility to change.
- Their evaluation of the immediate situation.
- Their anticipated consequences of the change.
- Their perception of what they have to lose and or gain.

It is important to recognise that not all key stakeholders are to be found within your immediate colleagues. Other barriers include organisational politics and conflict which sometimes cannot be easily identified or resolved. Therefore in order to progress with a change idea all the driving and restraining forces need to be identified (Lewin, 1951). Various types of forces that you will need to consider include:

- available resources/funding/costs;
- current targets;
- current and past practices;
- the vested interests of stakeholders;

- the attitudes of stakeholders and those who will be affected by the proposed change;
- regulations, policies and procedures (e.g. DH initiatives or local Trust policies);
- the organisational structures/traditions and/or culture;
- relationships;
- personal and/or group needs;
- the values of both the organisation and individuals;
- opportunities;
- productivity.

Focus upon a single aspect of care that you identified in the previous Stop and Think and chose a a recognised change management analysis tool from the NHS Improving Quality website (www.nhsiq.nhs.uk/resource-search/improvement-tools.aspx). Use your chosen tool to help you identify the driving and restraining forces that could impact upon any proposed change.

The identification of key stakeholders and their potential influence or resistance is somewhat crucial in helping to determine their fears and concerns as well as identifying potential difficulties. In order to be able to overcome resistance you will not only have to create interest in the proposed project you will also have to be prepared to face up to and win over the sceptics. Porter-O'Grady (2003) argues that leader or manager behaviour is the single most important factor in how people in an organisation accept change. The most successful change agents are those who possess the essential knowledge, skills and attributes for effective leadership and management.

Strategies to enhance change

By (2005) provides a useful critical review of organisational change management exploring the differences in approaches but concludes that there is still a lack of underpinning evidence to suggest the best approach in any given situation and suggests that more robust research is needed to evaluate organisational change management frameworks. This is particularly vital when considering change involving healthcare organisations. Traditional approaches – for example those suggested by Lewin (1951) and Bullock and Batten (1985) – are now viewed as simplistic and whilst some would argue that they are still relevant today, emergent approaches (e.g. Kanter et al., 1992; Kotter, 1996) acknowledging the complexity of working with individuals within multi-faceted organisations are considered more appropriate.

Lockitt (2004) suggests that there are five broad strategies for affecting change, each having its advantages, disadvantages and potential effects.

The *participative* strategy outlined in Table 8.9 reflects the view of Kouzes and Posner (2007) who maintain that having a leadership or management style which generates a shared purpose is the most effective strategy to ensure success. They identify the following five leadership behaviours which contribute to a leader's ability to engage and

Table 8.9 Strategies for affecting change

Strategy	Advantages	Disadvantages	Potential Effects
Directive: change is usually imposed by managers with little or no consultation with others (i.e. those affected).	Can be implemented quickly.	Fails to take into consideration the views and feelings of those involved in or affected by the change.	May lead to valuable information or ideas being missed. May cause resentment from staff and those affected.
Expert: management of change is seen as a problem-solving process that needs to be resolved by an 'expert'. Change is normally led by specialist project team or manager.	The 'experts' play a major role in finding the solution and often the solution can be implemented quickly as a small number of 'experts' are involved.	Those affected may have different views from those of the 'experts' and may not appreciate the solution being imposed or the outcomes of the changes made.	May cause resentment from staff and those affected.
Negotiating: recognises the willingness to negotiate and bargain in order to affect change.	Those affected by the change have an opportunity to have a say in what changes are made, how they are implemented and the expected outcomes, therefore feeling more involved and more supportive of the changes made.	Negotiating effectively takes time and the outcomes cannot be predicted.	Adjustments and concessions may be required in order to implement change therefore the final changes may not meet the total expectation of the change agent.
Educative: involves changing people's values and beliefs in order for them to fully support the proposed change. Involves a mixture of activities including persuasion, education, training and selection and led by in-house experts.	Encourages the development of a shared set of organisational values that individuals are willing and able to support.	Takes longer to implement change.	Involves a mixture of activities including persuasion, education, training and selection and is led by in-house experts.
Participative: involves all those affected by anticipated changes. Driven less by managers and more by groups or individuals within an organisation.	All views taken into account before change is made. Any changes made are more likely to be supported due to the involvement of all those affected. The commitment of individuals and groups within the organisation will increase as those individuals and groups feel ownership over the changes being implemented.	Can be time consuming and costly due to the number of meetings needed etc. Outcomes cannot be accurately predicted.	The organisation and individuals also have the opportunity to learn from this experience and will know more about the organisation and how it functions, thus increasing their skills, knowledge and effectiveness to the organisation.

Source: Lockett (2004)

empower others, some of which are considered crucial when attempting to affect change within the NHS and other healthcare settings:

- *Modelling the way* – Involves identifying and clarifying shared values (e.g. the application of evidence-based practice and the provision of an excellent standard of patient care) and then setting an example for others to follow. To be able to do this effectively requires an ability to identify new opportunities, the confidence to be able to speak up, to share fresh ideas and demonstrate commitment to supporting others in making the change by creating opportunities (e.g. setting interim goals to achieve small wins whilst working towards larger objectives using pilot studies or small trials).

- *Inspiring a shared vision* – Involves creating a shared picture of how things might be better with the change imposed. The leader needs to be able to inspire others by making the 'shared vision' appeal to a wider audience. Carefully exploring the interests and aspirations of others, listening to their views and finding a common ground to ensure that the 'vision' is shaped, shared and agreed by team members will help everyone involved to develop a strong sense of ownership. The ability to build coalitions of support and counter resistance to change is considered crucial to success (The Kings Fund, 2012) and the healthcare leader will play a key role in enabling others in the system to contribute their views, expertise and ideas.

- *Challenging the process* – Change often involves taking carefully considered risks and it is therefore important for a leader to be able to develop a supportive climate/culture (Larson and LaFasto, 1989) where trying out new approaches is considered normal and safe experimentation is encouraged (e.g. using an example from practice where a change when implemented did not work out). Mistakes and failures – whilst disappointing – are a key component of success as learning from these helps individuals to progress.

- *Enabling others to act* – Rogers (2003) suggested that a common process occurs as people adopt a new idea. He identified five categories of adopters of an innovation: innovators (eager and adventurous), early adopters (respected opinion leaders), early majority (may deliberate for some time), late majority (sceptical and cautious) and laggards (traditionalists who prefer to do things as they have always done) – all of whom will have an impact on success. It is clear that a variety of approaches may be needed to engage with all those involved as implementing the 'vision' will require collaboration over an extended period. Regularly reviewing and recognising the contribution of others as you go – encouraging, empowering and sometimes challenging all those involved – can help to develop confidence and competence and in turn generate an overall climate of trust. However, this will often require tolerance and empathy, showing sensitivity to the needs of others to make everyone feel included (Northouse, 2012).

- *Encouraging the heart* – Successfully managing change in healthcare organisations often involves a lot of hard work and dedication. People can frequently lose heart, particularly if there are no quick wins. Recognition of your own achievements and those of your colleagues (however small) helps to keep optimism and determination alive. Giving praise to others also shows that their support and commitment have been noticed and appreciated. This can involve something as simple as passing an encouraging comment or something a little more 'showy', such as public praise in team meetings, celebration events or 'telling the story'.

Bate et al. (2004) consider the act of connecting and engaging with others as crucial in order to effect change in healthcare settings. Their arguments (based upon *social movement theory*) are leading a new way of thinking that has helped to develop a number of wide-ranging initiatives aimed at speeding up the diffusion and adoption of innovation across the country in the hope of improving and sustaining patient outcomes. One such approach is the introduction of the NHS Change Model (NHS Improving Quality, 2013) which has been created to support the NHS and adopt 'a shared approach to leading change and transformation'. This model draws upon eight key components:

- Our shared purpose.
- Leadership for change.
- Spread of innovation.
- Improvement methodology.
- Rigorous delivery.
- Transparent measurement.
- System drivers.
- Engagement to mobilise.

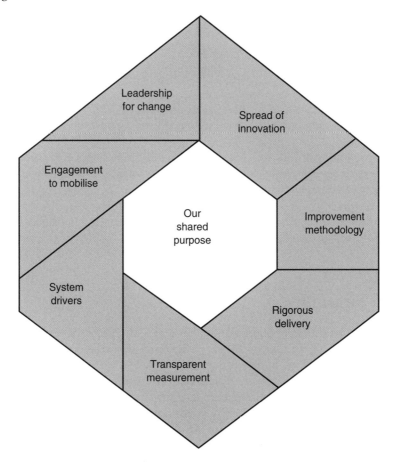

Figure 8.3   NHS Change Model

Available at: www.changemodel.nhs.uk

Source: NHS Improving Quality (2013).

By acknowledging the complexity of change management we recognise there is no prescribed linear order to the change process. Instead the framework encourages leaders of change to consider and focus upon a number of key interacting factors, ensuring that all the components are aligned for sustained success.

Whichever model or framework you choose to use, understanding the nature of the change or improvement you wish to make and the context in which you are working is important in determining your chosen approach. Having a clear understanding of the people, processes and organisational culture which will be affected by your change is considered crucial to success. Burnes (1996: 13) believes that 'successful change is less dependent on detailed plans and projections than on reaching an understanding of the complexity of the issues concerned and identifying the range of available options'. Whilst this seems a most sensible approach to take research demonstrates that such factors are often overlooked, ignored or underestimated by those wishing to implement change (Kotter, 1996; Fernandez and Rainey, 2006). It is vital to also remember that any changes to services should always take into account the needs of patients and clients first and foremost. Targets require constant monitoring and revising if necessary to remain valid and meaningful. Therefore evaluation is an essential part of this process whether or not the change has achieved the desired outcome.

ACTIVITY 8.5

- Make a list of the skills and attributes you think could be helpful when attempting to implement change within a healthcare setting and explain how and why they would be useful.
- Critically reflect upon your own change management skills and identify areas for personal development/improvement that will positively impact on multi-professional care delivery to service users.
- Consider how each of the 6Cs outlined in the Chief Nursing Officer's Strategy (Cummings and Bennett, 2012) relate to the role of leaders and managers in current healthcare settings.

Chapter summary

There is a huge cultural shift underway which places the needs of service users rather than those of the organisation at the very heart of services. The numerous current demands placed upon us as nurses sometimes challenge our ability to maintain – let alone improve – patient care. However, nurses in particular will remain the first line of defence in the safeguarding of quality care and patient protection. There is evidence to suggest that effective leadership is positively associated with improved patient outcomes (Wong et al., 2013). Therefore the need for strong, effective nurse leadership throughout the whole organisation has never been greater. However, leadership and management activities are complex and multifaceted, with many differing theories advocating essential skills, desirable attributes and approaches. It seems that the most effective leaders and managers are those who will be able to use an entire range of different skills in order to bring about the necessary service improvements. They will often rely on developing valuable relationships with others and applying well-developed leadership skills to underpin the use of recognised change management and quality improvement tools and techniques to improve care within their own sphere of influence.

Suggested further reading

1000 Lives Plus (2011b) *The Quality Improvement Guide: Nursing Edition*. Cardiff: 1000 Lives Plus.
Department of Health (2007) *Building a Safer NHS for Patients: Implementing an Organisation with a Memory*. London: DH.
Department of Health, Social Services and Public Safety (2011) *Quality 2020: A Ten-year strategy to Protect and Improve Quality in Health and Social Care in Northern Ireland*. Belfast: DHSSPS.
Gage, W. (2013) 'Using service improvement methodology to change practice', *Nursing Standard*, 27 (23): 51–7.
Healthcare Improvement Scotland (2013a) *Improvement and Implementation Support* Available at: www.healthcareimprovementscotland.org (last accessed 17 March 2015).
Healthcare Improvement Scotland (2013b) *Scottish Patient Safety Programme* Available at: www. healthcareimprovementscotland.org (last accessed 17 March 2015).
Huber, D.L. (2010) *Leadership and Nursing Care Management*. Missouri, IL: Elsevier.
Kouzes J.M. and Posner, B.Z. (2006) *A Leader's Legacy*. San Francisco, CA: Jossey Bass.
Northouse, P.G. (2013) *Leadership*, 6th edition. Thousand Oaks, CA: Sage.
NICE (2013a) *NICE Quality Standards and indicators* Available at: www.nice.org.uk/standards-and-indicators (last accessed 17 March 2015).
Royal College of Nursing (2003) *Clinical Governance: An RCN Resource Guide*. London: RCN.
Royal College of Nursing (2007) *Developing and Sustaining Effective Teams*. London: RCN. (A really useful guide which includes activities and tools to assist in team development.)
Royal College of Nursing (2011) *Accountability and Delegation: What You Need To Know*. London: RCN.
Scottish Government (2010) *The Healthcare Quality Strategy for NHS Scotland*. Edinburgh: Scottish Government.

Useful web-based resources

Healthcare Improvement Scotland: www.healthcareimprovementscotland.org.
Improving Quality Together NHS Wales: www.iqt.wales.nhs.uk/home
NHS Improving Quality (NHS IQ) NHS England : www.england.nhs.uk/ourwork/qual-clin-lead/nhsiq/
The Regulation and Quality Improvement Authority (Northern Ireland): www.rqia.org.uk/

References

Adair, J. (2009) *Effective Leadership: How to be a Successful Leader*. London: Pan Macmillan.
Almost, J. (2006) 'Conflict within nursing work environments: concept analysis', *Journal of Advanced Nursing*, 53(4): 444–53.
Almost, J., Doran, D.M., McGillis Hall, L.M. and Spence Laschinger, H.K. (2010) 'Antecedents and consequences of intra-group conflict among nurses', *Journal of Nursing Management*, 18: 981–992.
Bach, S. and Ellis, P. (2011) *Leadership, Management and Team Working in Nursing*. Exeter: Learning Matters.
Barr, J. and Dowding, L. (2012) *Leadership in Healthcare*, 2nd edition. London: Sage.

Bass, B.M. (1990) *Bass and Stodgill's Handbook of Leadership: Theory, Research and Managerial Application*, 3rd edition. New York: Free Press.

Batalden P.B. and Davidoff, F. (2007) 'What is "quality improvement" and how can it transform healthcare?', *Quality and Safety in Healthcare*, 16: 2–3.

Bate, P., Bevan, H. and Robert, G. (2004) *Towards a Million Change Agents: A Review of the Social Movements Literature: Implications for Large Scale Change in the NHS*. London: NHS Modernisation Agency.

Bennett, K. and Sawatzky, J.V. (2013) 'Building emotional intelligence: a strategy for emerging nurse leaders to reduce workplace bullying', *Nursing Administration Quarterly*, 37 (2): 144–51.

Bennis, W. (1994) *On Becoming a Leader*. Boston, MA: Addison-Wesley.

Bevan, H. (2013) *What Can Civil Rights Leaders Teach us about Strategy for Transformation?* [Online Blog]. Available at: www.hsj.co.uk/opinion/blogs/the-nhs-change-agent/the-nhs-change-agent/5003114.bloglead (last accessed 2 September 2013).

Blake, R. and Mouton, J. (1964) *The Managerial Grid: The Key to Leadership Excellence*. Houston, TX: Gulf.

Blanchard, K. and Johnson, S. (1982) *The One Minute Manager*. New York: William Morrow and Company.

Blanchard, K., Zigarmi, D. and Nelson, R. (1993) 'Situational Leadership after 25 years: a retrospective', *Journal of Leadership Studies*, 1 (1): 22–36.

Brinkert, R. (2010) 'A literature review of conflict communication causes, costs, benefits and interventions in nursing', *Journal of Nursing Management*, 18: 145–56.

Bullock, R.J. and Batten, D. (1985) '"It's just a phase we're going through": a review and synthesis of OD phase analysis', *Group and Organization Studies* , 10 (December): 383–412.

Burnes, B. (1996) 'No such thing as … a 'one best way' to manage organizational change', *Management Decision*, 34, 10: 11–18.

Burnes, B. (2004) *Managing Change: A Strategic Approach to Organisational Dynamics*, 4th edition. Harlow: Prentice Hall.

By, R.T. (2005) 'Organisational change management: a critical review, *Journal of Change Management*, 5 (4): 369–80.

Care Quality Commission (2010) *Essential Standards for Quality and Safety*. London: CQC.

Care Quality Commission (2012) *The State of Healthcare and Adult Social Care in England*. London: CQC.

Care Quality Commission (2014*) Barts NHS Trust Quality Report*. London: CQC.

Carsten, M.K., Uhl-Bien, M., West, B.J., Patera, J.L. and McGregor, R. (2010) 'Exploring social constructions of followership:a qualitative study', *The Leadership Quarterly*, 21: 543–62.

Carter, M., Thompson, N., Crampton, P., Morrow, G., Burford, B., Gray, C. and Illing, J. (2013) 'Workplace bullying in the UK NHS: a questionnaire and interview study on prevalence, impact and barriers to reporting', *British Medical Journal Open*, 3 (6): 1–12.

Chaleff, I. (2009) *The Courageous Follower: Standing up to and for Our Leaders*. San Francisco, CA: Berrett-Koehler.

Ciulla, J.B. (2003) *The Ethics of Leadership*. Belmont, CA: Wadsworth/Thompson Learning.

Coulter, A. (2012) *Leadership for Patient Engagement* [online]. Available at: www.kingsfund.org.uk/leadershipreview (last accessed 18 April 2012).

Cowden, T., Cummings, G. and Profetto-McGrath, J. (2011) 'Leadership practices and staff nurses intent to stay: a systematic review', *Journal of Nursing Management*, 19: 461–77.

Cummings, J. and Bennett, V. (2012) *Compassion in Practice: Nursing, Midwifery and Care Staff: Our Strategy*. Leeds: NHS Commissioning Board.

Department of Health (1998) *A First Class Service Quality in the New NHS*. London: DH. Available at: http://webarchive.nationalarchives.gov.uk/+/www.dh.gov.uk/en/publicationsandstatistics/publications/publicationspolicyandguidance/dh_4006902 (last accessed 26 March 2015).

Department of Health (2009) *The NHS Constitution for England*. London: DH.

Department of Health (2010a) *Equity and Excellence: Liberating the NHS*. London: DH.

Department of Health (2010b) *Liberating the NHS: Legislative Framework and Next Steps*. London: DH.

Department of Health (2012a) *The NHS Outcomes Framework 2013–14*. London: DH.

Department of Health (2012b) *The Public Health Outcomes Framework for England, 2013–2016*. London: DH.

Department of Health (2013) *Adult Social Care Outcomes Framework*. London: DH.

Dimond, B. (2005) *Legal Aspects of Nursing*, 4th edition. Harlow: Pearson Education.

Donabedian, A. (2005) 'Evaluating the quality of medical care 1966', *The Milbank Quarterly*, 83 (4): 691–729.

Duddle, M. and Boughton, M. (2007) 'Intra-professional relations in nursing', *Journal of Advanced Nursing*, 59(1), 29–37.

Fayol, F. (1916) *General and Industrial Management*. London: Pitman.

Fernandez, R. and Rainey, H.G. (2006) 'Managing successful organisational change in the public sector', *Public Administration Review*, March/April: 168–76.

Fiedler, F.E. (1967) *A Theory of Leadership Effectiveness*. New York: McGraw-Hill.

Francis, R. (2010) *Mid Staffordshire NHS Foundation Trust Inquiry*. London: HMSO.

Francis, R. (2015) *Freedom to Seak Up. An Independent Review into Creating an Open and Honest Reporting Culture in the NHS*. Available at: https://freedomtospeakup.org.uk/wp-content/uploads/2014/07/F2SU_web.pdf (last accessed 3 March 2015).

French, J.P.R. Jr. and Raven, B. (1960) 'The bases of social power'. In D. Cartwright and A. Zander (eds), *Group Dynamics*. New York: Harper & Row. pp. 607–23.

Friedman, R.A., Tidd, S.T., Currall, S.C. and Tsai, J.C. (2000) 'What goes around comes around: the impact of personal conflict style on work conflict and stress', *International Journal of Conflict Management*, 11: 32–55.

Goleman, D. (1995) *Emotional Intelligence: Why It Can Matter More Than IQ*. New York: Bantam.

Greenleaf, R.K. (1977) *Servant Leadership: A Journey into the Nature of Legitimate Power and Greatness*. New York: Paulist.

Hardacre, J., Cragg, R., Shapiro, J., Spurgeon, P. and Flanagan, H. (2011) *What's Leadership got to do with it?* London: The Health Foundation.

Hasson, F., McKenna, H.P. and Keeney, S. (2013) 'Delegating and supervising unregistered professionals: the student nurse experience', *Nurse Education Today*, 33 (3): 229–35.

Health and Safety Executive (2013) *Health and Safety in Human Health and Social Care in Great Britain 2013. Work-related Injuries and Ill Health*. Available at: www.hse.gov.uk/statistics/industry/healthservices (last accessed 22 February 2015).

Health and Safety Executive (2014) *Five Steps to Risk Assessment*. Belfast.

Hersey, P. and Blanchard, K.H. (1977) *Management of Organisational Behaviour: Utilising Human Resources*, 3rd edition. New Jersey: Prentice Hall.

Hersey, P. and Blanchard, K.H. (1988) *Management of Organizational Behavior*, 5th edition. New Jersey: Prentice Hall.

Hewison, A. and Griffiths, M. (2004) 'Leadership development in healthcare: a word of caution', *Journal of Health Organisation and Management*, 18 (6): 464–73.

Huber, D.L. (2010) *Leadership and Nursing Care Management*, 4th edition. Missouri, IL: Elsevier.

Hutchinson, D., Brown, J. and Longworth, K. (2012) 'Attracting and maintaining the Y Generation in nursing: a literature review', *Journal of Nursing Management*, 20 (4): 444–50.

Iles, V. and Sutherland, K. (2001) *Managing Change in the NHS: Organisational Change: A Review for Healthcare Managers, Professionals and Researchers*. London: London School of Hygiene and Tropical Medicine.

International Council of Nurses (2007) 'Positive practice environments: Quality workplaces = quality patient care'. Information and Action Tool Kit. Geneva, Switzerland: ICN

Kanter, R.M., Stein, B.A. and Jick, T.D. (1992) *The Challenge of Organizational Change*. New York: The Free Press.

Kennedy, I. (2001) Bristol Royal Infirmary Inquiry, 'The report of the public inquiry into children's heart surgery at the Bristol Royal Infirmary 1984–1995: Learning from Bristol'. London: HMSO.

Kotter, J.P. (1996) *Leading Change*. Boston, MA: Harvard Business School Press.

Kouzes, J. and Posner, B. (2007) *The Leadership Challenge*, 4th edition. San Francisco, CA: Jossey-Bass.

Langley, G.L., Nolan, K.M., Nolan T.W., Norman C.L. and Provost L.P. (2009) *The Improvement Guide: A Practical Approach to Enhancing Organizational Performance*, 2nd edition. San Francisco, CA: Jossey-Bass.

Large, S., Macleod, A., Cunningham, G. and Kitson, A. (2005) *A Multiple-case Study Evaluation of the RCN Clinical Leadership Programme in England*. London: Royal College of Nursing.

Larson, C.E. and LaFasto, F.M.J. (1989) *Teamwork: What Must Go Right, What Can Go Wrong*. London: Sage.

Leiter, M.P., Price, S.L. and Spence Lashinger, H.K. (2010) 'Generational differences in distress, attitudes and incivility among nurses', *Journal of Nursing Management,* 18: 970–80.

Lewin K. (1951) *Field Theory in Social Science*, New York: Harper and Row.

Lockitt, W. (2004) *Change Management*. Available at: www.scribd.com/doc/50615816/CHANGE-MANAGEMENT (last accessed 30 August 2013).

Lucas, B. and Buckley, T. (2009) 'Leadership for quality improvement– what does it really take?', *International Journal of Leadership in Public Services*, 5 (1): 37–46.

Luxford, K., Safran, D.B. and Delbanco, T. (2011) 'Promoting patient-centered care: a qualitative study of facilitators and barriers in healthcare organizations with a reputation for improving the patient experience', *International Journal for Quality in Healthcare*: 1–6.

Maintz, J. (2003) 'Defining and classifying clinical indicators for quality improvement', *International Journal for Quality in Healthcare*, 15 (6): 523–30.

Marquis, B.L. and Huston, C.J. (2006) *Leadership Roles and Management Functions in Nursing: Theory and Application*, 5th edition. Philadelphia: Lippincott.

Mayo, E. (1949) *Hawthorne and the Western Electrical Company: The Social Problems of an Industrial Civilisation*. London: Routledge and Kegan Paul.

McGregor, D. (1960) *The Human Side of Enterprise*. New York: McGraw Hill.

National Council of State Boards of Nursing (1997) *The Five Rights of Delegation*. Available at: www.dads.state.tx.us/qualitymatters/qcp/nursedelegation/fiverights.pdf (last accessed 3 March 2015).

National NHS Staff Survey Co-ordination Centre (2013) *Issues highlighted by the 2013 NHS Staff Survey England.*

National Quality Board (2013) *Quality in the New Health System: Maintaining and Improving Quality* (Final Report). Available at: www.gov.uk/government/uploads/system/uploads/attachment_data/file/213304/Final-NQB-report-v4-160113.pdf (last accessed 5 September 2013).

NHS Alliance (2003) *Vision in Practice Revisited: Holding the NHS at the Edge of Chaos*. Available at: www.nhsalliance.org/wp-content/uploads/2013/06/2003-Vision-in-Practice-revisited-holding-the-NHS-at-the-edge-of-chaos.1.pdf (last accessed 20 September 2013).

NHS Institute for Innovation and Improvement (2012) *Putting Patients First: The Productive Series*. NHS Institute for Innovation and Improvement. Available at: www.institute.nhs.uk/productives (last accessed 2 March 2015).

NHS Improving Quality (2013) *The NHS Change Model*. Available at: www.nhsiq.nhs.uk/capacity-capability/nhs-change-model.aspx (last accessed 3 March 2015).

NHS Institute for Innovation and Improvement (2013a) *Root Cause Analysis: Using the Five 'Whys' Approach*. Available at: www.institute.nhs.uk/quality_and_service_improvement_tools/quality_and_service_improvement_tools/identifying_problems_-_root_cause_analysis_using5_whys.html (last accessed 7 March 2014).

NHS Institute for Innovation and Improvement (2013b) *PDSA Cycle*. Available at: www.institute.nhs.uk/quality_and_service_improvement_tools/quality_and_service_improvement_tools/plan_do_study_act.html (last accessed 7 March 2014).

NHS Institute for Innovation and Improvement (2013c) *Six-stage Framework for Service Improvement*. Available at: www.institute.nhs.uk/quality_and_service_improvement_tools/ quality_and_service_improvement_tools/ (last accessed 7 March 2014).

NHS Leadership Academy (2014a) *Why does Leadership in the NHS Need to Change?* Available at: www.leadershipacademy.nhs.uk/about/ (accessed 19 November 2014).

NHS Leadership Academy (2014b) *Programmes-Developing Better Leaders, Delivering Better Care*. Available at: www.leadershipacademy.nhs.uk/programmes/ (accessed 19 November 2014).

NHS Leadership Academy (2014c) *Healthcare Leadership Model*. Available at: www.leadership academy.nhs.uk/resources/healthcare-leadership-model/ (last acessed 19 November 2014).

NHS Leadership Academy (2015) *Healthcare Leadership Model*. Available at: www.leadershipacademy. nhs.uk/resources/healthcare-leadership-model (last acessed 22 February 2014).

Northouse, P.G. (2012) *Introduction to Leadership Concepts and Practice*, 2nd edition. London: Sage.

Nursing and Midwifery Council (2010a) *Standards for Pre-registration Nursing Education (Competency Framework)*. Available at: www.nmc-uk.org/Educators/Standards-for-education/ (last accessed 18 February 2014).

Nursing and Midwifery Council (2010b) *Standards for Competence for Registered Nurses*. Available at: www.nmc-uk.org/Documents/Standards/Standards%20for%20competence.pdf. (accessed 19 November 2014).

Nursing and Midwifery Council (2015) *The Code: Professional Standards of Practice Behaviour for Nurses and Midwives*. London: NMC.

Olmstead, J (2013), The cure for workplace bullying, Nursing Management, 44(11): 53–55.

Olson, E.E. and Eoyang, G.H. (2001) *Facilitating Organizational Change: Lessons from Complexity Science*. San Francisco, CA: Jossey-Bass/Pfeiffer.

Onyett, S. (2012) 'Creating a culture to deliver compassionate care', *Nursing Times,* 108 (14/15).

Pearson, M.L., Upenieks, V.V., Yee, T. and Needleman, J. (2008) 'Spreading nursing unit innovation in large hospital systems', *Journal of Nursing Administration*, 38 (3): 146–52.

Porter-O'Grady, T. (2003) 'A different age for leadership, part 1', *Journal of Nursing Administration,* 33(10): 105–10.

Rogers, E.M. (2003) *Diffusion of Innovations*. New York: Free Press.

Royal College of Nursing (2003) *Clinical Governance: A RCN Resource Guide*. London: RCN.

Royal College of Nursing (2009) *Breaking Down Barriers, Driving Up Standards: The Role of the Ward Sister and Charge Nurse*. London: RCN.

Royal College of Nursing (2010) *The Principles of Nursing Practice*. Available at: www.rcn.org. uk/development/practice/principles (last accessed 21 February 2014).

Royal College of Nursing (2011) *Accountability and Delegation: What You Need To Know*. London: RCN.

Royal College of Nursing (2013) *Beyond Breaking Point*. London: RCN.

Scrivener R. et al. (2011) 'Accountability and responsibility: principle of nursing practice B', *Nursing Standard*, 25(29): 35–6.

Senge, P.M. (1990) *The Fifth Discipline: The Art and Practice of the Learning Organization*. London: Random House/Doubleday.

Sherwood, G. (2003) 'Leadership for a healthy work environment: caring for the human spirit', *Nurse Leader*, Sept/Oct: 36–40.

Sieloff, C.L. and Wallace Raph, S. (2011) 'Nursing theory and management (editorial)', *Journal of Nursing Management*, 19: 979–80.

Silber, M.B. (1993) 'The 'Cs' in excellence: choice and change', *Nursing Management,* 24 (9): 60–2.

Squires, M., Tourangeau, A., Spence Laschinger, H.K. and Doran, D. (2010) 'The link between leadership and safety outcomes in hospital', *Journal of Nursing Management*, 18: 914–25.

Stanley, D. (2010) 'Multigenerational workforce issues and their implications for leadership in nursing', *Journal of Nursing Management*, 18 (7): 846–52.

The Health and Social Care Act (2012). Available at: www.legislation.gov.uk/ukpga/2012/7/contents/enacted (last accessed 18 February 2014).

The Kings Fund (2011) *The Future of Leadership and Management in the NHS*. London: The Kings Fund.

The Kings Fund (2012) *Leadership and Engagement for Improvement in the NHS*. London: The Kings Fund.

Thomas, K.W. and Kilman, R.H. (1974) 'Developing a forced-choice measure of conflict behaviour: the "mode" instrument', *Educational and Psychological Measurement*, 37: 309–25.

Vitello-Cicciu, J.M. (2002) 'Exploring emotional intelligence: implications for nursing leaders', *Journal of Nursing Administration*, 32(4): 203–10.

Wong, C.A., Cummings, G.A. and Ducharme, L. (2013) 'The relationship between nursing leadership and patient outcomes: a systematic review update', *Journal of Nursing Management*, 21: 709–24.

Yukl, G., Gordon, A. and Taber, T. (2002) 'A hierarchical taxonomy of leadership behaviour: integrating a half century of behaviour research', *Journal of Leadership and Organizational Studies*, 9 (1): 15–32.

PART TWO

Caring for Adults in a Variety of Settings

This section of the book will help you to fully understand the various roles, responsibilities and functions of the adult nurse which take place in a variety of settings. In order to be able to deliver safe and effective care to meet the complex needs of adult patients it is essential that you gain in-depth knowledge of the common physical and mental problems encountered by adults as well as the evidence-based interventions, treatments and care that nurses can provide (NMC, 2010a).

As this book offers a broad rather than an in-depth approach it is also recommended that you access a wide range of alternative texts to ensure that you have a sound underpinning knowledge base of relevant anatomy and physiology in addition to knowledge from the life, behavioural and social sciences. You will also need to ensure that you have an in-depth knowledge and understanding of medical and surgical nursing in order to be able to respond appropriately to your patients' needs. Working in partnership with patients, families, groups, communities and organisations, the knowledge and understanding you develop as a result of reading this section will help you apply effective nursing care interventions which will meet a full range of complex health and dependency needs of the adult and their family during different life stages, including progressive illness, death and bereavement and help you to demonstrate the necessary knowledge and understanding for entry to the Nursing and Midwifery register as an adult nurse (NMC, 2010a).

9 Promoting Health

HELEN DAVIDSON

The aim of this chapter is to introduce you to the principles and practice of epidemiology, public health nursing and health promotion with individuals, families and communities. The activities included here will enable you to reflect upon your own health promotion skills and consider the range of opportunities available to promote health within a contemporary healthcare setting.

At this point you might be thinking that 'health promotion' is exclusively the domain of practice nurses, school nurses and health visitors. However, whilst health promotion is indeed a significant aspect of the community practitioner role (Baisch, 2009) it can also be applied across a range of settings with a variety of service users (Naidoo and Wills, 2009). There is an expectation that *all* nurses will work to promote health whenever the opportunity arises (NMC, 2010). Health promotion interventions can take a number of forms, and may be carried out with individuals, families or communities (NICE, 2007a; 2008; 2014). In addition, there is growing evidence of the effectiveness of health promotion across the lifespan (DH, 2011a; 2011b), including patients with dementia (Salva et al., 2009) and at the end of life (Street, 2007; Rosenberg and Yates, 2014). Therefore it is important to remember that individuals at all stages of life can benefit from health promotion and that health promotion is a key aspect of the adult nurse's role.

After reading this chapter you should be able to:

- Identify theories, models and approaches to health promotion and discuss how they can be adapted to meet the needs of individuals, groups and communities.
- Gain a basic understanding of how demographic health information and epidemiological data can inform national and global priorities for health and public health initiatives.
- Identify the tools and structures that underpin the assessment of health and healthcare needs, and consider the subsequent provision of health promotion initiatives and services.
- Explore the social determinants of health, inequalities in health and the role of the practitioner in contemporary public health practice.

The range of public health issues affecting populations on both a national and global level is vast (World Health Organization, 2002; Public Health England, 2013). However, this chapter will focus specifically on modifiable lifestyle behaviours/risk factors – particularly in relation to cardiovascular disease (CVD) and coronary heart disease, obesity, excessive alcohol consumption and sexual health – as these have significant implications for the health and well-being of the adult population across the UK (Health Protection Agency, 2009; Myint et al., 2011).

Related NMC competencies

An overarching requirement is that all nurses must:

… understand the public health principles, priorities and practice in order to recognise and respond to major causes and social determinants of health, illness and health inequalities. They must use a range of information and data to assses the needs of people, groups, communities and populations, and work to improve health, wellbeing and experiences of healthcare; secure equal access to health screening, health promotion and healthcare; and promote social inclusion (NMC 2010a: 18, NMC 2010b: 7). All nurses must support and promote the health, wellbeing, rights and dignity of people, groups, communities and populations. This includes people whose lives are affected by ill health, disability, ageing, death and dying. Nurses must understand how these activities influence public health and seek out every opportunity to promote health and prevent illness. (NMC, 2010a)

--------- To achieve entry to the register as an adult ---------
nurse you should be able to:

- Take every opportunity to encourage health-promoting behaviour through education, role-modelling, and effective communication.
- Understand how behaviour, culture, socioeconomic and other factors in the care environment and its geographical location can affect health, illness, health outcomes and public health priorities, taking this into account when planning and delivering care.
- Provide educational support, facilitation skills and therapeutic nursing interventions to optimise health and well-being.
- Use a range of information and data to assess the needs of people, groups, communities and populations, working to improve health, well-being and healthcare.
- Work in partnership with service-users, carers, families, groups, communities and organisations. You must promote health and well-being, while aiming to empower choices that promote self-care and safety.

(Adapted from the NMC Standards of Competence for Adult Nursing, 2010a, 2010b.)

Background

Historically, the health concerns of the day focused on infections and accidents (Rosen, 1993). Although these are still a concern today it is recognised that lifestyle is a major cause of morbidity and mortality (Upton and Thirlaway, 2010) and this has led to a growing emphasis on a number of UK public health strategies (for example, DH, 2012b; DHSSPS, 2014) and the role of the nurse in the implementation of these (RCN, 2012; DH, 2012b).

The evolution of public health (or 'population health') has demonstrated that there are a range of factors which influence the health of a population. These will be explored in more detail in order to help you to make the links between health promotion theory and adult nursing practice.

For health promotion interventions to be carried out effectively (for example, *health needs assessment*) you will need to understand the basic underlying principles (e.g., *population health* and *epidemiology*). Epidemiology studies the distribution of health events in particular populations (Last, 1988) and as such can be applied to the control of such events (Mulhall, 1996). These concepts will be discussed and clarified in more detail throughout the chapter.

It is also useful to explore the way public health has evolved over the years.

The four stages of public health

1. *Sanitary Reform 1848–1870s* Focued on: environmental issues and change.

During this time, Dr John Snow used the principles of epidemiology to identify the link between an outbreak of cholera and the use of the Broad Street water pump in London. This is a useful example of a population-based approach to health events, as the water pump was disabled by having its handle removed – thereby effectively ending the outbreak (Gunn and Masellis, 2008).

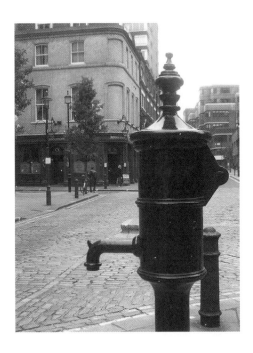

(Continued)

(Continued)

2. *Sanitary Science 1870–1930s* Focused on personal preventative measures.

Interestingly, the lifetime of Florence Nightingale spanned both stages (sanitary reform and sanitary science) and the principles of these stages are evident in the many accounts of her work (Bostridge, 2009).

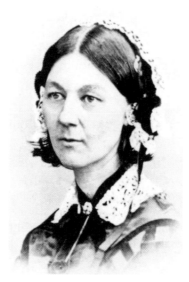

3. *Therapeutic Era 1930s–late 1970s* Focused on therapeutic interventions.

This stage saw a real increase in emphasis on hospital services and pharmaceutical approaches to medicine and health, although not all were in agreement that this would be the panacea for all health issues (McKeown, 1976).

4. *New Public Health: the 1980s to the present day* Focused on medical/social/environmental aspects, personal preventative measures and therapeutic intervention.

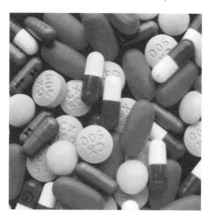

In 1974, the Lalonde highlighted the preventable aspects of ill-health. This was pre-sented via a framework called the 'Health Field Concept', which organised the various influences on health into four key areas: human biology, the environment, lifestyle and healthcare organisation. This concept can still be applied to modern-day public health policy and practice. For example, the effective promotion of 'healthy eating' would consider all of these four areas (DH, 2012a; 2012b).

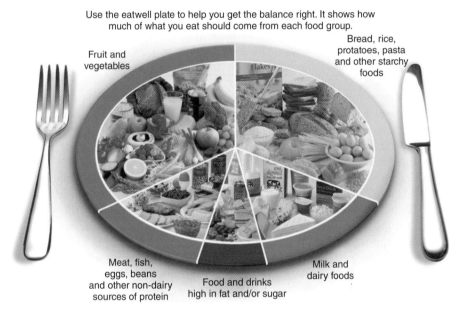

Figure 9.1   The eatwell plate

Source: Public Health England in association with Welsh Government, the Scottish Government and the Food Standards Agency Northern Ireland (2013). Available at: www.nhs.uk/Livewell/Goodfood/Documents/Eatwellplate.pdf

The evolution of public health has demonstrated the many determinants of health and the different approaches used to address the health issues of the day. In contemporary public health practice, the broad concept of health promotion is underpinned by princi-ples of 'equity', 'participation' and 'empowerment' (WHO, 1986; Davies and Macdowall et al., 2006). It is likely that you will come across these terms as you read around the general nursing literature. However, we should also consider these within the specific context of health promotion practice:

- *Equity* – It is important to consider this principle when thinking about the many determinants of health. For example, a population may share a similar level of access to healthcare services but have an unequal level of income or education.

Broadly speaking, this can have a negative impact on health. As outlined in Chapter 6, life expectancy can be (amongst other things) determined by the level of deprivation or affluence in a particular area (Marmot, 2010). In response to this, a number of health promotion initiatives aim to address 'inequalities in health' such as the provision of cookery lessons and food vouchers for low-income young families (DH, 2012a). Nevertheless, the issue of health inequalities continues to be important for modern Britain (Marmot, 2010).

- *Participation* – The involvement of service users is a significant feature of contemporary UK healthcare policy (for example, DH, 2010a; DHSSPS, 2014) and the views of patients, carers and communities are both desired and valued by the various stakeholders in public health policy (Griffiths et al., 2012). As adult nurses it can be easy to overlook the significance of family, friends and the wider community when working with individual patients, yet in many instances these 'hold the key' to achieving real results in health promotion (Koshy et al., 2010). A good example of this is the 'peer support' schemes available to breastfeeding mothers, where the main source of infant feeding support is another mother from the local community rather than the community nurse (Thomson et al., 2011). Nevertheless, the community nurse would still play a role here by referring mothers on to the peer support service and continuing to liaise with the local community.
- *Empowerment* – Much has been written about the concept of 'empowerment' (Tengland, 2007), with some authors asking if this is really achieved in healthcare (Mitcheson and Cowley, 2003). Nevertheless, within health promotion practice 'empowerment' is mainly about ensuring the service user has the resources, support and information required to make decisions about their own health and lifestyle (DH, 2010a). For example, many community nurses work with patients who express a desire to stop smoking but do not feel confident in taking control of their smoking behaviour. It is possible that the nurse would then work with the service user to help them identify the 'stage of change' they are at (Prochaska and Diclemente, 1986), as this can guide the motivational interviewing process undertaken by the nurse (Karatay et al., 2010). In addition, the community nurse could prescribe a tailored regimen of Nicotine Replacement Therapy, signpost the service user to additional smoking cessation services (DH, 2012a), and offer regular emotional support. Here, the community nurse can empower service users to reduce or stop their smoking at their own pace and on their own terms.

As you can see, the Department of Health (DH) has embraced these underlying concepts of health promotion within its numerous public health policies. Similarly, the World Health Organization (WHO) has been a driving force in the evolution of health promotion (Green and Tones, 2010) and has produced various declarations and statements (e.g. the Ottawa Charter (WHO, 1986), the Jakarta Declaration (WHO, 1997) and the Bangkok Charter (WHO, 2005)) offering an early definition of 'health promotion':

The process of enabling people to increase control over the determinants of health and thereby improve their health. (WHO, 1986)

Consider the definition 'health promotion' offered by the WHO:

- Do you think that this reflects the principles of 'equity', 'participation' and 'empowerment'?
- What do you think is meant by the terms 'health' and its 'determinants'?

What is health?

... a state of complete physical, mental and social well-being and not merely the absence of disease or infirmity. (WHO, 1946)

.... a positive concept emphasizing social and personal resources as well as physical capacities. Health is created and lived by people in the settings of their everyday lives. (WHO, 1990)

As this Stop and Think has demonstrated, adult nurses need to be aware of the resources that individuals, families and communities have access to when assessing their health needs and planning interventions. For example, if we are promoting healthy eating we should consider the individual or family budget, cultural issues and the quality of their food storage and preparation facilities. In addition, we need to think about the accessibility, availability and affordability of healthy food – as this can vary from place to place.Understanding the various determinants of health will help us anticipate and plan for targeted health promotion activity.

Dahlgren and Whitehead (1991) offer a useful visual representation of the various determinants of health (see Figure 9.1). Here they demonstrate that health is not solely dependent on healthcare services and that this is just one determinant of health. It could be argued therefore that the work of Dahlgren and Whitehead (1991) reflects the 'Health Field Concept' as presented by Lalonde (1974). That is, health is also affected by individuals themselves and their social and material resources, which are in turn influenced by healthcare policy (Naidoo and Wills, 2009). It is clear therefore that the nurse's role in health promotion is wide and far-reaching, and in many instances requires committed, joined-up working with other agencies (Green and Tones, 2010).

Due to the varied nature of the nurse's role in health promotion, it can sometimes be difficult to decide which approach to take when working with service users. Fortunately however a number of health promotion models have been created in order to make sense of and simplify the complexity of health promotion (Davies and Macdowell, 2006). Nurses can use these models to help select the most relevant type of health promotion activity, and decide whether the intervention is individually or collectively focused. We will look at some of the most commonly used models a little later in the chapter.

When we are thinking about the type of health promotion activity we might use, we need to consider whether the level of prevention we are aiming for is 'primary', 'secondary' or 'tertiary' (Loveday and Linsley, 2011). This is an important concept in health promotion theory as it helps both nurse and service user have realistic expectations of the planned intervention.

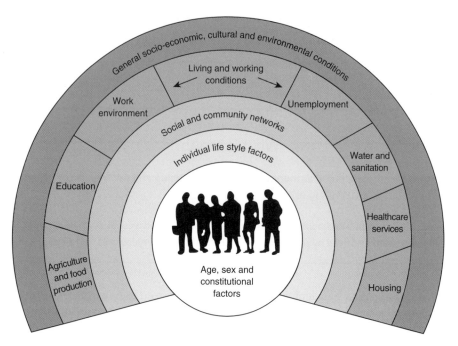

Figure 9.2   The main determinants of health
Source: Dahlgren and Whitehead (1991)

Levels of prevention

- Primary: to prevent the disease developing at all (the likely focus is population-wide).
- Secondary: to prevent the disease from progressing (the likely focus is those at risk but not unwell).
- Tertiary: to prevent the consequences of the disease.

STOP AND THINK

Consider the different scenarios below. Make a note of whether you think the level of prevention offered is primary, secondary or tertiary:

- The diabetes nurse specialist advises a 22-year-old female with Type 1 diabetes mellitus on her diet, insulin regimes and glucose monitoring.
- A 78-year-old male is given his annual influenza vaccination by the practice nurse.
- A 37-year-old female is offered annual mammograms after being identified as carrying the BRCA1 gene.

Was deciding on the level of prevention clear and straightforward or were some of the scenarios more difficult to appraise?

(Note: Do not worry if you found this Stop and Think challenging – in clinical practice cases can be more or less complex depending on factors such as age, gender, lifestyle and any other illnesses (or 'co-morbidities') a patient may have.)

As this Stop and Think has shown, deciding whether an intervention is primary, secondary or tertiary prevention is not as easy as it looks. For example, in areas such as cancer care, the distinctions are less clear (Silberstein and Parsons, 2010). Also, although a combination of approaches may have a significant effect on some disease outcomes there are other conditions, such as some musculoskeletal disorders, where there is a particular emphasis on primary prevention (Rozenfeld et al., 2010).

'Prevention is better than cure'. (Desiderius Erasmus)

Thus far we have established that the level of 'prevention' can vary depending on the patient's individual risk factors and current diagnosis. However this is not the only consideration in health promotion practice. Although nurses do carry out effective interventions within the healthcare setting, it is not the entire remit of their health promotion role. Adult nurses can have an impact on the health of individuals, families and communities within a range of settings (NICE, 2007b; 2008; 2014), whilst also influencing health policy on a local and national level (Naidoo and Wills, 2009). Here then health promotion models are particularly useful, as they identify the different levels of change:

- Individual behaviour change.
- Community development and action.
- Communication strategies.
- Organisational change.
- Public policy change.

For example, the Health Belief Model (Becker, 1974; Rosenstock, 1974) draws upon health psychology and focuses on individual belief systems in relation to lifestyle choices. An understanding of health psychology is a key part of effective health promotion as it can provide the practitioner with a range of tools to use. Some of these models are outlined in Table 9.1. Although these models differ, they all share the view that the individual's level of 'self-efficacy' or 'perceived control' may have an impact on the lifestyle decision he or she makes.

- As an adult nurse, think about how you could influence the patient's level of self-efficacy.
- How does this link to the practice of *empowerment*?

  Despite these models being applicable to work with individuals, they also consider the influence of the wider society. For example, the 'perceived severity' (Rosenstock, 1974) of a health issue (such as smoking) may be influenced by mass media campaigns (Borland and Balmford, 2003; Brown et al., 2014) and more informal social networks (Folland, 2008).

- As an adult nurse, how could you influence the 'perceived severity' of a particular health issue?

Table 9.1   An overview of models used in health psychology – and their application to health promotion

Nature of Model/ Approach	Author(s)	Key features
Health Belief Model	Rosenstock (1974), Becker (1974)	• Acknowledge the influence of demographics, social class, gender, age, internal and external cues • Perceived susceptibility and severity of the negative health outcome plays a key role • The perceived benefits and barriers to the behaviour change are also important • Specific 'cues to action' / perception of threat can contribute to a behaviour change • Levels of self-efficacy inform decision to change
Transtheoretical Model	Prochaska and Diclemente (1986)	• Suggest that change follows 'sequential' stages • Describe 'processes' which people typically use to facilitate change • Change can be predicted by consideration of the 'decisional balance' • Self-efficacy is described as the person's confidence in their ability to make changes This model has been applied to a variety of unhealthy behaviours (for example, smoking, alcohol consumption, exercise, diet, drug abuse) with evidence to suggest that health promotion programmes that are designed or tailored around each of the stages above are more effective (Noar et al., 2007).
Theory of Planned Behaviour	Ajzen (1991)	• An extension of the Theory of Reasoned Action (Ajzen and Fishbein, 1980) • Used to study cognitive determinants of health behaviours • Behaviour is determined by the strength of intention and the level of control a person perceives they have • Acknowledges the role of 'subjective norms' in influencing behaviour choices – that is, perceived social pressure to perform or not perform a behaviour (Ajzent, 1991)

From this Stop and Think you will see that the potential scope of health promotion activity is vast and goes beyond working with the individual. Therefore, in addition to models which focus on the individual, there are also 'collective' models such as Community Development Theory (Fawcett et al., 1995) which acknowledge the importance of harnessing the resources within a community.

At this point you may be thinking about the sheer number of theoretical models you could refer to – which may seem overwhelming. Table 9.2 summarises the main features of the most well-known 'Health Promotion' models. These models *specifically* focus on an area of health promotion and tend to acknowledge *both* individual and community approaches to public health interventions. Therefore 'Health Promotion' models are particularly useful as they tend to incorporate the many determinants of health with a combined approach to health promotion (Nutbeam and Harris, 2010).

Table 9.2   Models of health promotion: an overview

Nature of Model/Approach	Author(s)	Key features
'Mode of intervention' and 'Focus of intervention' criteria used to generate four models of health promotion activity	Beattie (1991)	• <u>Focus</u> of intervention may be *individual* or *collective* • <u>Mode</u> of intervention may be *authoritative* (top-down and expert-led) or *negotiated* (bottom-up, individual) • Health Promotion practice identified as: 　**Health persuasion** (authoritative, individual) 　**Legislative action** (authoritative, collective) 　**Personal counselling** (negotiated, individual) 　**Community development** (negotiated, collective)
Three overlapping spheres of activity: Health Education, Prevention and Health Protection	Tannahill (1990)	• **Health Education:** communication to enhance well-being and prevent ill-health through influencing knowledge and attitudes • **Prevention:** reducing or avoiding the risk of disease and ill health primarily through medical intervention • **Health Protection:** safeguarding population health through legislative, fiscal or social measures
Five Approaches to Health Promotion Activity	Ewles and Simnett (2003)	• **Medical approach:** treatment, for example drugs • **Behavioural approach:** providing advice and guidance • **Educational approach:** specific information and/or training provided • **Empowerment approach:** life skills approach, for example assertiveness and communication • **Social change approach:** appraisal of services available, lobbying, campaigning

Footnote: This table represents some of the health promotion models available. Further reading in relation to each specific model or approach is recommended.

Although there are only a selection of models presented here, you will see that there are a number of approaches to health promotion practice with a varied emphasis on each component:

- Consider which of these models appear particularly applicable to your own nursing practice? Why is this so?
- Try to identify three strengths and limitations for each model.

STOP AND THINK

The above Stop and Think demonstrates the utility of health promotion models in nursing practice on an individual, community and national level. It also helps to illustrate that that the scope of our practice as adult nurses goes beyond our immediate setting, with the potential for involvement in broader activity such as national campaigns and lobbying parliament (Naidoo and Wills, 2009). However, it is important to remain flexible and open-minded in terms of health promotion practice, as developments in both research and technology can significantly affect the lifestyle options available to individuals and communities (DH, 2010a).

Health needs assessment

So far we have considered the different approaches to health promotion. Before any health promotion activity is carried out however, there first needs to be an effective assessment of health needs – in terms of the individual, family and community. Assessment is an important element of the nursing process (Kozier, 2008) and this is often presented as an assessment of the individual, using frameworks such as the Activities of Daily Living Model (Roper et al., 2000) and more specific tools, for example a pressure area risk assessment tool (Waterlow, 1985).

STOP AND THINK

- What is a community health needs assessment?
- What knowledge and information would you need to be able to carry this out effectively?

A Community Health Needs Assessment is a process which systematically reviews the health of a population, and then informs on priorities and the allocation of resources (Cavanagh and Chadwick, 2005). Effective health promotion also requires a thorough knowledge of the health issues in any given community (Naidoo and Wills, 2009). Although this is particularly relevant to the work of community practitioners (Rowe et al., 2001), knowledge of an individual's local community is important for *all* nurses as this informs effective assessment and discharge planning across settings (Timby, 2012). Therefore we need to consider how community health needs are assessed and how the results inform practice.

The five stages of a Community Health Needs Assessment

1. Planning and beginning the process.
2. Identifying the health priorities.
3. Assessing a priority for action.
4. Action planning for change.
5. Moving on/project review.

(Adapted from Cavanagh and Chadwick, 2005: 20.)

It is helpful here to refer to Bradshaw's (1972) Taxonomy of Need when assessing the health of a community:

- *Normative* – an agreed standard that is laid down by an expert professional body, i.e. as defined by professionals.
- *Felt* – as perceived by individuals (a subjective view of need).

- *Expressed* – demanded or felt need turned into action.
- *Comparative* – exists when two groups of people with the same condition receive an unequal provision of services (i.e. the variation between different population groups).

A good community assessment includes standard measurements such as epidemiological data and the views of service users.

Think back over the last few months about any assessment (individual, family or community) that you have encountered.
   Consider the following:

- Was this assessment based on normative needs?
- Were 'other' needs discovered ('expressed', 'felt')?
- What do you think are the challenges in discovering 'expressed' and 'felt' needs?

STOP AND THINK

Health needs assessment is not always straightforward, yet it is a key aspect of service planning (Green and Tones, 2010). We have to make sure therefore that the appropriate modes of assessment are used and the people involved know about the significant health issues in a community and can make changes happen (DH, 2010a).

Modes of assessment – Community Health Needs

There are three main perspectives:

- The epidemiological perspective.
- The health economist's perspective – i.e. is the health promotion intervention 'clinically effective' and 'cost effective'?
- The sociological perspective – i.e. the health issue is considered from a sociological perspective, including a consideration of health inequalities.

We will focus now on the epidemiological perspective, as epidemiological data can help us identify the main health issues in a particular area (Mulhall, 1996). Epidemiological data include morbidity and mortality rates, census data and deprivation scores (Naidoo and Wills, 2009). Let us clarify these terms in a little more detail, as an understanding of these will help us acknowledge their role in a community health needs assessment:

- *Mortality rates* – the rates of death within a defined population over a defined time-frame.
- *Morbidity rates* – the 'incidence' and 'prevalence' of a particular disease, condition or event within a defined population.

─────── The difference between 'incidence' and 'prevalence' ───────

As a nurse you will come across these terms very frequently and at times it will seem that they are used almost interchangeably. There is however a notable difference between the two, with implications for your role as an adult nurse.

'Incidence' refers to the number of new cases of a particular disease, condition or event in a particular population (usually within the previous year).

'Prevalence' refers to the total number of cases in a particular population (at a set point or period in time), some of which may have been diagnosed for a number of years.

STOP AND THINK

What can *incidence* rates tell us about our health promotion practice?

- *Census data* can demonstrate the social and economic differences between populations. Sources include the Office of National Statistics (ONS) data.
- The *Index of Multiple Deprivation* (IMD) measures various indicators to obtain a score of relative deprivation (i.e. affluence).

Therefore there is a range of factors to consider when assessing community health needs and as adult nurses it is reassuring for us to know that this information may be obtained from a range of sources, as there are a number of interested stakeholders. Nevertheless, although population health is a regional, national and global concern (WHO, 2002), the role of the nurse in everyday practice can be significant. For example, a five-minute conversation with a patient prior to discharge can help signpost them towards resources of which they would otherwise be unaware. A useful example of this is sexual health screening services for the over-55 age group (DH, 2013).

Alternatively, depending on the setting, adult nurses could form longer-term relationships with service users and therefore be able to implement more focused health promotion strategies. This may involve the facilitation of a 'patient support' group with diabetic patients (Gillett et al., 2010), the delivery of a cardiac rehabilitation programme within the community (Taylor et al., 2010) or motivational interviewing as part of a smoking cessation package (Karatay et al., 2010).

Therefore the approach to health promotion can vary depending on the patient, setting and resources available. In this respect, health promotion can be either 'planned' – that is, as part of a wider public health initiative (RCN 2012) – or 'opportunistic' – in other words, delivered as the need arises – *Making Every Contact Count: MECC* (RCN, 2012; DH, 2012a).

STOP AND THINK

- When do you have the opportunity to incorporate health promotion within your every-day nursing practice? List three examples.

Once you have completed this Stop and Think keep your results handy as we will now con-sider the effectiveness of different approaches in a variety of situations and settings.

Prisons

Watson et al. (2004) identified the tension that exists between the correctional aspects of being in prison (such as separation from society and confinement), to the healthcare issues which may arise in prison (for example, mental health issues, bullying and com-municable diseases). As a nurse working within a prison setting, you may come across challenges to effective health promotion. Nevertheless, Exworthy et al. (2001) suggested that the principle of 'equivalence of care' is not wholly applicable, as prisons are not equivalent to the outside, civilian community in some areas.

This is evident in the primary care provision in prisons, and interestingly, the number of consultations within a prison setting is much higher than the community equivalents (Watson et al., 2004). As an adult nurse working within such settings, there is therefore the opportunity to implement more involved health promotion strategies, with the scope to evaluate the success of these.

Travelling communities

Van Cleemput et al. (2007) highlighted the specific cultural beliefs which inform many travellers' health behaviours, including a low expectation of healthcare services, clear rules regarding what is 'pure' and 'impure' and a notable 'fear of death'. The beliefs regarding 'pure' and 'impure' extended to the uptake of vaccinations, whilst the 'fear of death' meant that a general anaesthetic was avoided, as this was considered to be a 'lit-tle death' (Van Cleemput et al., 2007). Lehti and Mattison (2001) also discussed the hierarchical order within the travelling community according to age and gender, with specific implications for sexual health promotion.

STOP AND THINK

Considering the examples given above, identify the potential health needs (and any chal-lenges to health promotion) within the following settings:

- Prisons.
- Travelling communities.
- Your workplace/placement setting or geographical area.

What steps could be taken to overcome these challenges?

It is clear that the setting can really inform the adult nurse's approach to health promotion. This is not the only consideration however, as some health promotion initiatives are informed by wider policy, which will now be addressed in more detail.

Policy and health promotion

Before we consider the policy context, it would be useful to think about what we mean when we talk about 'policy' as it is another term which is frequently used in nursing practice. In general, a policy is a statement of a decision about a goal in healthcare and a plan for achieving that goal (Earle et al., 2007). For example, to prevent a flu epidemic in older people, a programme for inoculating that population is developed and implemented. Examples of policies include the National Institute for Health and Clinical Excellence (NICE) guidelines, and government White Papers (for example *Equity and Excellence*: DH, 2010a). A White Paper is an official government report which sets out the government's policy on a matter that is presented to parliament. Acts, on the other hand, are laws, for example the *Clean Air Act* (1956), the *Smoking (Northern Ireland) Order* (HMSO, 2006) or the *Tobacco and Primary Medical Services (Scotland) Act* (Scottish Government, 2010). These are usually preceded by a White Paper (Masterson, 2011).

London's Great Smog (1952) and the Clean Air Act (1956)

London's Great Smog in 1952 occurred between the 5th and 9th of December 1952 (Davis and Bates, 2002). This resulted in 12,000 immediate deaths and a further 6,000 subsequent deaths (Bell et al., 2004). Despite these shocking figures, the government was initially reluctant to act. Nevertheless, in 1956 the *Clean Air Act* banned emissions of black smoke (Naidoo and Wills, 2009).

The impact of the *Clean Air Act* on many private households influenced the debate about public health, individual choice and the scope of government intervention.

You may come across this 'nanny state' debate today – 'individual autonomy' versus the 'needs of a population' continues to be a tension in health promotion practice.

- Can you think of any examples of this?

In addition to the tension described above, there are a number of different challenges to the implementation of health promotion policy. Laws and policies are often insufficient as stand-alone agents to change health behaviour. For example, despite the *Health Act* (2006) and subsequent smoking ban, quit rates are low (DH, 2010b) and there are inequalities in smoking rates across social groups (National Audit Office, 2010).

Psychological theory suggests that people have to want to stop smoking (Prochaska and DiClemente, 1986) and hence there will be a group of people who do not want to stop smoking for a range of reasons (Buck and Frosini, 2012). An important consideration therefore in a smoking cessation policy is how this group of people are accessed and targeted.

The acknowledgement of health promotion in the policy context can be found as early as 1997, for example in *The New NHS: Modern, Dependable* (DH, 1997).

Each government launched their main 'flagship' health policy, which set out their long-term vision for the NHS. The current coalition government in England produced *Equity and Excellence: Liberating the NHS* (DH, 2010a) which emphasised patients being at the heart of everything the NHS does, including public health practice.

STOP AND THINK

- Reflect upon your current abilities within health promotion, do you think you have any areas for improvement?
- Have a closer look and review your answers to the previous Stop and Think (opportunities for health promotion) and ask yourself 'How does my practice incorporate the recommendations of public health policy?'

The last Stop and Think activity should have helped you to think about your role as an adult nurse and how you can contribute to the health needs of the population as identified by local and central government. In addition to the government policies which address a range of health issues, there are also those which address specific issues, or lifestyle factors, such as alcohol use (The Scottish Government, 2009; 2010; DHSSPS, 2011) and smoking (DH, 2011b; The Scottish Government, 2013).

Interestingly, the following four lifestyle factors are associated with nearly half of the overall 'illness burden' in the developed world (WHO, 2002):

- Excessive alcohol use.
- Smoking.
- Poor diet, including low consumption of fruit and vegetables.
- Low levels of physical activity.

These factors often occur together (NHS Information Centre, 2012), and there is a growing interest in the reasons for this (Buck and Frosini, 2012), much like the co-existence of different illnesses in patients with long-term conditions and 'co-morbidities' (DH, 2014). As the 'clustering' of unhealthy behaviours can have a compound effect on patients' health outcomes (Khaw et al., 2008), these can also have implications for the approach to health promotion practice and the nurse's role in this (RCN, 2012). It is noteworthy that some studies have demonstrated a greater prevalence of multiple risk factors in groups with a lower socio-economic status (Poortinga, 2007; Tobias et al., 2007; Shankar et al., 2010).

Lifestyle and public health

As adult nurses we come across a range of health issues (both acute and long term) which can be influenced in part by lifestyle choices (ONS, 2011). For example, a clear and well-known example of this is the link between smoking, lung cancer (Doll and Hill, 1950) and chronic obstructive pulmonary disease (Fletcher and Peto, 1977). Similarly, alcohol, diet, drug use and physical activity can all play a significant role in health outcomes for adults across the lifespan (Fuller, 2011). As these lifestyle behaviours often occur together (Littleton et al., 2007), this can often have a compound effect on the health of an individual (Buck and Frosini, 2012).

Although alcohol intake is a recognised aspect of the British culture and lifestyle (HMSO, 2012), the first national strategy for England was only published relatively recently (The Prime Minister's Strategy Unit, 2003). Nevertheless, there have been updates since then (Home Office, 2007; HMSO, 2012) replicated in similar policies across the UK (The Scottish Government, 2009; DHSSPS, 2011). Excess alcohol intake has been linked to a range of public health and social issues (Hughes et al., 2008), with an increased incidence of crime (Chaplin et al., 2011) and hospital admissions when binge drinking has occurred (HMSO, 2012). At first glance we could assume that binge drinking is only a small part of our national lifestyle, yet *half* of the total alcohol consumption in this country is attributed to binge drinking (HMSO, 2012).

Therefore, a number of strategies have been put forward to address this issue. For example, Babor et al. (2003) argue that pricing is the most effective strategy to reduce the harm done by alcohol consumption and a number of proposals have been put forward to address irresponsible promotions of cheap alcohol (HMSO, 2012). Similarly, strategies to address the use of drugs have also been publicised (DH, 2007; The Scottish Government, 2008). What does this mean however for us as adult nurses? We have to remember that our role is to promote health when working with individuals, groups and communities (NMC, 2015), whilst also remaining non-judgemental of individual lifestyle choices (Jarvis et al., 2005).

ACTIVITY 9.1

Find out more about motivational interviewing. You can access some of the following websites or articles or books suggested below:

1. Wagner, C. and Ingersol, K.S. (2012) *Motivational Interviewing in Groups*. London: Guildford.
2. Miller, W.R. and Rollnick, S. (2012) *Motivational Interviewing: Helping People Change*. London: Guildford.
3. Miller, W.R. and Rollnick, S. (2009) Ten things that motivational interviewing is not, *Behavioural and Cognitive Psychotherapy*, 37: 129–40.
4. Copello, A., Velleman, R. and Templeton, L. (2005) Family interventions in the treatment of alcohol and drug problems, *Drug and Alcohol Review*, 24: 369–85.

Make a list of the key elements you consider important and then reflect upon how these might influence your work with:

- individuals;
- families;
- groups.

Would your approach differ depending on the lifestyle behaviour being addressed? (Keep your results handy as you may return to this later in the chapter.)

Despite the need to consider the co-existence of unhealthy behaviours, this does not mean that we should immediately reject any intervention which focuses on just one behaviour (for example smoking). Indeed it may be that co-existing unhealthy behaviours *do* need to be addressed 'one at a time', as success in one lifestyle change may empower and motivate an individual to make other changes (Paiva et al., 2012). That said, this is an area where work is ongoing and no doubt you will encounter similar issues in practice.

We have already acknowledged the value in looking at health issues and lifestyle behaviours, both in clusters and on an individual basis. We will now look at the specific areas of obesity, cardiovascular disease/coronary heart disease (CVD/CHD), sexual health and alcohol misuse in more detail. These areas are all affected by *at least one* of the four lifestyle behaviours as outlined by the WHO (2002), and as such can be effectively targeted for health promotion intervention.

Table 9.3   Lifestyle problems in the UK

Health issue	Scale of the problem	Associated lifestyle behaviours – examples
Obesity	Between 1993 and 2012: % of obese women increased from 16.4% to 25.1% % of obese men increased from 13.2% to 24.4% (Health and Social Care Information Centre, 2014)	• Low level of physical activity • Poor diet
Cardiovascular disease/coronary heart disease (CVD/CHD)	Leading cause of death in developed countries, including England (PHE, 2013) 1,877,518 (3.5% prevalence), Scotland: 228,074 (4.4% prevalence), Wales: 128,114 (4% prevalence), and Northern Ireland: 75,027 (4% prevalence) (British Heart Foundation, 2014).	• Poor diet • Smoking • Low level of physical activity
Sexual health	Rates of infectious syphilis highest since the 1950s Nearly 50% of pregnancies are unplanned (DH, 2013)	• Excessive alcohol use increases likelihood of risk taking behaviour (Corte and Sommers, 2005)

Let us now take a closer look at these health issues, and the possible health promotion interventions which could be implemented.

Obesity

Whilst obesity is an increasing problem, we must also consider safety, comfort, dignity and respect with regard to the nursing care of this group. Obesity can have a range of consequences on both physical and mental health (PHE, 2013) and as such it is never too late to start or continue any intervention for addressing obesity.

 LUCY AND PAUL

Lucy is a 27 year old with a BMI (Body Mass Index) of 35. (Note that BMI is weight in kg/height in metres, squared). She is married to Paul, 31, who has a BMI of 21. Both Lucy and Paul are smokers. Lucy works as a receptionist but has recently had a long period of absence due to back pain. Paul is a long distance lorry driver who works erratic hours. Lucy has attended the asthma clinic with the practice nurse, and has asked for advice regarding healthy weight loss and has disclosed that she and Paul would like to start a family.

(Continued)

(Continued)

- What are Lucy's main health needs?
- What are the key influencing factors?
- As a newly qualified staff nurse, what would be your approach to promoting Lucy's health in this scenario?
- Can you always rely on the BMI as an accurate indicator of obesity?

There is a range of factors which contribute to obesity, whether this is due to diet (WHO, 2002), inactivity (NICE, 2013a; 2013b) or alcohol intake (Shelton and Knott, 2014). In addition the impact of obesity can have far-reaching consequences, for both the individual and the family (Flodgren et al., 2010). This is evident within this scenario, as there could be a possible impact on fertility (Pasquali et al., 2007) in addition to an increased risk of heart disease (Yusuf et al., 2001, 2004) and diabetes (Daousi et al., 2006). The good news, however, is that there are a number of health promotion strategies to use in cases such as this. For example, as an adult nurse the work you do with Lucy and Paul could be on an individual, family or community basis (Naidoo and Wills, 2009) and target a range of lifestyle issues. For example, motivational interviewing could be implemented as part of an individual smoking cessation programme (Karatay et al., 2010), with the additional benefit of Lucy and Paul supporting each other. In turn, this would facilitate an improvement in the ability to exercise (DH, 2011a), in which case a referral to a community diet and exercise programme (NICE, 2008; DHSSPS, 2012) would be beneficial.

It must be noted however that care must be taken when evaluating the success of certain initiatives, as any data gathered must be a valid measure of their impact (Flodgren et al., 2010). For example, you may have already come across the difficulty with BMI as a 'universal' measurement. That is, some individuals with a 'high' BMI may simply have a higher muscle mass (Shah and Braverman, 2012) and/or be from a different ethnic group (NICE, 2013b) as opposed to being 'obese'. In such instances additional measurements such as 'waist to height ratio' should also be considered (NICE, 2013b), as well as a broader, holistic assessment of the individual (Roper et al., 2000).

CVD/CHD

CVD and CHD are the leading causes of death in developed and developing countries (WHO, 2002), although there are differences by population due to the epidemiological transition and environmental factors due to the culture and industrialisation, genetic factors and urbanisation (Yusuf et al., 2001). In 2010, 180,000 people died from CVD and 8,000 due to CHD (ONS, 2011). Nevertheless, the overall incidence, acute hospitalisations and mortality for CHD have been declining – although death rates are falling more slowly in younger age groups (ONS, 2011). Mortality from CHD in England is highest in the North West region (ONS, 2011).

Risk factors

What is a risk factor?

- A factor (a characteristic, action) that increases the risk of a specific condition or event.
- In CHD/CVD the risk factors include smoking, abnormal lipids (cholesterol and triglycerides), hypertension, diabetes, abdominal obesity, psychosocial factors, age, gender, and genetics (Yusuf et al., 2004).

(Note also that factors can be *protective* as well, and in CVD/CHD include the consumption of fruits and vegetables, moderate alcohol intake and regular physical activity: Yusuf et al., 2004.)

You can see that a knowledge of both risk and protective factors can help a nurse to deliver targeted and effective health promotion and the general statistics in relation to CHD and CVD appear to be positive. However, as CHD/CVD continues to be a national and global concern (WHO, 2002; Buck and Frosini, 2012) we must continue to deliver health promotion in this area as part of our adult nursing role.

 JEAN

You are due to assess a 60-year-old woman, Jean, who has been referred to you as part of a community rehabilitation programme. She suffered a myocardial infarction two weeks ago. Jean is retired, and lives with her husband Andy, also retired. Andy is well and they have one son, Martin, who lives in Australia. Jean is generally well, although both she and Andy smoke 20 cigarettes a day:

- What assessment tools would you use to ascertain Jean's health needs?
- What health promotion initiatives could be accessed which may benefit Jean?

Case Scenario

The above Case Scenario demonstrates the multifactorial nature of CVD and CHD (WHO, 2002; Tolstrup et al., 2014) and the implications of this for health promotion practice. The importance of a case-specific assessment is apparent here, as it would appear that the evidence for home- and centre-based cardiac rehabilitation services demonstrates a broadly equal level of effectiveness (Taylor et al., 2010). Therefore, further exploration of factors such as personal preference and convenience would enable the adult nurse to implement an appropriate health promotion initiative (Naidoo and Wills, 2009). (See the suggested Further Reading and useful resources at the end of this chapter.)

Sexual health

Sexual health needs vary according to factors such as age, gender, sexuality and ethnicity, and some groups are particularly at risk of poor sexual health. It is crucial that individuals are able to live their lives free from prejudice and discrimination. However, while individuals' needs may vary, there are certain core needs that are common to everyone. (DH, 2013: 4)

Although there is a growing awareness of sexual health within the UK, there are a number of ongoing issues in England, for example:

- Rates of infectious syphilis are at their highest since the 1950s (DH, 2013).
- STIs have increased in older people.
- STI testing rates among young men remain low (Knight et al., 2012).
- HPV and other STI rates continue at a level which requires effective behavioural intervention (Shephard et al., 2014).

 RICHARD AND DAVID

Case Scenario

Richard and his partner David have both attended the sexual health clinic as part of the local screening services for MSM (men who have sex with men). Both Richard and David attend the clinic for their results and state that they are happy to obtain their results together. When you access the records you see that David has tested positive for chlamydia but Richard hasn't.

- What are the wider issues involved here?
- How could you overcome these challenges to health promotion?
- What nursing skills would be required in this scenario?

Now consider the many factors which may affect or inform sexual health. This may include religious beliefs, social norms, drug and alcohol use, and issues of vulnerability, coercion and abuse.

- What strategies could you employ as an adult nurse to address these factors, as part of your nursing assessment?

Sexual health is an extremely important and personal issue which can have a profound impact on an individual's physical and emotional well-being (NICE, 2007b). Although sexual health promotion is an important aspect of adult nurses' work with younger clients (Knight et al., 2012; Shephard et al., 2014), it should be considered across the adult lifespan (Matzo et al., 2013) as sexuality is a key aspect of the self (Roper et al., 2000).

Summary

It is clear that there are many different issues to consider when promoting health, but perhaps the most important principle to remember as an adult nurse is: to promote health whenever the opportunity arises – as even five minutes can make a difference (DH, 2012a). The importance of a nurse's role in health promotion has moved to the forefront of the

NHS conscience and this is evident in a range of publications (RCN, 2012; DH, 2012a). All adult nurse are expected to be accountable, compassionate practitioners (Griffiths et al., 2012), and this is equally applicable to health promotion practice, regardless of the setting.

As an adult nurse you will need to refer to the best available evidence to inform your health promotion practice. As you qualify, these transferable skills will also help you to appraise the effectiveness of your interventions – with individuals, families and communities (NICE, 2007a; 2007b; 2008; 2014).

Suggested further reading

Department of Health, Social Services and Public Safety (2012) *A Fitter Future for All: Framework for Preventing and Addressing Overweight and Obesity in Northern Ireland 2012–2022*. Belfast: DHSSPS.

Evans, D., Coutsaftiki, D. and Fathers, C.P. (2011) *Health Promotion and Public Health for Nursing Students*. Exeter: Learning Matters.

Hawtin, M. and Percy-Smith, J. (2007) *Community Profiling: A Practical Guide* (2nd edition). Maidenhead: Open University Press/McGraw-Hill Education.

Hubley, J. and Copeman, J. (2008) *Practical Health Promotion*. Cambridge: Polity.

Linsley, P., Kane, R. and Owen, S. (eds) (2011) *Nursing for Public Health: Promotion, Principles and Practice*. Oxford: Oxford University Press.

NICE (2014) *Behaviour Change: Individual Approaches: NICE Public Health Guidance 49*, London: National Institute for Health and Clinical Excellence.

Piper, S. (2010) *Health Promotion for Nurses: Theory and Practice*. London: Routledge.

Royal College of Nursing (2013) *Rights, Risks and Responsibilities in Service Redesign for Vulnerable Groups*. London: RCN.

The Scottish Government (2010) *The Sexual Health and Blood Borne Virus Framework 2011–15*. Edinburgh: The Scottish Government.

The Scottish Government (2014) *The Quality Principles Standard Expectations of Care and Support in Drug and Alcohol Services*. Edinburgh: The Scottish Government.

Useful resources

Association of Public Health Observatories. Available at: www.apho.org.uk

Faculty of Public Health. Available at: www.fph.org.uk

Health Development Agency. Available at: www.hda-online.org.uk/

National Library for Health. Available at: www.library.nhs.uk

National Obesity Forum. Available at: www.nationalobesityforum.org.uk/

National Obesity Observatory. Available at: www.noo.org.uk

National Institute for Health and Clinical Excellence (NICE). Available at: www.nice.nhs.uk

Solutions for Public Health. Available at: www.sph.nhs.uk

The Information Centre for Health and Social Care. Available at: www.hscic.gov.uk/public-health

UK Public Health Association. Available at: www.ukpha.org.uk

References

Ajzen, D. (1991) 'The theory of planned behaviour', *Organisational Behavior and Human Decision Processes*, 50: 179–211.

Ajzen, D. and Fishbein, M. (1980) *Understanding Attitudes and Predicting Social Behaviour*. Englewood Cliffs, NJ: Prentice-Hall.

Babor, T., Caetano, R., Casswell, S., Edwards, G., Giesbrecht, N. and Graham, K. (2003) *Alcohol: No Ordinary Commodity: Research and Public Policy*. Oxford: Oxford University Press.

Baisch, M.J. (2009) 'Community health: an evolutionary concept analysis', *Journal of Advanced Nursing*, 65: 2464–76.

Beattie, A. (1991) 'Knowledge and control in health promotion: a test case for social policy and theory'. In J. Gabe, M. Calnan and M. Bury (eds), *The Sociology of the Health Service*. London: Routledge.

Becker, M.H. (ed.) (1974) 'The Health Belief Model and personal health behaviour', *Health Education Monographs*, 2: 324–473.

Bell, M.L., Davis, D.L. and Fletcher, T. (2004) 'A retrospective assessment of mortality from the London Smog episode of 1952: the role of influenza and pollution', *Environmental Health Perspectives*, 112 (1): 6–8.

Borland, R. and Balmford, J. (2003) 'Understanding how mass media campaigns impact on smokers', *Tobacco Control*, 12 (2), suppl 2: ii–45.

Bostridge, M. (2009) *Florence Nightingale: The Woman and Her Legend*. Harmondsworth: Penguin.

Bradshaw, J. (1972) 'A taxonomy of social need', *New Society* (March): 640–3.

British Heart Foundation (2014) *Prevalance of CHD, Stroke and Hypertension, by Health Authority, England, Scotland, Wales and N.Ireland 2010/2011*. British Heart Foundation Statistics. Available at: www.bhf.org.uk/research/heart-statistics (last accessed 3 December 2014).

Brown, J., Kotz, D., Michie, S., Stapleton, J., Walmsley, M. and West, R. (2014) 'How effective and cost effective was the national mass media smoking cessation campaign 'Stoptober'?', *Drug and Alcohol Dependence*, 135: 52–8.

Buck, D. and Frosini, F. (2012) *Clustering of Unhealthy Behaviours Over Time: Implications for Policy and Practice*. London: The Kings Fund.

Cavanagh, S. and Chadwick, K. (2005) *Summary: Health Needs Assessment at a Glance*. London: Health Development Agency/NICE.

Chaplin, R., Flatley, J. and Smith, K. (2011) *Crime in England and Wales 2010/11*. Home Office Statistical Bulletin 10/11. London: The Home Office.

Clean Air Act (1956) 'Parliament of the United Kingdom'. In J. Naidoo and J. Wills (eds) (2009) *Foundations for Health Promotion*, 3rd edition. London: Bailliere Tindall/Elsevier. p.174.

Corte, C.M. and Sommers, M.S. (2005) 'Alcohol and risky behaviors', *Annual Review of Nursing Research*, 23: 327–60.

Dahlgren, G. and Whitehead, M. (1991) *Policies and Strategies to Promote Social Equity in Health*. Stockholm: Institute for Future Studies.

Daousi, C., Casson, I.F., Gill, G.V., MacFarlane, I.A., Wilding, J.P.H. and Pinkney, J.H. (2006) 'Prevalence of obesity in type 2 diabetes in secondary care: association with cardiovascular risk factors', *Postgraduate Medical Journal*, 82: 280–4.

Davies, M. and Macdowall, W. (2006) *Health Promotion Theory*. Maidenhead: Open University Press.

Davis, D.L. and Bates, D. (2002) 'A look back at the London Smog of 1952 and the half century since', *Environmental Health Perspectives*, December.

Department of Health (1997) *The New NHS: Modern, Dependable*. London: HMSO.

Department of Health (2007) *Drug Misuse and Dependence: UK Guidelines on Clinical Management*. London: HMSO.

Department of Health (2010a) *Equity and Excellence: Liberating the NHS*. London: HMSO.

Department of Health (2010b) *Health Profile of England 2009*. London: HMSO.

Department of Health (2010c) *Healthy Lives, Healthy People: Our Strategy for Public Health in England*. *London*: HMSO.

Department of Health (2011a) *Healthy Lives, Healthy People: A Call to Action on Obesity in England*. London: HMSO.

Department of Health (2011b) *Healthy Lives, Healthy People: A Tobacco Control Plan for England*. London: HMSO.

Department of Health (2012a) *Government Response to NHS Future Forum's Second Report.* London: HMSO.

Department of Health (2012b) *The Public Health Outcomes Framework for England, 2013–2016.* London: HMSO.

Department of Health (2013) *A Framework for Sexual Health Improvement in England.* London: HMSO.

Department of Health (2014) *Better Care for People With 2 or More Long Term Conditions.* London: HMSO.

Department of Health, Social Services and Public Safety (2011) *New Strategic Direction for Alcohol and Drugs (Phase 2) 2011–2016: A Framework for Reducing Alcohol and Drug Related Harm in Northern Ireland.* Belfast: DHSSPS.

Department of Health, Social Services and Public Safety (2012) *A Fitter Future for All: Framework for Preventing and Addressing Overweight and Obesity in Northern Ireland 2012–2022.* Belfast: DHSSPS.

Department of Health, Social Services and Public Safety (2014) *Making Life Better: A Whole System Strategic Framework for Public Health 2013–2023.* Belfast: DHSSPS.

Doll, R. and Hill, A.B. (1950) 'Smoking and carcinoma of the lung – a preliminary report', *British Medical Journal*, 30: 738–47.

Downie, R.S., Fyfe, C. and Tannahill, A. (1990) *Health Promotion: Models and Values.* Oxford: Oxford University Press.

Earle, S., Lloyd, C.E., Sidell, M. and Spur, S. (2007) *Theory and Research in Promoting Public Health.* London: Sage.

Ewles, L. and Simnett, I. (2003) *Promoting Health,* 5th edition. London: Baillière Tindall.

Exworthy, T., Wilson, S. and Forrester, A. (2001) Beyond equivalence: prisoners' right to health, *The Psychiatrist*, 35: 201–2.

Fawcett, S.B., Paine-Andrews, A., Francisco, V.T., Schultz, J.A., Richter, K.P., Lewis, R.K., Williams, E.L., Harris, K.J., Berkley, J.Y., Fisher, J.L. and Lopez, C.M. (1995) 'Using empowerment theory in collaborative partnerships for community health and development', *American Journal of Community Psychology*, 23 (5): 677–97.

Fletcher, C. and Peto, R. (1977) 'The natural history of chronic airflow obstruction', *British Medical Journal*, 1: 1645–8.

Flodgren, G., Deane, K., Dickinson, H.O., Kirk, S., Alberti, H., Beyer, F.R., Brown, J.G., Penney, T.L., Summerbell, C.D. and Eccles, M.P. (2010) 'Interventions to change the behaviour of health professionals and the organisation of care to promote weight reduction in overweight and obese adults (Review)', The Cochrane Collaboration. Chichester: Wiley.

Folland, S. (2008) 'An economic model of social capital and health', *Health Economics, Policy and Law*, 3 (4): 333–48.

Fuller, E. (2011) *Smoking, Drinking and Drug use among Young People in England in 2010.* Information Centre for Health and Social Care, England.

Gillett, M., Dallosso, H.M., Dixon, S., Brennan, A., Carey, M.E., Campbell, M.J., Heller, S., Khunti, K., Skinner, T.C. and Davies, M.J. (2010) 'Delivering the diabetes education and self management for ongoing and newly diagnosed (DESMOND) programme for people with newly diagnosed type 2 diabetes', *British Medical Journal*, 341. Available at: http://dx.doi.org/10.1136/bmj.c4093(last accessed 28 July 2014).

Green, J. and Tones, K. (2010) *Health Promotion: Planning and Strategies,* 2nd edition. London: Sage.

Griffiths, J., Speed, S., Horne, M. and Keeley, P. (2012) '"A caring professional attitude": what service users and carers seek in graduate nurses and the challenge for educators', *Nurse Education Today*, 32: 121–7.

Gunn, S.W. and Masellis, M. (2008) *Concepts and Practice of Humanitarian Medicine.* Springer.

Health Act (2006) (c 28) Parliament of the United Kingdom. London: HMSO.

Health and Social Care Information Centre (2014) *Statistics on Obesity, Physical Activity and Diet, England 2014.* Available at: www.hscic.gov.uk/catalogue/PUB13648 (last accessed 28 July 2014).

Health Protection Agency (2009) *Sexual Health: Chlamydia Rates Continue to Rise*. Available at: www.statistics .gov.uk/cci/nugget.asp?id=412 (last accessed 28 July 2014).

HMSO (2006) The Smoking (Northern Ireland) Order 2006. London: HMSO.

HMSO (2012) *The Government's Alcohol Strategy*. London: HMSO.

Home Office (2007) *Safe, Sensible and Social: The Next Steps in the National Alcohol Strategy*. London: The Home Office.

Hughes, K., Anderson, Z., Morleo, M. and Bellis, M.A. (2008) 'Alcohol, nightlife and violence: the relative contributions of drinking before and during nights out to negative criminal justice outcomes', *Addiction*, 103 (1): 60–5.

Jarvis, T.J., Tebbutt, J., Mattick, R.P. and Shand, F. (2005) *Treatment Approaches to Drug and Alcohol Dependence: An Introductory Guide*, 2nd edition. Chichester: Wiley.

Karatay, G., Kublay, G. and Emiroglu, O.N. (2010) 'Effect of motivational interviewing on smoking cessation in pregnant women', *Journal of Advanced Nursing*, 66 (6): 1328–37.

Khaw, K.T., Wareham, N., Bingham, S., Welch, A., Luben, R. and Day, N. (2008) 'Combined impact of health behaviours and mortality in men and women: the EPIC-Norfolk prospective population study', *Public Library of Science Medicine*, 5(1): 39–47.

Knight, R., Shoveller, J.A., Oliffe, J.L., Gilbert, M., Frank, B. and Ogilvie, G. (2012) 'Masculinities, "guy talk" and "manning up": a discourse analysis of how young men talk about sexual health', *Sociology of Health and Illness*, 34 (8): 1246–61.

Koshy, P., Mackenzie, M., Tappin, D. and Bauld, L. (2010) 'Smoking cessation during pregnancy: the influence of partners, families and friends on quitters and non-quitters', *Health and Social Care in the Community*, 18 (5): 500–10.

Kozier, B. (2008) *Fundamentals of Nursing: Concepts, Process and Practice*. London: Pearson.

Lalonde, M. (1974) *A New Perspective on the Health of Canadians: A Working Document*. Ottawa: Government of Canada.

Last, J.M. (1988) *A Dictionary of Epidemiology*, 2nd edition. New York: Oxford University Press.

Lehti, A. and Mattison, B. (2001) 'Health, attitude to care and pattern of attendance among gypsy women – a general practice perspective', *Family Practice*, 18 (4): 445–8.

Littleton, J., Barron, S., Prendergast, M. and Nixon, S.J. (2007) 'Smoking kills (alcoholics): shouldn't we do something about it?', *Alcohol and Alcoholism*, 42: 167–73.

Loveday, I. and Linsley, P. (2011) 'Implementing interventions: delivering care to individuals and communities'. In P. Linsley, R. Kane and S. Owen (eds), *Nursing for Public Health: Promotion, Principles and Practice*. Oxford: Oxford University Press. pp. 134–43.

MacDowall, W., Bonell, C. and Davies, M. (2006) *Health Promotion Practice*. Maidenhead: Open University Press.

Marmot, M. (2010) *Fair Society, Health Lives*. The Marmot Review. Available at: www. instituteofhealthequity.org/projects/fair-society-healthy-lives-the-marmot-review (last accessed 28 July 2014).

Masterson, A. (2011) 'The importance of nursing to public health: the political and policy context'. In P. Linsley, R. Kane and S. Owen (eds), *Nursing for Public Health: Promotion, Principles and Practice*. Oxford: Oxford University Press. pp. 89–97.

Matzo, M., Pope, L.E. and Whalen, J. (2013) 'An integrative review of sexual health issues in advanced incurable disease', *Journal of Palliative Medicine*, 16 (6): 686–91.

McKeown, T. (1976) *The Role of Medicine: Dream, Mirage or Nemesis?* London: Nuffield Provincial Hospitals Trust.

Mitcheson, J. and Cowley, S. (2003) 'Empowerment or control? An analysis of the extent to which client participation is enabled during health visitor/client interactions using a structured health needs assessment tool', *International Journal of Nursing Studies*, 40 (4): 413–26.

Mulhall, A. (1996) *Epidemiology, Nursing and Healthcare: A New Perspective*. Basingstoke: Macmillan.

Myint, P.K., Smith, R.D., Luben, R.N., Surtess, P.G., Wainwright, N.W., Wareham, N.J. and Khaw, K.T. (2011) 'Lifestyle behaviours and quality-adjusted life years in middle and older age', *Age and Ageing*, 40 (5): 589–95.

Naidoo, J. and Wills, J. (2009) *Foundations for Health Promotion,* 3rd edition. London: Bailliere Tindall/Elsevier.

National Audit Office (2010) *Tackling Inequalities in Life Expectancy in Areas with the Worst Health and Deprivation.* London: HMSO.

NHS Information Centre (2012) *The Health Survey for England.* Available at: www.ic.nhs.uk (last accessed 28 July 2014).

NICE (2007a) *Behaviour Change: the Principles for Effective Interventions NICE Public Health Guidance 6.* London: National Institute for Health and Clinical Excellence.

NICE (2007b) *One to One Interventions to Reduce the Transmission of Sexually Transmitted Infections (STIs) Including HIV, and to Reduce the Rate of under 18 Conceptions, Especially Among Vulnerable and At Risk Groups.* London: National Institute for Health and Clinical Excellence.

NICE (2008) *Community Engagement NICE Public Health Guidance 9.* London: National Institute for Health and Clinical Excellence.

NICE (2013a) *Physical Activity: Brief Advice for Adults in Primary Care, NICE Public Health Guidance 44.* London: National Institute for Health and Clinical Excellence.

NICE (2013b) *Assessing Body Mass Index and Waist Circumference Thresholds for Intervening to Prevent Ill Health and Premature Death Among Adults from Black, Asian and Other Minority Groups in UK', NICE Public Health Guidance 46.* London: National Institute for Health and Clinical Excellence.

NICE (2014) *Behaviour Change: Individual Approaches, NICE Public Health Guidance 49.* London: National Institute for Health and Clinical Excellence.

Noar, S.M., Benac, C.N. and Harris, M.S. (2007) 'Does tailoring matter? Meta-analytic review of tailored print health behavior change interventions', *Psychological Bulletin,* 4: 673–93.

Nursing and Midwifery Council (2010a) *Standards for Pre-registration Nursing Education.* London: NMC.

Nursing and Midwifery Council (2010b) *Standards for Competence for Registered Nurses.* Available at: www.nmc-uk.org/Documents/Standards/Standards%20for%20competence.pdf (last accessed 19 November 2014).

Nursing and Midwifery Council (2015) *The Code* Professional Standards of Practice and Behaviour for Nurses and Midwives. London: NMC.

Nutbeam, D. and Harris, E. (2010) *Theory in a Nutshell: A Guide to Health Promotion Theory.* Australia: McGraw-Hill.

Office of National Statistics (2011) *Statistics on CHD and CVD in England.* London: ONS.

Paiva, A.L., Prochaska, J.O., Yin, H.G., Rossi, J.S., Redding, C.A., Blissmer, B., Robbins, M.L., Velicer, W.F., Lipschitz, J., Amoyal, N., Babbin, S.F., Blaney, C.L., Sillice, M.A., Fernandez, A., McGee, H. and Horiuchi, S. (2012) 'Treated individuals who progress to action or maintenance for one behaviour are more likely to make similar progress on another behaviour: coaction results of a pooled data analysis of three trials', *Preventive Medicine,* 54 (5): 331–4.

Pasquali, R., Patton, L. and Gamberini, A. (2007) "Obesity and infertility": current opinion in endocrinology', *Diabetes and Obesity,* 14 (6): 482–7.

Poortinga, W. (2007) 'The prevalence and clustering of four major lifestyle risk factors in an English adult population', *Preventive Medicine,* 44 (2): 124–8.

Prime Minister's Strategy Unit (2003) *Alcohol Misuse: How Much Does It Cost?* London: Prime Minister's Strategy Unit.

Prochaska, J.O. and Diclemente, C.C. (1986) 'Towards a comprehensive model of change'. In W.R. Miller and N. Heather (eds), *Treating Addictive Behaviors: Processes of Change.* New York: Plenum. pp. 3–27.

Public Health England (PHE) (2013) *Our Priorities for 2013/14.* London: HMSO.

Roper, N., Logan, W.W. and Tierney, A.J. (2000) *The Elements of Nursing.* Edinburgh: Churchill Livingstone.

Rosen, G. (1993) *A History of Public Health.* Baltimore: John Hopkins University Press.

Rosenberg, J.P. and Yates, P. (2014) 'Health promotion in palliative care: the case for conceptual congruence', *Critical Public Health*, 20 (2): 201–10.

Rosenstock, I.M. (1974) 'Historical origins of the health belief model', *Health Education Monographs*, 2: 328–35.

Rowe, A., McClelland, A. and Billingham, K. (2001) *Community Health Needs Assessment: An Introductory Guide for the Family Health Nurse in Europe*. Geneva: World Health Organization.

Royal College of Nursing (2012) *Going Upstream: Nursing's Contribution to Public Health: RCN Guidance for Nurses*. London: RCN.

Rozenfeld, V., Ribak, J., Tsamir, J. and Carmeli, E. (2010) 'Prevalence, risk factors and preventive strategies in work-related musculoskeletal disorders among Israeli physical therapists', *Physiother Res Int*, 15 (3): 176–84.

Salva, A., Andrieu, S., Fernandez, E., Schiffrin, E.J., Moulin, J., Decarli, B., Guigoz, Y. and Vellas, B. (2009) 'Health and nutritional promotion program for patients with dementia (NutriAlz study): design and baseline data', *J Nutr Health Ageing*, 13 (6): 529–37.

The Scottish Government (2008) *The Road to Recovery: A New Approach to Tackling Scotland's Drug Problem*. Edinburgh: The Scottish Government.

The Scottish Government (2009) *Changing Scotland's Relationship with Alcohol: A Framework for Action*. Edinburgh: The Scottish Government.

The Scottish Government (2010) *Tobacco and Primary Medical Services (Scotland) Act 2010* (asp 3). Edinburgh: The Scottish Government.

The Scottish Government (2013) *Creating a Tobacco-Free A Generation. Tobacco Control Strategy for Scotland*. Edinburgh: The Scottish Government.

Shah, N.R. and Braverman, E.R. (2012) 'Measuring adiposity in patients: the utility of Body Mass Index (BMI), Percent Body Fat, and Leptin', *PLoS ONE*, 7 (4):e33308.doi:10.1371/journal.pone.0033308.

Shankar, A., McMunn, A. and Steptoe, A. (2010) 'Health-related behaviours in older adults: relationships with socioeconomic status', *American Journal of Preventive Medicine*, 35 (3): 219–24.

Shelton, S.J. and Knott, C.S. (2014) 'Association between alcohol calorie intake and overweight and obesity in English adults', *American Journal of Public Health*, 104 (4): 629–31.

Shephard, J.P., Frampton, G.K. and Harris, P. (2014) 'Interventions for encouraging sexual behaviours intended to prevent cervical cancer' (Review), The Cochrane Collaboration. Chichester: Wiley.

Silberstein, J.L. and Parsons, J.K. (2010) 'Prostate cancer prevention: concepts and clinical recommendations', *Prostate Cancer and Prostatic Disease*, 13 (4): 300–6.

Street, A.F. (2007) 'Leading the way: innovative health promoting palliative care', *Contemporary Nurse*, 27 (1): 104–6.

Tannahill, A. (1990) In R.S. Downie, C. Fyfe and A. Tannahill (1990) *Health Promotion: Models and Values*. Oxford: Oxford University Press.

Taylor, R.S., Dalal, H., Moxham, T. and Zawada, A. (2010) 'Home-based versus centre-based cardiac rehabilitation', *Cochrane Database of Systematic Reviews*. (Issue 1), Cochrane Collaboration. Chichester: Wiley.

Tengland, P. (2007) 'Empowerment: a goal or a means for health promotion?', *Medicine, Healthcare and Philosophy*, 10 (2): 197–207.

Thomson, G., Crossland, N. and Dykes, F. (2011) 'Giving me hope: women's reflections on a breastfeeding support service', *Maternal and Child Nutrition*, 8: 340–53.

Timby, B.K. (2012) *Fundamental Nursing Skills and Concept*, 10th edition. USA: Lippinicott Williams and Wilkins.

Tobias, M., Jackson, G., Yeh, L.C. and Huang, K. (2007) 'Do health and unhealthy behaviours cluster in New Zealand?', *Australian and New Zealand Journal of Public Health*, 31 (2): 155–63.

Tolstrup, J.S., Hvidtfeldt, U.A., Flachs, E.M., Spiegelman, D., Heitmann, B.L., Balter, K., Goldbourt, U., Hallmans, G., Knekt, P., Liu, S., Pereira, M., Stevens, J., Virtamo, J. and Feskanich, D. (2014) 'Smoking and risk of coronary heart disease in younger, middle-aged, and older adults', *American Journal of Public Health*, 104(1): 96–102.

Upton, D. and Thirlaway, K. (2010) *Promoting Healthy Behaviour: A Practical Guide for Nursing and Healthcare Professionals*. London: Pearson Education.

Van Cleemput, P., Parry, G., Thomas, K., Peters, J. and Cooper, C. (2007) 'Health-related beliefs and experiences of gypsies and travellers: a qualitative study', *Epidemiology and Community Health*, 61: 205–10.

Waterlow, J. (1985) *The Waterlow Pressure Area Risk Assessment Chart*. Available at: www.judy-waterlow/the-waterlow-score-card.htm (last accessed 28 July 2014).

Watson, R., Stimpson, A. and Hostick, T. (2004) 'Prison healthcare: a review of the literature', *International Journal of Nursing Studies*, 41: 119–28.

World Health Organization (1946) *Definition of Health*. Geneva: WHO.

World Health Organization (1986) *Ottawa Charter for Health Promotion: An International Conference on Health Promotion*. Geneva: WHO.

World Health Organization (1990) *Definition of Health*. Geneva: WHO.

World Health Organization (1997) *Jakarta Declaration*. Geneva: WHO.

World Health Organization (2002) *The World Health Report 2002: Reducing Risks, Promoting Healthy Life*. Geneva: WHO.

World Health Organization (2005) *The Bangkok Charter*. Geneva: WHO.

Yusuf, S., Hawken, S., Ounpuu, S., Dans, T., Avezum, A., Lanas, F., McQueen, M., Budaj, A., Pais, P., Varigos, J. and Lisheng, L. (2004) 'Effect of potentially modifiable risk factors associated with myocardial infarction in 52 countries (the INTERHEART study): case-control study', *The Lancet*, 364 (9438): 937–52.

Yusuf, S., Reddy, S., Ounpuu, S., and Anand, S. (2001) 'Global burden of cardiovascular diseases, part 1: general considerations, the epidemiological transition, risk factors, and impact of urbanization', *Circulation*, 104: 2746–53.

10 Supportive Care: Caring for Adults with Long-Term Conditions

JUDITH ORMROD AND DIANNE BURNS

Introduction

This chapter aims to offer an introduction to the role of the adult nurse in supporting individuals who are living with a chronic illness or a long-term condition (LTC).

Chronic illness was defined by The Commission on Chronic Illness (1956) as

> …pathological changes in the body that are non-reversible, permanent or leave residual disability: they may be characterised by periods of recurrence and remission and they generally require extended periods of supervision, observation, care & rehabilitation.

However, definition has been simplified in more recent years by the Department of Health (2005), referring to any chronic illness as a 'long-term health condition which cannot at present be cured, but can be controlled by medication and other therapies'.

Reading and completing the activities in the previous chapter you will be aware of the adult nurse's public health role and the importance of identifying and reducing recognised risk factors, and educating patients and their families to help them stay healthy, thereby preventing or minimising (as far as possible) the impact on health of many long-term conditions. This chapter will help you to build on this knowledge, requiring you to draw upon it when considering the role of the nurse in supporting patients suffering from a variety of long-term conditions.

Whilst it is beyond the remit of this chapter to include every single LTC you might encounter during your pre-registration programme, we intend to focus upon some common conditions, since it could be argued that many of the associated issues/problems encountered by patients are shared across a wide spectrum of conditions.

After reading this chapter you should be able to:

- Identify and discuss the common problems encountered by individuals living with an LTC.
- Recognise the adult nurse's role in supporting individuals (and their carers) living with long-term conditions in the UK.
- Identify treatment and care pathways that provide the evidence base used to underpin your practice.

(Continued)

(Continued)

- Identify relevant government policies which aim to support self-management, personalised care planning and working in partnership with patients and carers.
- Understand how the concepts of *patient empowerment, shared decision making* and *concordance* can be used to inform the adult nurse's role in partnership working.

Related NMC competencies

The overarching NMC requirement is that adult nurses must:

> … work in partnership with people who have long term conditions, their families and carers to provide therapeutic nursing interventions, optimise health and well-being, facilitate choice and maximise self-care and self management … adult nurses must also be able to work with other health and social care professionals and agencies, in all settings to ensure that decisions about care are shared. (NMC, 2010a: 19, 2010b: 10)

———— To achieve entry to the register as an adult ———— nurse you should be able to:

- Promote the rights, choices and wishes of all people, paying particular attention to equality, diversity and the needs of an ageing population.
- Ascertain and respond to the physical, social and psychological needs of people, groups and communities.
- Understand and apply current legislation to all service users, paying special attention to the protection of vulnerable people, including those with complex needs arising from ageing, cognitive impairment, long-term conditions and those approaching the end of their life.
- Promote the concept, knowledge and practice of self-care with people with long-term conditions, using a range of communication skills and strategies to help.
- people to make choices about their healthcare needs, and involving families and carers where appropriate to maximise their ability to care for themselves.

(Adapted from the NMC Standards of Competence for Adult Nursing, 2010a, 2010b.)

Background

The incidence of chronic illness across the UK currently presents a significant cost burden for the economy and the healthcare system. In England approximately 15 million people (one in three of the population) are living with a long-term condition (ONS, 2011; DH, 2012). Similarly in Wales it is estimated one in three of all adults have at least one LTC (DHSSPSNI, 2012), whilst in Scotland and Northern Ireland these figures rise to 40% and 42% (Gray and Leyland, 2013).

Moreover, it is expected that these figures will rise further in the future (DH, 2012) as a result of an increasingly ageing population, increasing obesity levels, low levels of physical

activity, the effects of tobacco/alcohol consumption, and improving treatments and interventions which allow individuals to survive previously fatal events (see Figure 10.1).

Snell et al. (2011) suggest that by 2030 the number of older people with personal care
needs (e.g. washing and dressing) is expected to rise from 2.5 million to 4.1 million (an
increase of 61%).

The burden of living with an LTC affects the most disadvantaged in society. It is estimated that those belonging to social class V have a 60% higher prevalence of LTCs and
a 60% higher severity as we have highlighted in the previous chapter. There also appears
to be clear links between LTCs, lifestyle factors, deprivation and wider determinants of
health (WHO, 2011). These lifestyle risk factors include tobacco use, high cholesterol
(hypercholesterolemia), high blood pressure (hypertension), obesity/poor diet, alcohol
abuse, exposure to certain infectious diseases and physical inactivity. Other factors such
as socio-economic status, social isolation, access to adequate education and health literacy, together with an environmental disadvantage, should also be taken into account.

Those living with an LTC may experience disadvantage in opportunities in education,
employment and income (Salway et al., 2007). They are also more likely to experience
psychological problems, particularly stress and depression. Experiencing stress over a
long period of time is detrimental to immunity and may increase the likelihood of an
increased disease burden and prolonged recovery (Keller et al., 2000). Moreover, people
living with long-term depression are also at risk of developing co-morbidities (HM
Government/Department of Health, 2011). Therefore, when providing ongoing support
to patients with LTCs it is important for you to be able to recognise the associated
multi-factorial causes and also the opportunities available to help your patients/clients
to minimise or alleviate such risks.

Furthermore, whilst the human cost to individuals who are living with an LTC may be
large, the economic burden is huge. It has been estimated that the most frequent users of
healthcare services are those people living with an LTC – 50% of all GP appointments
and 70% of all inpatient bed days are taken up by people living with an LTC in England.
Within the primary and acute care budget for England 70% is spent on people living
with at least one LTC. Rather surprisingly this corresponds to one in three of the population, accounting for two-thirds of the money spent (ONS, 2011).

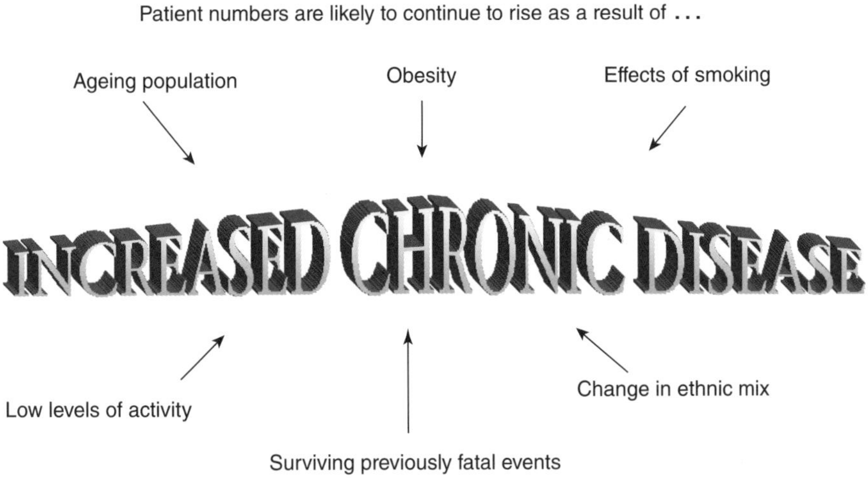

Patient numbers are likely to continue to rise as a result of . . .

Ageing population   Obesity   Effects of smoking

INCREASED CHRONIC DISEASE

Low levels of activity   Surviving previously fatal events   Change in ethnic mix

Figure 10.1   Causes of increased chronic disease

According to the World Health Organization (2011), non-communicable diseases (e.g. cardiovascular diseases, cancers, diabetes and chronic lung diseases) are the leading causes of death globally. In 2008, 17 million deaths were attributed to cardiovascular diseases, 7.6 million to cancers, and 4.2 million to respiratory diseases, including asthma and chronic obstructive pulmonary disease. Diabetes caused an additional 1.3 million deaths. Figure 10.2 illustrates the leading causes of death (England and Wales) in 2012, whilst Figure 10.3 highlights the incidence of disease across the population of England and Wales in 2012.

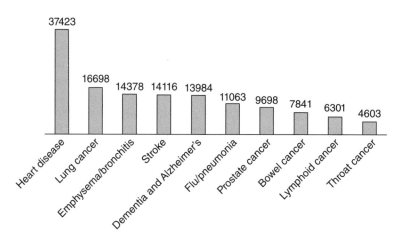

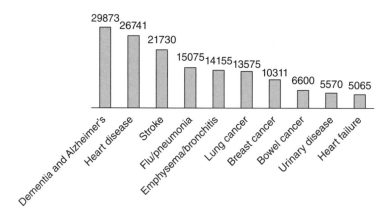

Figure 10.2   Leading cause of deaths in England and Wales in 2012

Source: ONS Part of Mortality Statistics : Deaths Registered in England and Wales (Series DR), 2012 Release (ONS, 2013)

Note: These graphs are based on data from England and Wales in 2012. The numbers at the top of the columns show the actual number of deaths in that year.

Heart and circulatory disease

Circulatory diseases are the primary cause of death globally (WHO, 2011). In addition to the 7.6 million deaths attributed to coronary heart disease (CHD), there are also another 6.2 million due to stroke or cerebrovascular disease (CVD). Coronary heart disease is caused when the heart's blood vessels become narrowed or blocked due to the development of fatty deposits (*atheroma*) on the vessel walls. An individual may be unaware they have CHD until they experience chest pain during exercise which is relieved by rest (angina), or suffer severe chest pain which is not relieved by rest, together with nausea and breathlessness (myocardial infarction). This occurs due to the complete blockage of one or more coronary arteries. Although CHD is preventable and the incidence is falling across the UK, it remains a leading cause of illness and death (ONS, 2013, 2014), particularly in Scotland (e.g. approximately 8,000 deaths per year) where there is a high prevalence of associated risk factors such as smoking, poor diet and physical inactivity (Information Services Division Scotland, 2014). Furthermore, it is estimated that 2.7 million UK residents are living with the condition, and whilst the majority are men, women over the age of 50 have a similar chance to that of men of developing the condition.

Cerebrovascular disease affects the blood vessels supplying the brain and can lead to a stroke, transient ischaemic attacks (TIA), subarachnoid haemorrhage and/or vascular dementia. This is due to the build-up of fatty deposits or atheroma on the intima layer of the blood vessels supplying the brain. Alternatively blood clots or thrombi travelling to the brain (often from the left side of the heart in the presence of *atrial fibrillation*) lead to an occlusion in a smaller cerebral blood vessel. A stroke occurs when there is insufficient blood to an area of the brain due to a blood clot, the narrowed lumen of blood vessels, or a bleed. The flow of blood and hence oxygen is prevented from reaching those areas of the brain the blood vessel supplies. A less common cause of stroke is a subarachnoid haemorrhage due to a ruptured aneurysm (vessel weakness usually at the point of bifurcation) within the cerebral circulation. Whilst cerebrovascular disease tends to affect adults, children can also be affected.

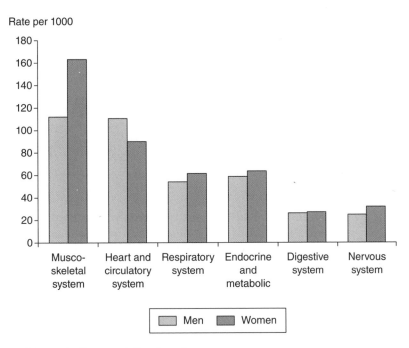

Figure 10.3   Disease in the population (2012)
Source: General Lifestyle Survey-Office for National Statistics (2012)

Hypertension (high blood pressure) is one of the most preventable causes of premature illness and death across the UK (NICE, 2011). It is a common condition, affecting at least 50% of adults over the age of 60 and is a major risk factor for stroke, heart disease, heart failure, chronic kidney disease and cognitive decline. Although the exact cause is unknown, several factors are thought to play a part including obesity, smoking, insufficient exercise, stress, high salt intake, alcohol consumption and genetic pre-disposition.

ACTIVITY 10.1

Access and read the resources identified below:

1. DH (2000) *The National Service Framework for Coronary Heart Disease*. London: DH. Available at www.gov.uk.
2. DH (2007) *The National Stroke Strategy*. DH: London.
3. DH (2013) *Cardiovascular Disease Outcomes Strategy: Improving Outcomes for People with or at Risk of Cardiovascular Disease*. London: DH. Available at www.gov.uk.

Using the resources above:

- identify lifestyle factors which contribute to hypertension, CHD and CVD;
- outline the development of hypertension, CHD and CVD;
- list the symptoms of hypertension, CHD and CVD;
- list the treatment options/aims for each condition;
- list the short- and long-term complications for hypertension, CHD and CVD.

Access the following article: Hopp, F.P., Thornton, N. and Martin, L. (2010) The lived experience of heart failure at the end of life: a systematic literature review, *Health Soc Work*, 35 (2):109–17.

Make a note of the key issues faced by patients. Keep your notes handy – we will return to these later.

Cancer

Cancer can develop at any age but it is most commonly diagnosed in older people aged 75 years and above. The risk of developing cancer over the age of 50 is 1 in 35 for men and 1 in 20 for women (Cancer Research UK, 2014). The incidence of cancer is predicted to rise in all regions of the world over the next few decades, with lung, breast, colorectal, stomach and liver cancers causing the majority of cancer deaths (WHO, 2011). In 2011, cancers accounted for 30 per cent of all deaths (Office for National Statistics, 2012). Cancer is often a greatly feared condition: it occurs when cells specific to one area of the body grow and reproduce uncontrollably. These cancerous cells can then spread to other areas of the body including other organs, causing *metastases*.

ACTIVITY 10.2

Go to the Cancer Research UK website at http://publications.cancerr
then undertake the following:

1. Review the incidence of cancer the UK.
2. Write down a list of the common cancers affecting individuals in the UK, noting any differences you find between the male and female mortality rates.
3. Make a note of all of the precipitating factors related to the cancers identified above.
4. Compare the death rates above with those from previous years.

What are your findings? What do you consider to be the influencing factors in the differences between these rates ?

Now access the following reports:

1. Macmillan Cancer Support Report (2013) *Cured but at What Cost? Long Term Consequences of cancer and its treatment.* Available at www.macmillan.org.uk/
2. NHS Wales (2013) *Wales Cancer Patient Experience Survey.* Cardiff: NHS Wales.

Make a note of the key issues faced by patients who have survived cancer. As previously keep your notes handy – we will return to these later.

Respiratory disease

Chronic obstructive pulmonary disease (COPD) is a progressive and life-threatening lung disease which leads to dyspnoea, primarily due to airway obstruction. It is estimated 64 million people worldwide are living with COPD (WHO, 2015). Within the UK it is thought over 3 million people are living with the disease but only 900,000 have been diagnosed. Additionally, asthma affects over 5 million people in the UK (Asthma UK, 2004). It is a commonly occurring LTC which often commences in childhood.

ACTIVITY 10.3

Access the following resources:

1. NICE (2010) *Chronic Obstructive Pulmonary Disease: Management of Chronic Obstructive Pulmonary Disease in Adults in Primary and Secondary Care (Partial Update), Clinical Guideline 101.* Manchester: NICE.
2. British Thoracic Society/Scottish Intercollegiate Guidelines Networks (2014) *Asthma Guidelines.* Available at www.brit-thoracic.org.uk/document-library/clinical-information/asthma/btssign-asthma-guideline-2014/

(Continued)

(continued)

Using the above documents as supporting evidence:

- Outline the main differences between Asthma and COPD.
- What lifestyle factors contribute to the onset of Asthma/COPD?
- Make a list of the symptoms of Asthma and COPD.
- Identify the short- and long-term complications of poorly controlled Asthma/COPD.

Now have a look at the following articles: Barnett, M. (2005) Chronic obstructive pulmonary disease: a phenomenological study of patients' experiences, *Journal of Clinical Nursing*, 14 (7): 805–12.

Write down the key issues faced by these patient – we will return to your notes later.

Diabetes

Diabetes Mellitus is a chronic and lifelong condition which occurs when an individual's blood glucose becomes elevated. Either the pancreas does not produce enough of the hormone insulin which facilitates the transport of glucose into the cells of the body or the body is unable to effectively use the insulin produced.

In the UK approximately 2.9 million people are living with the condition and an estimated 850,000 with undiagnosed diabetes. There are two main types: Type 1 and Type 2 (T2DM). By 2025 it is estimated that this number will rise to over 4 million (Diabetes UK, 2013).

ACTIVITY 10.4

Access the following resources:

1. Department of Health (2001) *The National Service Framework for Diabetes.* Available at www.gov.uk
2. NICE (2014) *Diabetes Pathway.* Available at http://pathways.nice.org.uk/pathways/diabetes
3. Diabetes UK (2013) *State of the Nation 2013: England.* London: Diabetes UK.

Using the above documents undertake the following:

- Identify the factors which contribute to the onset of Type 1 and Type 2 diabetes.
- Outline the main symptoms of undiagnosed or poorly controlled diabetes.
- Summarise the main treatment aims and make a list of the short- and long-term complications of Type 1 and Type 2 Diabetes Mellitus. Now consider the following question.

Why do you think that the management of diabetes continues to be a major challenge for the NHS?

Chronic liver disease

Liver disease is the fifth most common cause of death in the UK. Over the last ten years there has been a five-fold increase in the development of *cirrhosis* in 35 to 55 year olds and deaths from liver disease appear to be rising steadily (ONS, 2008). Causes of liver disease can vary but include alcohol misuse, infection (Hepatitis B and C) and obesity (British Liver Trust, 2014).

ACTIVITY 10.5

1. Access the following websites to find out more about liver disease and its management –
   British Liver Trust website: www.britishlivertrust.org.uk
2. Download a copy of 'Living with Liver Disease' and identify potential issues faced by patients.
3. Review the following clinical guidelines: Society of Gastroenterology (2009) *Management of Patients with Chronic Liver Disease.* Available at www.bsg.org.uk/
4. Royal College of Nursing (2013) *Caring for People with Liver Disease: A Competency Framework for Nursing.* London: RCN.

According to the British Society of Gastroenterology (2009), liver disease is now the fifth most common cause of death in the UK, largely as a result of lifestyle factors such as obesity, harmful alcohol use and hepatitis infection.

Chronic kidney disease

Chronic Kidney Disease (CKD) is a term used to describe abnormal kidney function and/or structure. It is common, frequently unrecognised, and often exists together with other conditions (for example, cardiovascular disease and diabetes). In England in 2008/09 there were 1,739,443 people aged 18 and over registered with CKD, though since some individuals remain undiagnosed the UK prevalence is likely to be higher (East Midlands Public Health Observatory and NHS Kidney Care, 2010).

ACTIVITY 10.6

1. Access the NHS Kidney Care (2010), *Kidney Disease Facts and Figures.* East Midlands Public Health Observatory and NHS Kidney Care East Midlands, and then do the following:

- Make a list of the risk factors associated with the development of CKD.
- Outline the associated health burdens and complications of CKD.

2. Review the Department of Health's (2009 and 2010) *National Service Framework (NSF) for Renal Services Parts 1 and 2* and NICE (2014) *Chronic Kidney Disease: Early Identification and Management of Chronic Kidney Disease in Adults in Primary and secondary Care. NICE Guideline CG 182.* Available at www.nice.org.uk
3. Access the following article: Caress, A.-L, Luker, K.A. and Owens, A.G. (2001) A descriptive study of meaning of illness in chronic renal disease, *Journal of Advanced Nursing,* 33(6): 716–27. Make a note of the key issues faced by patients with CKD.

Long-term neurological conditions

Neurological conditions collectively affecting ten million people across the UK account for 20% of all acute hospital admissions (DH, 2005). Examples include dementia/Alzheimer's, epilepsy, Multiple Sclerosis, Parkinson's Disease, stroke and traumatic brain injury and myalgic encephalomyelitis (CFS/ME). At any one time, it is estimated that 350,000 people with a long-term neurological condition will need support with their daily living (DH, 2005).

ACTIVITY 10.7

Find out more about how common neurological conditions affect people in the UK by accessing the following guidelines:

1. Department of Health (2005) *National Service Framework for Long Term Conditions.* London: DH.
2. Scottish Intercollegiate Guidelines Network (2013) 'Diagnosis and pharmacological management of Parkinson's disease: a national clinical guideline'. Available at www.sign.ac.uk/pdf/sign113.pdf
3. NICE (2003) *Multiple Sclerosis: Management of Multiple Sclerosis in Primary and Secondary Care.* London: NICE.

You can also find out more about specific conditions at the websites identified below:

- Multiple Sclerosis Society: www.mssociety.org.uk
- Parkinson's UK: www.parkinsons.org.uk
- Alzheimer's Society: www.alzheimers.org.uk
- Epilepsy Society :www.epilepsysociety.org.uk/
- ME Association: www.meassociation.org.uk/
- Action for ME: www.actionforme.org.uk/

Make a list of the potential problems encountered by patients suffering from a neurological LTC (remember to include physical/motor, sensory, cognitive, communication, psychosocial and emotional effects).

Chronic Muscular Skeletal Conditions (MSK)

The term 'musculoskeletal' describes conditions which affect the joints, muscles and bones. Whilst the prevalence of MSK conditions tends to increase with age, they can affect any age group and account for 40% of all disabilities across the UK. Conditions include those caused by an abnormal inflammatory process (e.g. Rheumatoid Arthritis and Ankylosing Spondylitis), general 'wear and tear' (e.g. osteoarthritis), and bone disease (Osteoporosis). Fibromyalgia is a common condition characterised by widespread muscle and joint pain and stiffness.

ACTIVITY 10.8

Go to the Arthritis Research UK website and download the following article:
   Ryan et al. (2013) *The Absent Professional.* London: Arthritis UK.
   Available at www.arthritisresearchuk.org/health-professionals-and-students/the-absent-health-professional.aspx

- Make notes on the report's key findings.
- Now think about what adult nurses could do to help.

As an adult nurse, it is important that you continue to update your knowledge and understanding, making sure that the care you deliver is based upon best available evidence. Having undertaken all of the activities in this book thus far, you should have a good level of knowledge and understanding of the common long-term conditions that affect individuals living in the UK, and the lifestyle factors that often contribute to the onset of some of these conditions. This knowledge and understanding prove crucial when we focus upon the role of the adult nurse in supporting patients later in this chapter.

Living with a long-term condition: the patient experience

Most people have to learn to 'live with' rather than 'die from' a chronic illness (Verbrugge and Jette, 1994). Therefore we need to consider the psychosocial impact that living with a long-term condition can have on individuals and their families.

STOP AND THINK

- What percentage of the patients you have met have been living with either one or more LTC?

Using the notes you have made when undertaking the previous activities consider the potential impact that an LTC has on job prospects, lifestyle, and relationships with family or significant others, as well as the physical, psychological and behavioural aspects of life. This is a good opportunity to explore some of these issues with your patients too (although you will need to do this sensitively).
   Make a list of as many impact factors you can think of (including those that you identified earlier). Points you might want to consider include the following:

- If your patients/clients were admitted to hospital, what factors led to their admission (e.g. a link to hospital or community care provision)?
- Are there any contributing factors which may have led to other admissions?

(Continued)

(Continued)

- If a patient/client was based in a community setting, what care was required and how often was the intervention undertaken?

Try also to consider how the LTC may have affected either their ability to work or their choice of job if working. Also consider how an LTC can affect lifestyle, hobbies, holidays taken, family and social interaction.

ACTIVITY 10.9

Now access the following website: www.healthtalkonline.org

- Listen to some of the patient accounts of how various long-term conditions can affect the lives of patients on a day-to-day basis.
- Compare their accounts with the issues you have identified above.

Over the years researchers have sought to describe patients' lived experiences of living with chronic illness or a long-term condition (Caress et al., 2001; Crumbie and Lawrence, 2002; Barnett, 2005; Claessens et al., 2005; Salway et al., 2007; Tierney et al., 2008; Clancy et al., 2009; Lempp et al., 2009; Hopp et al., 2010), and although many of these studies focus on a specific disease or condition, there are a number of frequently occurring issues and symptoms which appear to be present no matter what the diagnosis or condition may be. Most commonly, these include:

- *symptoms* (e.g. tiredness/fatigue, increasing disability, anxiety or depression);
- *perceived loss* (in terms of independence and social activity linked to increasing disability affecting daily activities, occupation, confidence, self-worth/value, intimacy, role within family, control, individuality);
- *feelings* (e.g. fear, frustration, blame, denial, and sometimes anger).

Fatigue

Fatigue is commonly experienced by people suffering from a variety of chronic illnesses (not just those identified as suffering from CFS/ME: for more specific information about this condition see the suggested Further Reading at the end of the chapter).

The concept of fatigue was initially used in the sixteenth century to describe a tedious duty, though nowadays fatigue is regarded as feeling tired for 'no reason'. Barsevick et al. (2010) have described it as being subjective; a feeling unrelated to being tired after exercise and being relieved after rest. It may be regarded as exhaustive, unpredictable in its course, and affecting cognitive ability. Fatigue is often described as multi-dimensional and disabling, affecting the quality of life of those living with it. Negative emotions such as anxiety, numbness and vulnerability may also be experienced, and are likely to have an impact on social relationships and family life, often leading to withdrawal and social isolation. Wilson et al. (2011) considered the concept of chronic fatigue within their qualitative study of 43 individuals who were living with chronic fatigue. Participants were predominately female and aged 45 or older. A thematic analysis of the interview transcripts identified two main themes, that of managing energy and redefining the self. Overall the study suggested that gaining an understanding of how each individual conceptualises their own unique experience would be a good starting point for nurses, allowing them to tailor interventions that would best suit their patients rather than merely suggesting strategies for successful living.

Chronic insomnia

Chronic insomnia is defined as a difficulty initiating and/or maintaining sleep, early waking and sleep which is non-restorative, together with daytime fatigue and poor concentration lasting over six months (American Academy of Sleep Medicine, 2005; Matin and Benca, 2012). Chronic insomnia is often found in individuals suffering from chronic illness (Taylor et al., 2007; Lempp et al., 2009). However, according to Williams et al. (2013) it may be difficult to determine the cause since predisposing conditions precipitating circumstances and perpetuating factors may be included. Examples include:

- A person who has an anxious personality trait may predispose to sleep problems, resulting in hyper arousal.
- A precipitating event (maybe a decline in health).
- A stressful event.
- Insomnia that is maintained by perpetuating factors, such as having a nap during the day or having an extended lie-in.
- Use of prescribed medications, alcohol or other stimulants (e.g. caffeine).
- Pain.

The exclusion of primary sleep disorders is important. A primary sleep disorder is defined as:

> ... one that arises out of the physiological processes of sleep for example obstructive sleep apnoea, restless legs syndrome. (Clinical Practice Guidelines Working Group, 2010)

This may involve a the patient keeping a sleep diary which aims to highlight patterns of insomnia, prescribed medication such as hypnotics and instances of rebound insomnia (Gottlieb et al., 2005).

Mental health issues

The impact of poor mental health is well documented. Globally, depression is the second leading cause of years lived with disability, affecting around 150 million people worldwide (Vos et al., 2012). Those living with an LTC are two to three times more likely to experience mental ill health such as anxiety and depression than those in the general population. It has also been suggested that at least 30% of those living with an LTC will develop mental ill health (Cimpean and Drake, 2011).

Biessels et al. (2006) found that individuals with CVD and diabetes were also at increased risk of developing mild cognitive impairment, vascular dementia and Alzheimer's disease. Furthermore, the relationship between mental and physical health is a complex one. Prince et al. (2007) have suggested there is a combination of environmental, psychological, biological and behavioural factors involved. The relationship between physical and mental health is not linear, and those who primarily experience a mental health problem are at increased risk of developing a long-term physical illness such as cardiovascular diseases, stroke and Type 2 diabetes mellitus. In one US study (Goldberg, 2010) the rates of depression were found to be double in those living with a diagnosis of hypertension, coronary heart disease and heart failure, and three times the incidence in those people living with COPD. A number of other studies have highlighted how depression can exacerbate the distress, pain, sleeplessness and fatigue experienced by many people living with an LTC. There also appears to be a strong correlation between heart disease (such as a myocardial infarction) and depression, both in the immediate diagnostic period and up to a year after diagnosis (Lesperance et al., 2009). Ultimately it appears that those living with two or more LTCs are much more likely to have depression than a healthy person.

However some would argue that this aspect of care is often overlooked, and many of the patients suffering from chronic medical conditions and co-occurring depression or anxiety are never diagnosed or treated for their psychiatric conditions (Cepoiu et al., 2008; Melek and Norris, 2008). The impact of this can be a reduced quality of life, poorer self-care and adverse health behaviours, as well as poorer health outcomes and overall prognosis (Naylor et al., 2012). Mental health problems can also negatively impact upon a person's ability to self manage their condition (HMG/DH, 2011). Salway et al. (2007) suggest that positively adapting to chronic illness requires both mental adjustments and the ability to gain control by developing coping strategies, and that patients may need additional support from adult nurses and other external sources in order to positively adapt to their changed health status.

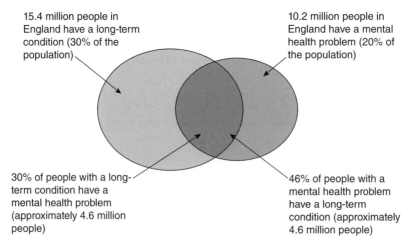

15.4 million people in England have a long-term condition (30% of the population)

10.2 million people in England have a mental health problem (20% of the population)

30% of people with a long-term condition have a mental health problem (approximately 4.6 million people)

46% of people with a mental health problem have a long-term condition (approximately 4.6 million people)

Figure 10.4   The overlap between long-term conditions and mental health problems (Naylor et al., 2012)

Social isolation and loneliness

Loneliness is a complex concept and a variety of definitions exist. It may be regarded as social loneliness or isolation whereby contact with friends and social networks are limited, or as emotional isolation or a feeling of not being in time or in connection with other human beings (Holmes et al., 2000). This definition links with earlier work by Bowlby and Weiss (1973) who considered loneliness from a social and psychological perspective and suggested it to consist of two dimensions, emphasising the core experience rather than the intensity of the relationships. The experience of loneliness among the very old (Kirkevold et al., 2012) has been regarded in positive terms, for example a feeling of being free, as well as the more negative connotation of being abandoned and feelings of fear and sadness. Alternatively, Killeen (1998) considered the concept of loneliness as a continuum, with the most positive attributes being feelings of connectedness and the most negative being alienation and powerlessness as displayed by social and self-isolation.

However, despite the plethora of definitions there is reticence on the part of many people to acknowledge that they are lonely, possibly due to the degree of stigma attached to it but also that it is an expected part of growing old. A number of studies throughout the world have identified that approximately 40% of people aged 65 and over describe themselves as lonely (Victor and Yang, 2012; Victor and Bowling, 2012). Predisposing factors include living alone, experiencing social and physical losses (for example, having difficulties getting out of the house) and also chronic health problems which may be physical and/or psychological (Victor and Bowling, 2012). In an interview study carried out in the UK, Australia and Norway, Kirkevold et al. (2012) identified differences between those who considered themselves 'lonely' and 'not lonely'. The study involved 78 individuals, with 55 women and 23 men aged 65 and above. The themes identified from interviews with the 'not lonely' group included accepting losses and moving on, staying committed to activities, staying connected to other people, and being able to create a meaningful life in one's own company. The group who regarded themselves as 'lonely' emphasised the themes such as being caught in loneliness and isolation, being overpowered by accumulating losses, being unable to carry on with activities, being isolated from other people, and considering that a life alone is an empty life. These differences appeared to be dependent on how the participants understood and dealt with losses. However, as Kirkevold et al. (2012) point out they did not assess for indictors of depression in the participants who contributed to this study.

It appears crucial for nurses to be able to identify those who are lonely, although this may be problematic due to the degree of stigma attached to the concept. There is obviously a need for nurses to facilitate discussion once a rapport has been established with an individual living with a chronic condition. Individuals who have experienced major losses (for example, being widowed or having a chronic health condition) are at risk of loneliness. An early indicator is the difference in everyday activities, although the need to assess for low mood is also important since changes in everyday activities are one indicator of depression.

In July 2000 the UK government published the NHS Plan (DH, 2000), establishing a strategy for the provision of high quality services focusing on a number of chronic diseases through the implementation of a series of National Service Frameworks (NSFs). The various NSFs outline both the actions needed to be taken to reduce the incidence of specific diseases and the treatment and care which should be provided for patients.

Therefore you will no doubt recognise how important it is for healthcare professionals to be able to recognise, diagnose, instigate and evaluate treatment alongside improved patient access to high quality services. Moreover, the National Service Framework (NSF) for Long Term Conditions (DH, 2005) highlights the importance of a 'person-centred' approach to care provision, and sets out the way in which all healthcare professionals are expected to support patients to live as independently as possible by:

- giving people choice, through services planned and delivered around their individual needs;
- coordinating partnership working between health and social services and other local agencies.

Underpinned by a Health and Social Care Framework (DH, 2005) (see Figure 10.5), the NSF for LTC stresses the need for patients to have access to the relevant information necessary to be able to make an informed choice about their treatment.

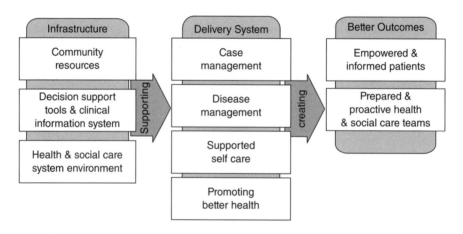

Figure 10.5   The NHS and Social Care Long Term Conditions Model

Source: Department of Health (2005)

Supported self-care

Around 80% to 90% of all care for people with long-term conditions is undertaken by patients themselves and their families (Entwistle and Cribb, 2013). *Self-care* is defined by the Department of Health (2009: 4) as:

> ... people taking responsibility for their own health and well-being. It includes staying fit and healthy, taking action to prevent illness and accidents, using medicines effectively, treating minor ailments appropriately, and seeking professional help when necessary.

Supported self-care requires a healthcare professional to support patients in making decisions that will help them effectively manage their long-term condition.

The Department of Health (2009) suggests that this involves offering patients timely information and support to empower them to take an active role in maintaining their health. Similarly, the Long Term Conditions Alliance Scotland (LTCAS) defines self management as:

> ... the successful outcome of the person and all appropriate individuals and services working together to support him or her to deal with the very real implications of living the rest of their life with one or more long term condition. (Scottish Government, 2009: 2)

The supported self-care approach requires adult nurses to provide information, care and encouragement for patients in order to help them understand and manage their illness themselves, make informed decisions about their care, and engage in healthy behaviours. It also includes working to enhance a patient's capacity for self management, providing support to ensure that they have more control of their conditions and therefore their life. Evidence suggests that supported self-care can result in beneficial health outcomes for people and more appropriate use of health and social care services (DH, 2009). However, self management also involves the patient coming to terms with and effectively dealing with the consequences of their condition/s. This requires the patient having the confidence and ability to problem solve and make decisions about their care in partnership with healthcare professionals (we will explore this aspect again later in the chapter). Furthermore, there is no one single approach advocated. Corben and Rosen (2005) argue that individuals often have different ways of coping with an LTC and not everyone will want to be actively involved in managing their own condition, though it is necessary to recognise that a patient's willingness to be involved might also fluctuate over time and depending upon the circumstances.

Disease management is defined as a system of co-ordinated, multidisciplinary healthcare interventions for people with long-term conditions, the aim of which is to ensure that patients are monitored regularly and defined outcomes/indicators are achieved in order to reduce the risk of health deterioration (Dusheiko et al., 2011). Disease management strategies are targeted at those patients at lower risk of admission to hospital and are usually delivered within a community setting (often by GPs, practice nurses, pharmacists, and other healthcare workers). For example, nurses working in general practice often aim to improve the health of individual patients with chronic conditions via monitoring (e.g. checking the blood sugar levels of patients with diabetes, the blood pressure of patients with hypertension) and/or providing lifestyle advice for smokers or the obese. In 2004, a 'pay for performance' incentive scheme, the Quality and Outcomes Framework (QOF) (Health and Social Care Information Centre, 2013b), was introduced by the UK government as part of the new GP contract for the delivery of primary care in England, in the hope that this would stimulate an improvement in the way chronic disease was managed.

ACTIVITY 10.10

Access the Health and Social Care Information Centre Website and search for the Quality Outcomes Framework results for one of the GP practices (perhaps your own if you live in England): www.qof.hscic.gov.uk/index.asp

- Make a list of the clinical areas covered.
- How do the QOF results of your own GP practice compare against other GP practices in your area?
- What do you think might account for any differences?

Now consider the potential impact of the QOF on nursing practice.

- What challenges might adult nurses face when collecting QOF data during a patient consultation/visit?
- Make a list of potential organisations and professional/non-professionals that could be involved in supporting patients with an LTC.
- What skills would an adult nurse require to be able to work effectively with the multi-disciplinary team?

According to Steel and Willems (2010) the positive impact of the QOF remains patchy and inconclusive, and there have been some concerns related to the potential neglect of non-incentivised disease areas and 'gaming', whereby GP practices might remove patients with an LTC from their register or alter levels of reporting to influence the results (Maresso, 2013). There are also concerns that an 'information collecting' or 'box-ticking' approach can negatively impact upon the notion of patient-centred care (Upton et al., 2011; Phillips, 2013).

Case management

Hutt et al. (2004) describe case management as 'the process of planning, co-ordinating and reviewing the care of an individual'. The intended focus is aimed at patients who are the most vulnerable, who have highly complex needs or multiple LTCs (multiple morbidity), and are therefore at greater risk of admission to hospital. A case management approach is used to anticipate and co-ordinate health and social care, with the aim of reducing hospital admissions and/or length of hospital stay, improving care outcomes for patients, and enhancing the patient experience. Ross et al. (2011) suggest that case management involves:

- case-finding;
- assessment;
- care planning;
- care co-ordination (usually undertaken by a case manager in the context of a multi-disciplinary team).

There is some evidence to suggest that ongoing and personalised case management can improve care and reduce inpatient and outpatient costs (Roland et al., 2012).

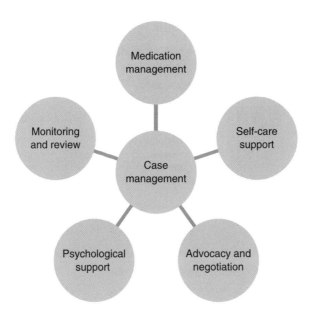

Figure 10.6   Case management

However, case management is not always implemented in a cost-effective way or for the benefit of patients and carers (Ross et al., 2011; Roland et al., 2012). Purdy (2010) argues that other approaches are more beneficial (i.e. patient self management, continuity of GP care, and the integration of primary/secondary care and health/social care). In particular, those patients who have more than one LTC as well as older patients often face an increasingly fragmented and 'specialised' response (Department of Health/Long Term Conditions, 2012). You may well have noticed this yourself, especially in terms of patients you may come across who have experienced multiple admissions to hospital over the last 12 months.

Therefore, in contrast to the reactive, disease-focused and clinically-driven care of the recent past, *integrated care* models are now being explored as a means of meeting the challenges of changing disease burdens (Goodwin et al., 2013a, 2013b).

Coulter et al. (2013) propose the use of a co-ordinated 'House of Care Model' (see Figure 10.7) which aims to deliver holistic patient-centred preventative and proactive care in England by 'taking as its starting point the active involvement of patients in developing their own care plans through a shared decision-making process with clinicians' (Coulter et al., 2013: 2)

Establishing a collaborative approach with active client/patient involvement is considered crucial. Another key aspect of the model is to ensure that the care planning for individuals and commissioning for local populations are closely linked. The aim is for local services, community resources, social and healthcare – together with more traditional health services – to work together (Coulter et al., 2013). Furthermore, it is argued that the whole health and social care system should be interdependent.

The aim is for planning, implementation and evaluation of care to be an ongoing process and that the healthcare provider is able to recognise the personal strengths and the lived experiences of the patient. This requires time, especially for those individuals who may be living with multiple LTCs where longer appointment times are necessary. It is hoped that by using integrated health and social care planning, care is personalised, the patient is an active participant, and sufficient support is offered for self-management.

IT: clinical record of care planning

Test results / agenda
setting prompts:
beforehand

Know your population

Contact numbers and
safety netting

Organisational
processes

'Prepared' for
consultation

Consultation skills
/ attitudes

Information/
Structured
education

**Collaborative
care
planning
consultation**

Integrated,
multidisciplinary
team & expertise

Engaged,
informed patient

HCP committed to
partnership working

Senior buy-in &
local champions
to support & role
model

Emotional &
psychological
support

Commissioning
– The foundation

Commissioning the menu
(including Non Traditional
Providers)

Commissioning care
planning

Metrics and
monitoring

Figure 10.7   The House of Care Model
Source: Coulter et al. (2013)

It is also crucial that the health and social care is co-ordinated and crosses team and geographical boundaries so that care planning moves away from a reactive illness model of care towards a proactive one which aims to help individuals stay active as long as possible (King's Fund, 2012).

ACTIVITY 10.11

Access the following document: Naylor et al. (2013) *Transforming Our Healthcare System: Ten Priorities for Commissioners*. Available at www.kingsfund.org.uk/publications/articles/transforming-our-health-care-system-ten-priorities-commisioners
    Identify the ten priorities for Healthcare Commissioners which are needed to transform the healthcare system.

The Mandate for NHS England (DH, 2014) and the *NHS Constitution* (DH, 2013c) aim to ensure everyone who is living with an LTC (either primarily physical or psychological) has their wishes regarding care respected and an agreed single personalised care plan formulated.

Patient empowerment and partnership working

People with an LTC are now increasingly working in partnership with health and social care professionals, taking an active role in managing their condition. However, many say that they want to be listened to and be more involved in decisions about their care. They also want access to information to help them make those decisions, and more support in developing the confidence to manage and understand their condition/s, particularly in relation to medications and treatments and general health advice (DH, 2006; Ipsos Mori, 2011).

ACTIVITY 10.12

Take a look at the National Voices report focusing on what patients, service users and carers say they want: Integrated Care: What do Patients, Service Users and Carers Want? Available at www.nationalvoices.org.uk

In your role as an adult nurse, how might you begin to address these needs in your everyday practice?

Partnership working is a fundamental aspect of the adult nurse's role. Therefore an adult nurse must be able to develop an inclusive and mutually beneficial relationship with patient/clients and carers in order to improve the quality and experience of care.

In the past a paternalistic/maternalistic relationship (reflecting a medical model of care) often meant that patients were expected to accept a passive role in any healthcare encounter, whereby the doctor/nurse would tell patients what they needed and patients would submissively accept this. Nowadays however, the power-relationship between healthcare professionals and patients should be more equal (see Figure 10.8).

The concept of patient 'empowerment' has many facets which can differ depending upon on whether this is applied to a community, organisational or individual context.

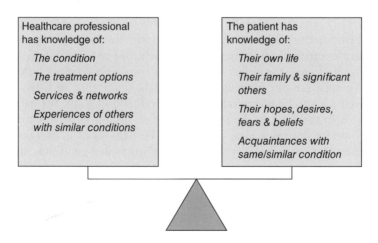

Figure 10.8   The balance of power in the patient-professional relationship

Source: Crumbie and Lawrence (2002)

However, in this case we refer to it as being suggestive of the nurse handing over or 'giving power' to the patient. It is a process which aims to change the nature and distribution of power in the nurse-patient therapeutic relationship, with the intention to increase the patient's control over their own health. Patients become active partners in the management of their own condition (e.g. planning care, deciding upon and evaluating treatment options). By acknowledging that the patient is an expert in terms of their own experience and condition, a more equal and facilitative relationship is established.

STOP AND THINK

Reflecting on the care that you provided to one of your patients recently – think about what you did and how you did it.

- Was it possible to take every opportunity to empower your patient? If so how? If not, why not?
- How did this impact upon the care provided?

We have established that working in partnership should involve acknowledging and respecting a patient's views, circumstances, and preferences for care. Yet research findings suggest that true collaboration or 'power-sharing' appears to be rare and this can act as a barrier to patient participation in care. Examples of 'overt' power and persuasion can still be found (Upton et al., 2011). Barriers to partnership working can include a nurse's (or patient's) lack of confidence, experience, or a perceived lack of time, as well as the attitude of the healthcare professional and/or patient (Millard et al., 2006; Wilson et al., 2006; Zoffmann and Kirkevold, 2005 and 2007; Upton et al., 2011). We also need to ensure that we take account of cultural differences.

How can we work to empower patients?

Dowling et al. (2011) suggest that in order to be able to empower patients, we ourselves must first feel empowered. We must also be able to communicate effectively and be willing to surrender 'control' to our patients. Conversely, our patients will need to be motivated to change and have the ability to engage in the empowerment process. To make this happen we must see our patients as individuals, make time to listen to their concerns, and develop a good understanding of their values and goals. We will also have to ensure that we help them access the information they need in order for them to be able to make appropriate decisions about their care. Perhaps most importantly, there is a need to regard the person as an individual who is living with a condition but not defined by it.

Zoffmann and Kirkevold (2012) suggest that the use of a Guided Self Determination (GSD) model can assist healthcare practitioners in helping patients to identify, express and share the unique and unexpected difficulties they face whilst living with an LTC. Using a life-skills approach, the five-stage process involves:

1. The establishment of an I–you-sorted relationship.
2. Self-exploration.
3. Self-understanding.

4. Action.
5. Feedback from action.

Zoffmann and Kirkevold argue that use of the model has helped nurses establish meaningful therapeutic relationships with their patients, raise awareness of the 'life versus
disease conflicts' faced by both patient and nurse, and in doing so, has helped to overcome many of the barriers to empowerment.

ACTIVITY 10.13

Access a copy of the Department of Health (2009) document *Your Health Your Way* and
write down your answers to the following questions:

- Identify the five core aims of the document.
- Now thinking about each of these in turn, what will you need to do to ensure that as an
  adult nurse you will be able to support patients with LTCs in the future?

There is a wide range of initiatives aimed at supporting self-care, varying from the provision of information and education to develop technical skills, to proactive strategies
aimed at changing behaviour and increasing self efficacy. All of these approaches are
important but there is evidence to suggest that adopting proactive strategies is the most
effective (De Silva, 2011).

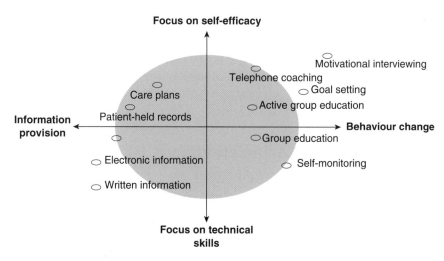

Figure 10.9   Continuum strategies to support self-management

Source: The Health Foundation (2011)

Providing health information

The NHS Constitution (DH, 2013c) sets out a commitment to offer easily accessible,
reliable and relevant information to enable people to participate fully in healthcare decisions

and support them in making choices. In the previous chapter we explored the role of the adult nurse in helping patients to make healthy lifestyle choices, particularly in terms of taking adequate exercise, good nutrition, and the avoidance of unhealthy behaviours such as excessive alcohol consumption and smoking. There is also a clear need to ensure patients are able to access the information and support needed in order to gain the knowledge and confidence to communicate effectively with healthcare workers. This could include the provision of written or electronic information, videos/DVDs, online courses, patient-held records or care plans, and the use of web-based technologies (Kuijpers et al., 2013) such as the internet or *e-health* initiatives (e.g. NHS Information Prescriptions – www.nhs.uk/information prescriptions, and E-learning for Healthcare – www.e-lfh.org.uk). Evidence suggests that self-management behaviours can be facilitated through the exchange of health information and disease experience (Willis, 2013).

ACTIVITY 10.14

1. Find out where you can access information that will help improve your own knowledge and understanding of each LTC and how best to support your patients.
2. Make a list of local and national sources of information that would be useful for patients to help improve their knowledge and understanding of their LTC.
3. Consider the pros and cons associated with utilising the internet or e-resources (for healthcare professionals and patients).
(Do remember to include all public, private and voluntary sources.)

One of the key issues faced by healthcare professionals today is that patients often have unlimited access to sources of information about health, illness treatment and care, including web-based chat or bulletin boards and social networking sites.

• How could this impact upon the quality of information or advice given ?
• As an adult nurse, how can you advise and support your patients accordingly?

Tools and self-monitoring devices

Tools and self-monitoring devices can help individuals play an integral role in monitoring their LTC (De Silva, 2011). This can involve the monitoring of physiological measurements (e.g. blood pressure or blood glucose/cholesterol levels) via electronic devices or written self-management plans which assist patients to self-medicate and self-refer when appropriate. Moreover the use and impact of telehealthcare is an initiative currently attracting a lot of interest, particularly in terms of exploring associated cost implications (Rogers et al., 2011; Car et al., 2012; Henderson et al., 2013) and benefits to patients and healthcare professionals (Verhoeven et al., 2007; Milligan et al., 2011). The term 'telehealthcare' relates to the real-time monitoring of physiological data (which can include remote professional assistance) though there is a limited evidence base for their effectiveness. Examples include closed circuit TV/video conferencing, the use of email and remote monitoring. Other approaches such as *M-health* involve the use of mobile apps or personalised systems downloaded to phones or personal computers which are used for the personal monitoring of chronic conditions. These systems can communicate with remote call centres, thereby providing data for a professional review. McLean et al. (2013) point out that longer-term studies are needed to determine the long-term benefit of such approaches.

Make a list of the equipment and tools you have come across that assist your patients to self-care and maintain their independence:

- Do you (and your patients) know how to use these properly?
- Are there any other devices or tools that they might be able to access?
- How would your patients gain access to these?

(Remember that in addition to devices related to health and social care, you should consider the contribution of other aids and adaptations that can be accessed via the voluntary and private sector.)

STOP AND THINK

The voluntary and community sector has a key role in terms of providing advice and information about equipment and tools to help people self-care and maintain their independence. Housing and care services, such as home improvement agencies, will install aids and adapt and repair people's homes to help them live independently (DH, 2009).

Skills training and support networks

As previously mentioned LTCs appear to disproportionately affect those with lower socio-economic status and poorer health literacy. Whilst there is a need for skills training and continuing support to help people engage with healthcare professionals, nurses and other healthcare professionals also need to support the collaborative process and encourage patients into being better-informed active participants. For some individuals referral to a self- help group or a lay-led educational programme such as the *Expert Patient Programme* (EPP) may be beneficial. A literature review carried out by Entwistle and Cribb (2013) suggests that proactive, behaviourally-focused self-management support can have a positive impact on clinical symptoms, attitudes and behaviours, patient quality of life and the use of healthcare resources. Self-management programmes such as EPP have been shown to reduce costs and improve health (Kennedy et al., 2007; Rogers et al., 2008; Expert Patients Programme, 2010; Sibbald et al., 2010), though Wilson and Brooks (2007) highlight the need to ensure that programmes such as these are able to attract individuals from a variety of backgrounds and cultural groups. Reported positive patient outcomes include reductions in depression, anxiety, pain and fatigue, fewer GP visits and increased use of cognitive symptom management techniques, for example goal-setting, exercise and relaxation. Similarly the professionally-led DESMOND (Davies et al., 2008) and DAFNE (Leelarathna et al., 2011) programmes for those people living with Diabetes Mellitus have enabled collaborative care planning. Voluntary groups and charities also play an important role in helping to support patients and their families. In one study involving patients living with diabetes, Due-Christensen et al. (2012) reported major benefits in terms of patients 'feeling less alone' and reducing diabetes-related and psychological distress.

However, further improvements are necessary. The Mental Health Foundation (2012) has called for improvements in the access, quality and professional support provided to peer support schemes aimed at addressing the mental health needs of patients with LTCs, an aspect of care which is often overlooked.

STOP AND THINK

What programmes, courses or voluntary groups are available to patients in your area?

- What referral criteria are used?

Consider how you might use this information to help you to support patients with LTCs in your workplace.

Personalised Care Planning (PCP)

Personalised Care Planning is defined by the Department of Health as:

> ... addressing an individual's full range of needs, taking into account their health, personal, social, economic, educational, mental health, ethnic and cultural background and circumstances. It recognises that there are other issues in addition to medical needs that can affect a person's total health and well-being. (Department of Health, 2009: 4)

PCP involves helping people with an LTC to identify *their* desired outcomes and then setting agreed goals, action planning, problem solving, and providing information and access to additional support and treatments where necessary to help them achieve those goals. The process of developing a care plan can help people understand the aims of the care and support they are receiving, as well as any actions they may need to take if their condition worsens (i.e. emergency or crisis planning). The benefits of having a care plan include greater *concordance* with agreed treatment plans and an increased sense of control for patients.

The personalised care planning journey has three distinct phases:

- Preparing.
- Planning.
- Maintaining.

It is a process which will call upon your numerous skills and developing knowledge base.

STOP AND THINK

- What skills do you have that will assist you in supporting patients through this process?
- What new knowledge and skills might you need to access in order to develop and/or review an individual plan?

Developing a personal care plan in partnership with patients and carers will call upon all of the skills, attributes, values and behaviours outlined in previous chapters that are considered crucial when attempting to build a therapeutic relationship. The process involves discussion, negotiation, shared decision making, and review. Care plans (written or otherwise) should include information on the individuals' concerns, their well-being needs, actions, goals, information relating to support organisations, and any other specific needs they may have.

 MURIEL

Muriel lives with her 76-year-old husband Clive in a ground floor maisonette in an inner city area. Clive has been living with COPD and Type 2 diabetes for over 28 years and had to retire early (at 50) from his job as a joiner due to increased breathlessness and his poorly controlled diabetes. Since that time he has, until recently, enjoyed socialising with his friends, trying to keep his allotment going (he enjoys growing West Indian vegetables and peppers), and has remained the patriarch of his extended family. Muriel has tried to support her husband both physically and emotionally whilst still taking on some cleaning jobs in the city. Clive admits to being rather stubborn in regard to his dietary control, alcohol intake and occasional cigarette smoking – however the development of an ulcer on his right leg has led to a prolonged period of physical inactivity, disturbed sleep and increasing social isolation. Clive confides in you that he has been feeling tired, lonely, isolated and depressed which has resulted in his 'comfort eating'. He is becoming increasingly breathless and tells you that he still occasionally has a secret cigarette in the back garden. His grandchildren visit after school and try and keep him company, but both Muriel and Clive wonder (for different reasons) if he will be able to resume his previous levels of activity. In your role as an adult nurse, you have been asked to provide support for Muriel and Clive:

- How would you assess the bio-psychosocial needs of this family?
- What do you consider to be the main areas of concern?
- What information might Clive and Muriel (and you) need in order to ensure an evidence-based approach to care?
- How could you encourage personalised care planning, working in partnership and self-management?
- Are there any issues connected with Muriel being a carer for Clive as well as working part-time? How may this dual role affect Muriel physically, emotionally and socially?
- Compare your answers by discussing this case scenario with your mentor and/or other colleagues in practice. Is there anything they would do differently?

Case Scenario

You will no doubt have identified a number of key issues that need addressing in order to improve Clive's health. However, first and foremost the most important thing to do would be to begin to try to build a therapeutic relationship with Clive and Muriel. To do this, you will need to make time to communicate effectively with them in order to establish their key concerns. Clive exhibits a number of physical illnesses, exacerbating symptoms and unhealthy lifestyle choices. He also reports a deterioration in his mental health and social activity. As nurses, we are often driven by the need to 'make things better' and so there is a temptation to jump right in and begin to plan the care *we* think is needed to address all of the health issues we have identified. Yet, by *listening* carefully to Clive and Muriel, you will be able to ascertain *their* priorities for care. You will then need to consider what valid and reliable assessment tools you might use to assist in this process. For example, how might you assess Clive's sleeping difficulties, fatigue, loneliness and emotional distress?

By assessing and discussing Clive's needs in more depth and providing information about how identified issues could be addressed, you can empower Clive to take an active role in improving his health and any agreed interventions are more likely to be successful. For example:

- Use an holistic approach to assessment to ensure that social and psychological factors are also taken in to account.
- Refer to local/national national guidelines and evidence-based care pathways.
- Explore how access to a wider multi-agency team, private or voluntary agencies could help.
- Negotiate and agree a culturally sensitive, person-centred action plan.

Muriel's needs should also be considered. Carers can often feel overlooked and as an adult nurse you will be responsible for ensuring that she also receives individualised information, advice and support, thereby adopting a family- rather than patient-focused approach.

The role of carers

A carer, as defined by HM Government, is an individual who:

> … spends a significant proportion of their life providing unpaid support to family or friends. This could be caring for a relative, partner or friend who is ill, frail, disabled or has mental health or substance misuse problems. (HM Government, 2008: 20)

Immediate family members are often seen as a primary resource for managing the impact of long-term ill health across all cultures and groups (Salway et al., 2007), though we should remember that cultural concepts of caring are not universal.

In 2011 there were around six million carers across England and Wales. Many of these report a significant negative impact on their own health as a result (Office for National Statistics, 2011). According to Carers UK (2014), 45% of these have given up work to care for family members or friends, 49% struggle financially, and 61% have faced depression because of their caring role. Adult nurses play a vital role in ensuring that the health needs of carers are addressed so that they are able to maintain their own health and well-being. For example, a separate assessment of a carer's needs can help to identify potential interventions and support (e.g. education/training, financial assistance, local support groups or respite needs) that can help to sustain their caring role. This assessment should also include questions about a carer's willingness and ability to continue caring. In 2008 the UK government document, *Carers at the Heart of 21st-Century Families and Communities: A Caring System on Your Side: A Life of Your Own* (HM Government, 2008), set out a framework for developing ongoing support for carers. Updated in 2010, the aim of the policy was to ensure that the needs of carers are recognised and that carers are given the help and support they require to maintain their own health and well-being.

What support services are available to carers in your area (e.g. financial entitlement, respite care/carer breaks, and all other forms of support available in the locality)?

- How can you use this knowledge to provide information and support to carers?

Integrated care

Many patients with a LTC will require support from a range of professionals. As an adult nurse you will need to be able to work in partnership with other organisations and services (including those in the statutory, voluntary, community and independent sectors) in order to ensure streamlined and integrated care delivery. This may include working across organisational boundaries between statutory, voluntary, community and independent sectors, demanding effective communication and collaborative multi-agency working skills. Guthrie et al. (2012) argue that current clinical guidelines which focus on single conditions do little to assist healthcare practitioners in supporting people with multiple LTCs and suggest that clinical guidelines are adapted in future to take account of *multi-morbidity*, emphasising the need to ensure an individual personalised approach is taken.

While there is no single definitive model of integrated care, the Expanded Chronic Care Model (Barr et al., 2003) highlights the essential components of care, suggesting that the best outcomes for patients are achieved when these components are integrated, joint professional working is accomplished and a patient-centred approach is adopted – thus moving away from the more traditional 'single disease slio' approach which can sometimes result in duplication or patients 'falling through the gaps' as they attempt to navigate their way through the complex array of health and social care services via a series of un-co-ordinated interactions or patient pathways.

 PATRICK

Patrick, a 79-year-old man, lives with his wife Sally. They have known each other since childhood and have been married for more than fifty years. Patrick is admitted to hospital after suffering a Cerebral Vascular Accident (CVA). His left side is weakened and he has a catheter in situ. He is able to stand and walk for short distances with the aid of a frame. Patrick is able to understand what is being said to him but he sometimes has difficulty expressing himself as a result of *dysphasia* caused by the CVA. During his time in hospital he has been diagnosed with Type 2 diabetes. Sally has been recently diagnosed with Parkinson's disease. Patrick is her main carer and they have no children. They live in a house with stairs where the only bathroom and toilet are upstairs. They both want to stay together in their own home.

- What are the overall health and social needs that you would need to consider in order to plan for Patrick's discharge?
- Which other healthcare professionals and organisations would need to be involved?
- How would you reach an agreed plan of care?

The term 'revolving door syndrome' is often used for the re-admission of patients to hospital within a few days of their discharge. Whilst some of these re-admissions may be difficult to prevent, often they are a result of poor communication, a fragmented care system, or inadequate discharge planning. In 2013 the Royal Voluntary Service (RVS, 2013) found that 150,000 older people had no support on returning home from hospital, and for those that did get some kind of help a fifth didn't receive essential continuing support. Not surprisingly, therefore, 15.3% of those aged over 75 were admitted to hospital again within 28 days of discharge (Health and Social Care Information Centre, 2013a).

Effective discharge planning

Most patients with LTCs will be cared for in a community setting. However there will be occasions when admission or transfer to and from acute, intermediate or respite care will be required. Individualised discharge planning has been identified as having the potential to reduce a length of stay in hospital and re-admission rates (Shepperd et al., 2013). To ensure continuity of care, the Department of Health (2010) has outlined ten key steps involved in the *transfer of care* process:

1. Start planning for discharge or transfer before or on admission.
2. Identify whether the patient has simple or complex discharge and transfer planning needs, involving the patient and carer in your decision.
3. Develop a clinical management plan for every patient within 24 hours of admission.
4. Co-ordinate the discharge or transfer of care process through effective leadership and the handover of responsibilities at ward level.
5. Set an expected date of discharge or transfer within 24–48 hours of admission, and discuss this with the patient and carer.
6. Review the clinical management plan with the patient each day, take any necessary action, and update progress towards the discharge or transfer date.
7. Involve patients and carers so that they can make informed decisions and choices that will deliver a personalised care pathway and maximise their independence.
8. Plan discharges and transfers to take place over seven days to deliver continuity of care for the patient.
9. Use a discharge checklist 24–48 hours prior to a transfer.
10. Make decisions to discharge and transfer patients each day.

Planning a patient's discharge or transfer from any care setting is an important part of personalised care planning and will ensure that individuals and their families continue to be supported. As an adult nurse you must be able to liaise effectively with patients, their families and all other agencies involved to achieve a smooth transition of care (NMC, 2010a, 2010b, 2015). Safe and effective discharges/transfers rely on robust decision-making processes and reaching a consensus with patients, families and carers as well as other members of the multidisciplinary team. Patients with LTCs often have complex needs and as such this process is reliant on therapeutic engagement and a shared philosophy of care where ethical principles are identified as vital to the nursing endeavour, in terms of doing good, avoiding harm, promoting autonomy, and affording justice.

The *Common Assessment Framework* (CAF) or *Single Assessment Process* (SAP) is a generic multidisciplinary assessment tool aimed at improving the sharing of information between health and social care support agencies.

ACTIVITY 10.15

Find out more about the CAF/SAP and how they can improve the care of patients by accessing the following websites:

- NHS Networks: www.cpa.org.uk/sap/caf_more_about.html
- HM Government: https://www.gov.uk/enabling-integrated-care-in-the-nhs

Chapter summary

This chapter has encouraged you to find out more about common long-term conditions that affect adults across the UK and the evidence-based interventions which aim to help patients manage their conditions. We have explored the impact that many long-term conditions have on both our patients and their families. We have also examined some of the contemporary approaches aimed at providing help and support to patients, carers and families in our role as adult nurses. The concept of patient-centred supported self-care, and the importance of integrated care provision in order to deliver good quality effective nursing care, have also been highlighted.

Suggested further reading

Burns, D., McGough, A. and Bennett, C. (2012) 'Chronic fatigue syndrome or myalgic encephalomyelitis (CFS/ME)', *Nursing Standard*, 26 (25): 48–56.

Clayton, E.W. et al. (2015). *Beyond Myalgic Encephalomyelitis/Chronic Fatigue Syndrome. Redefining an Illness* (Report Brief). US Institute of Medicine. Washington. Available at: www.edu/Reports/2015/ME-CFS.aspx (last accessed 2 March 2015).

Denny, E. and Earle, S. (2009) *The Sociology of Long Term Conditions*. Basingstoke: Palgrave Macmillan.

Department of Health (2011) *No Health Without Mental Health: A Cross Government Mental Health Outcomes Strategy for People of All Ages*. London: DH.

Egan, G. (2006) *The Skilled Helper. A Problem-management and Opportunity Development Approach to Helping*. Chicago, IL: Wadsworth.

Griffin, J. (2010) *The Lonely Society*. London: The Mental Health Foundation. Available at: www.mentalhealth.org.uk/publications/the-lonely-society/ (last accessed 18 March 2015).

Lloyd, C.E. and Heller, T. (eds) (2011) *Long-term Conditions: Challenges in Health and Social Care*. London: Sage.

Northern Ireland: Department of Health, Social Services and Public Safety (2012), *Living with Long Term Conditions: A Policy Framework*. Belfast: DHSSPS.

Useful resources

Department of Health: www.gov.uk/government/policies/improving-quality-of-life-for-people-with-long-term-conditions (improving quality of life for people with long term conditions policy page)

Expert Patient Programme: www.nhs.uk/NHSEngland/AboutNHSservices/doctors/Pages/expert-patients-programme.aspx

Integrated Care and Support Exchange (ICASE): www.icase.org.uk (a learning community focused on integrated care and support that helps you to make connections, share information and find answers to key challenges)

National Voices: www.nationalvoices.org.uk/ (a registered charity which stands up for the rights of patients, service users and carers)

NHS Information Centre for Health and Social Care Data Collections: www.hscic.gov.uk/searchcatalogue

NHS Information Prescriptions: www.nhs.uk/informationprescriptions

NHS Institute for Innovation and Improvement 'Joined Up Care' Resources: www.institute.nhs.uk/qipp/joined_up_care/joined_up_care_homepage.html (a suite of products and tools to help create seamless care between services)

Office for National Statistics – Health and Social Care: www.ons.gov.uk

The Health Foundation Self Management Resource Centre: http://selfmanagementsupport.health.org.uk/

References

American Academy of Sleep Medicine (2005) *Diagnostic and Coding Manual: The International Classification of Sleep Disorders,* 2nd edition. Westchester, PA: AASM.

Asthma UK (2004) *Where Do We Stand? Asthma in the UK Today.* Available at: www.asthma.org.uk (last accessed 14 August 2014).

Barnett, M. (2005) 'Chronic obstructive pulmonary disease: a phenomenological study of patients' experiences' , *Journal of Clinical Nursing,* 14: 805–12.

Barr, V.J., Robinson, S., Marin-Link, B., Underhill, L., Dotts, A., Ravensdale, D. and Salivaras, S. (2003) 'The Expanded Chronic Care Model: an integration of concepts and strategies from population health promotion and the Chronic Care Model' , *Hosp Q,* 7(1): 73–82.

Barsevick, A.M., Cleelan, C.S., Manning, D.C., O'Mara, A.M., Reeve, B.B., Scott, J.A., Sloan, J. and AASCPRO (Assessing Symptoms of Cancer Using Patient Reported Outcomes) (2010) 'ASCPRO recommendations for the assessment of fatigue as an outcome in clinical', *Journal of Pain Symptom Management,* 39: 1086–99.

Biessels, G.J., Stackenborg, S., Brunner, E., Brayne, C. and Scheltens, P. (2006) 'Risk of dementia in diabetes mellitus: a systematic review', *The Lancet Neurology,* 5(1): 64–7.

Bowlby and Weiss, R.S. (1973) *Loneliness: The Experience of Emotional and Social Isolation.* Cambridge, MA: MIT Press.

British Liver Trust (2014) *Pioneering Liver Health.* Available at: www.britishlivertrust.org.uk (last accessed 31 August 2014).

British Society of Gastroenterology (2009) *Management of Patients with Chronic Liver Disease.* Available at: www.bsg.org.uk/clinical/commissioning-report/management-of-patients-with-chronic-liver-diseases.html (last accessed 20 November 2014).

Cancer Research UK (2014) *Cancer Statistics for the UK.* Available at: www.cancerresearchuk.org/cancer-info/cancerstats/keyfacts/Allcancerscombined/ (last accessed 31 August 2014).

Car, J., Huckvale, K. and Hermens, H. (2012) 'Telehealth for long term conditions', *British Medical Journal,* 344: e4201. Available at: www.bmj.com/content/344/bmj.e4201.full.pdf (last accessed 29 August 2014).

Carers UK (2014) *State of Caring.* Available at: www.carersuk.org/stateofcaring (last accessed 28 August 2014).

Caress, A.-L., Luker, K.A. and Owens, R.G. (2001) 'A descriptive study of meaning of illness in chronic renal disease', *Journal of Advanced Nursing,* 33(6): 716–27.

Cepoiu, M., McClusker, J., Cole, M.G., Sewitch, M., Belzile, E. and Ciampi, A. (2008) 'Recognition of depression by non-psychiatric physicians – a systematic literature review and meta-analysis', *Journal of General Internal Medicine,* 23(1): 25–36

Cimpean, D. and Drake, R.E. (2001) 'Treating co-morbid medical conditions and anxiety/depression', *Epidemiology and Psychiatric Sciences,* 20 (2): 141–50.

Claessens, P., Moons, P., Dierckx de Casterle, B., Cannaerts, N., Budts, W. and Gewillig, M. (2005) 'What does it mean to live with a congenital heart disease? A qualitative study on the lived experiences of adult patients', *European Journal of Cardiovascular Nursing*, 4: 3–10.

Clancy, K., Hallett, C.E. and Caress, A. (2009) 'The meaning of living with chronic obstructive pulmonary disease', *Journal of Nursing and Healthcare of Chronic Illness*, 1(1): 78–86.

Clinical Practice Guidelines Working Group (2010) *Guideline to Adult Insomnia: Assessment to Diagnosis*. Available at: www.topalbertadoctors.org/download/440/insomnia_assessment_guideline.pdf (last accessed 20 August 2014).

Commission on Chronic Illness (1956) *Guides to Action on Chronic Illness*. New York: National Health Council.

Corben, S. and Rosen, R. (2005) *Self-management for Long-term Conditions: Patients' Perspectives on the Way Ahead*. London: The King's Fund.

Coulter, A., Roberts, S. and Dixson, A. (2013) *Delivering Better Services for People With Long-Term Conditions: Building the House of Care*. London: The King's Fund.

Coventry, P., Hays, R., Dickens, C., Bundy, C., Garrett, C., Cherrington, A. and Chew-Graham, C.A. (2011) 'Talking about depression: barriers to managing depression in people with long term conditions in primary care', *BMC Family Practice*, 12 (10): 1–11.

Crumbie, A. and Lawrence, J. (eds) (2002) *Living with a Chronic Condition: A Practitioner's Guide*. London: Elsevier.

Davies, M.J., Heller, S., Skinner, T.C., Campbell, M.J., Carey, M.E., Cradock, S., Fallosso, H.M., Daly, H., Doherty, Y., Eaton, S., Fox, C., Oliver, L., Rantell, K., Rayman, G.M. and Khunti, K. (2008) 'Effectiveness of the diabetes education and self management for ongoing and newly diagnosed (DESMOND) programme for people with newly diagnosed type 2 diabetes: cluster randomised controlled trial', *British Medical Journal*, 33(7642): 491–95.

De Silva, D. (2011) *Helping People Help Themselves*. London: The Health Foundation.

Department of Health (2000) *The NHS Plan: A Plan for Investment, A Plan for Reform*. London: DH.

Department of Health (2005) *National Service Framework for Long Term Conditions*. London: DH.

Department of Health (2006) *Our Health, Our Care, Our Say: A New Direction for Community Services*. London: DH.

Department of Health (2009) *Your Health, Your Way: A Guide to Long Term Conditions and Self-care: Information for Healthcare Professionals*. Leeds: DH.

Department of Health (2010) *Ready to Go: Planning the Discharge and the Transfer of Patients from Hospital and Intermediate Care*. Leeds: DH.

Department of Health (2013a) *Improving Quality of Life for People Living with Long Term Conditions*. Available at: www.gov.uk/government/policies/improving-quality-of-life-for-people-with-long-term-conditions. London: DH.

Department of Health (2013b) *The Mandate: A Mandate from the Government to the NHS Commissioning Board*: April 2013 to March 2015. Available at www.gov.uk/DH.

Department of Health (2013c) *The NHS Constitution*. London: DH.

Department of Health (2014) *The Mandate: A Mandate from the Government to NHS England: April 2014 – March 2015*. Availabe at: www.gov.uk/government/uploads/system/uploads/attachments_data/file/383495/2902896_DoH_Mandate (last accessed 22 February 2015).

Department of Health/Long Term Conditions (2012) *Long Term Conditions Compendium of Information*, 3rd edition. Available at: www.gov.uk/government/uploads/system/uploads/attachment_data/file/216528/dh_134486.pdf (last accessed 31 August 2014).

Department of Health, Social Services and Public Safety Northern Ireland (2012) *Living With Long Term Conditions: A Policy Framework*. Belfast: DHSSPNI.

Diabetes UK (2013) *State of the Nation 2013: England*. London: Diabetes UK.

Dowling, M., Murphy, K., Cooney, A. and Casey, D. (2011) 'A concept analysis of empowerment in chronic illness from the perspective of the nurse and the client living with chronic obstructive pulmonary disease', *Journal of Nursing and Healthcare in Chronic Illness*. doi:10.111/j.1752-9824.2011.011123x

Due-Christensen, M., Zoffmann, V., Hommel, E. and Lau, M. (2012) 'Can sharing experiences in groups reduce the burden of living with diabetes, regardless of glycaemic control?', *Diabetic Medicine*, 29(2): 251–56.

Dusheiko, M., Gravelle, H., Martin, S., Rice, N. and Smith P.C. (2011) *Does Better Disease Management in Primary Care Reduce Hospital Costs?* York: University of York, The Centre for Health Economics.

East Midlands Public Health Observatory and NHS Kidney Care (2010) *Kidney Disease Facts and Figures* (September). East Midlands Public Health Observatory.

Entwistle, V.A. and Cribb, A. (2013) *Enabling People to Live Well: Fresh Thinking about Collaborative Approaches to Care for People with Long-term Conditions*. London: The Health Foundation.

Expert Patients Programme (2010) *Self-care Reduces Costs and Improves Health: The Evidence*. Available at: www.expertpatients.co.uk/sites/default/files/publications/self-care-reduces-cost-and-improves-health-evidence.pdf (last accessed 28 August 2014).

Goldberg, D. (2010) 'The detection and treatment of depression in the physically ill', *World Psychiatry*, 9(1): 16–20.

Goodwin, N., Sonola, L., Thiel, V. and Konder, D.L. (2013a) *Co-ordinated Care for People with Complex Chronic Conditions: Key Lessons and Markers for Success*. London: The King's Fund.

Goodwin, N., Smith, J., Davies, A., Perry, C., Rosen, R., Dixon, A. and Ham, C. (2013b) *Integrated Care for Patients and Populations: Improving Outcomes by Working Together*. London: The King's Fund. Available at: www.kingsfund.org.uk/publications/integrated-care-patients-and-populations-improving-outcomes-working-together (last accessed 28 August 2014).

Gottlieb, P.J., Punjabi, N.M., Newman, A.B., Resnick, H.E., Redline, S., Baldwin, C.M. and Nieto, F.J. (2005) 'Association of sleep time with diabetes mellitus and impaired glucose tolerance', *Archives of International Medicine*, 165 (8): 863–7.

Gray, L., and Leyland, A. (2013) 'Long-term conditions'. In *Scottish Health Survey* 2012: Volume 1 Main Report. The Scottish Government Health Directorate.

Guthrie, B., Payne, K., Alderson, P., McMurdo, M.E.T. and Mercer, S.W. *(2012)* 'Adapting clinical guidelines to take account of multimorbidity', *British Medical Journal*, 345 (e6341–e6341: ISSN 0959-535X: doi:10.1136/bmj.e6341).

Health and Social Care Information Centre (2013a) *Hospital Episode Statistics: Emergency Readmissions to Hospital within 28 Days of Discharge: Financial Year 2011/12*. Leeds: HSCIC. Available at: www.hscic.gov.uk/catalogue/PUB12751/hes-emer-read-hosp-28-days-disc-2002-2012-rep.pdf (last accessed 2 September 2014).

Health and Social Care Information Centre (2013b) *The Quality Outcomes Framework 2012–13*. Available at www.hscic.gov.uk/qof (last accessed 2 September 2014).

Henderson, C., Knapp, M., Fernandez, J., Beecham, J., Hirani, S.P., Cartwright, M., Rixon, L., Beynon, M., Rogers, A., Bower, P., Doll, H., Fitzpatrick, R., Steventon, A., Bardsley, M., Hendy, J., Stanton, P. and Newman, D. (2013) 'Cost effectiveness of telehealth for patients with long term conditions (Whole Systems Demonstrator telehealth questionnaire study): nested economic evaluation in a pragmatic, cluster randomised controlled trial', *British Medical Journal*, 22 March: 346: f1035. Available at: www.bmj.com/content/346/bmj.f1035.full.pdf (last accessed 29 August 2014).

HM Government (2008) *Carers at the Heart of 21st-century Families and Communities: 'A caring system on your side. A life of your own'*. London: Department of Health.

HM Government/Department of Health (2011) *No Health Without Mental Health: A Cross Government Mental Health Outcomes Strategy for People of All Ages*. London: DH.

Holmes, K., Ericsson, K. and Winblad, B. (2000) 'Social and emotional loneliness among non-demented and demented elder people', *Archives of Gerontology and Geriatrics*, 31: 17–7193.

Hopp, F.P., Thornton, N. and Martin, L. (2010) 'The lived experience of heart failure at the end of life: a systematic literature review', *Health Soc Work*, 35 (2): 109–17.

Hutt, R., Rosen, R. and McCauley, J. (2004) *Case-managing Long-term Conditions: What Impact does it Have in the Treatment of Older People?* London: The King's Fund.

Information Services Division Scotland (2014) *Heart Disease Statistics Update: Year Ending 31 March 2013*. Available at: https://isdscotland.scot.nhs.uk/Health-Topics/Heart-Disease/Publications/2014-01-28/2014-01-28-Heart-Disease-Summary.pdf?43513125182 (last accessed 31 August 2014).

Ipsos Mori (2011) *Long Term Health Conditions 2011: Research Study*. Leeds: Ipsos MORI.

Keller, S. E., Schleifer, S. J., Bartiett, J.A., Shiflett, S.C. and Rameshwar, P. (2000) 'Stress, depression, immunity and health'. In K. Goodkin and A.P. Visser (eds), *Psychoneuroimmunology: Stress, Mental Disorders, and Health*. Washington: American Psychiatric Press. pp. 1–25.

Kennedy, A., Reeves, D., Bower, P., Lee, V., Middleton, E., Richardson, G., Gardner, C., Gately, C. and Rogers, A. (2007) 'The effectiveness and cost effectiveness of a national lay-led self-care support programme for patients with long-term conditions: a pragmatic randomised controlled trial', *Journal of Epidemiology and Community Health*, 61: 254–61. doi: 10,1136/jecj2006.053538.

Killeen, C. (1998) 'Loneliness: an epidemic in modern society', *Journal of Advanced Nursing*, 28 (4): 762–70.

Kirkevold, M., Moyle, C., Wilkinson, C., Meyer, J. and Hauge, S. (2012) 'Facing the challenge of adapting to a life "alone" in old age: the influence of losses', *Journal of Advanced Nursing*, 69 (2): 394–403.

Kuijpers, W., Groen, W.G., Aaronson, N.K. and van Harten, W.H. (2013) 'A systematic review of web-based interventions for patient empowerment and Physical Activity in chronic diseases: relevance for cancer survivors', *Journal of Medical Internet Research*, 15(2): e37.

Leelarathna, L., Ward, C., Davenport, K., Donald, S., Housden, A., Finucane, F.M. and Evans, M. (2011) 'Reduced insulin requirements during participation in the DAFNE (dose adjustment for normal eating) structured education programme', *Diabetes Res Clin Pract*, 92(2): e34–6. doi: 10.1016/j.diabres.2011.01.001.

Lempp, K.H., Hatch, S.L., Carville, S.F. and Choy, E.H. (2009) 'Patients' experiences of living with and receiving treatment for fibromyalgia syndrome: a qualitative study', *BMC Musculoskeletal Disorders*, 10 (24).

Lesperance, F., Frasure Smith, N., Talajic, M. and Bourassa, M.G. (2002) 'Five year risk of cardiac mortality in relation to initial severity and one year changes in depression symptoms after myocardial infarction', *Circulation*, 105(9): 1049–53.

Maresso, A. (2013) 'The quality and outcomes framework in England', *Eurohealth*, 19(2): 9.

Matin, C. and Benca, R. (2012) 'Chronic insomnia', *The Lancet*, 379: 1129–41.

McLean, S., Sheikh, A., Cresswell, K., Nurmatov, U., Mukherjee, M., Hemmi, A. and Pagliari, C. (2013) 'The impact of telehealthcare on the quality and safety of care: a systematic overview', *PLos One*, 8 (8). e71238. doi: 10.1371/ journal.pone.007.1238.

Melek, S. and Norris, D. (2008) *Chronic Conditions and Co-morbid Psychological Disorders*. Seattle: Milliman.

Mental Health Foundation (2012) *Developing Peer Support for Long Term Conditions (Final Report)*. Edinburgh: Mental Health Foundation.

Millard, L., Hallett, C.E. and Luker, K.A. (2006) 'Nurse-patient interaction and decision-making in care: patient involvement in community nursing', *Journal of Advanced Nursing*, 55 (2): 142–50.

Milligan, C., Roberts, C. and Mort, M. (2011) 'Telecare and older people: who cares where?', *Social Science & Medicine*, 72 (2011): 347e354.

National Institute for Health and Care Excellence (2011) *Hypertension: Clinical Management of Primary Hypertension in Adults [CG127]*. Available at: www.nice.org.uk/guidance/cg127/chapter/introduction (last accessed 20 November 2014).

Naylor, C., Parsonage, M., McDaid, D., Knapp, M., Fossey, M. and Galea, A. (2012) *Long-term Conditions and Mental Health: The Cost of Co-morbidities*. London: The King's Fund. Available at: www.kingsfund.org.uk/publications/long-term-conditions-and-mental-health (last accessed 13 March 2014).

Nursing and Midwifery Council (2010a) *Standards for Pre-registration Nursing Education.* Available at: http://standards.nmc-uk.org (last accessed 11 November 2014).

Nursing and Midwifery Council (2010b) *Standards for Competence for Registered Nurses.* Available at: www.nmc-uk.org/Documents/Standards/Standards%20for%20competence.pdf. (last accessed 11 November 2014).

Nursing and Midwifery Council (2015) *The Code: Professional Standards of Practice and Behaviour for Nurses and Midwives.* London: NMC.

Office for National Statistics (2008) *Health Service Quarterly*, Winter, 40, p59–60

Office for National Statistics (2011) *2011 Census: Unpaid Care Snapshot.* London: ONS.

Office for National Statistics (2012) *Deaths Registered in England and Wales (Series DR)*, 2011. Available at: www.ons.gov.uk/ons/dcp171778_284566.pdf (last accessed 22 February 2015).

Office for National Statistics (2013) *General Lifestyle Survey, 2011 Report.* Available at: www.ons.gov.uk/ons/rel/ghs/general-lifestyle-survey/2011/index.html (last accessed 31 August 2014).

Office for National Statistics (2014) *Deaths Registered in England and Wales, 2013.*

Phillips, A. (2013) 'Intuitive practice and skill development in diabetes care', *Practice Nursing*, 24 (9): 445–7.

Prince, M., Patel, V., Saxena, S., Maj, M., Maselko, J., Phillips, M.R. and Rahman, A. (2007) 'No health without mental health', *The Lancet*, 370 (9590); 859–77.

Purdy, S. (2010) *Avoiding Hospital Admissions: What does the Research Evidence Say?* London: The King Fund.

Rogers, A., Kennedy, A., Bower, P., Gardner, C., Gately, C., Lee, V., Reeves, D. and Richardson, G. (2008) 'The United Kingdom Expert Patients Programme: results and implications from a national evaluation', *MJA*, 189(10): S21–S24.

Rogers, A., Kirk, S., Gately, C., May, C. and Finch, T. (2011) 'Established users and the making of telecare work in long term condition management: implications for health policy', *Social Science and Medicine*, 72(7): 1077–84.

Roland, M., Lewis, L., Steventson, A., Abel, G., Adams, J., Bardsley, M., Brerton, L., Chitnis, X., Conklin, A., Staetsky, L., Tunkel, S. and Ling, T. (2012) 'Case management for at-risk elderly patients in the English integrated care pilots: observational study of staff and patient experience and secondary care utilisation', *International Journal of Integrated Care.* Available at: www.ijic.org/index.php/ijic/article/view/850/1771 (last accessed 28 August 2014).

Ross, S., Curry, N. and Goodwin, N. (2011) *Case Management: What it is and How it can Best be Implemented.* London: The King's Fund. Available at: www.kingsfund.org.uk/publications/case-management (last accessed 21 August 2014).

Royal Voluntary Service (2013) *Avoiding Unhappy Returns: Radical Reductions in Readmissions achieved with Volunteers.* Cardiff: RVS. Available at: www.royalvoluntaryservice.org.uk/Uploads/Documents/Get%20involved/avoiding_unhappy_returns.pdf (last accessed 2 September 2014).

Salway, S., Platt, L., Chowbey, P., Harriss, K. and Bayliss, E. (2007) *Long Term Ill Health, Poverty and Ethnicity.* York: Joseph Rowntree Foundation.

Shepperd, S., Lannin, N.A., Clemson, L.M., McCluskey, A., Cameron, I.D. and Barras, S.L. (2013) 'Discharge planning from hospital to home', *Cochrane Database of Systematic Reviews*, Issue 1. Art. No.: CD000313. doi:10.1002/14651858.CD000313.pub4.

Sibbald, B., Rogers, A., Lester, H., Harrison, P., Checkland, K., Sutton, M., Campbell, S. and Roland, M. (2010) *National Primary Care Research and Development Centre Final Report: 2005–2010.* Manchester: National Primary Care Research and Development Centre.

Snell, T., Wittenberg, R., Fernandez, J.L., Malley, J., Comas-Herrera, A. and King, D. (2011) Discussion Paper: *Future Demand for Social Care, 2010 to 2030: Projections of Demand for Social Care and Disability Benefits for Younger Adults in England: Report to the Commission on Funding of Care and Support*, PSSRU 2800/2. Available at: www.pssru.ac.uk/pdf/DP2880-3.pdf (last accessed 2 September 2014).

Steel, N. and Willems, S. (2010) 'Research learning from the UK Quality and Outcomes Framework: a review of existing research', *Quality in Primary Care*, 18(2):117–25.

Taylor, D.J., Mallory, L.J., Lichstein, K.L., Durrence, H.H., Riedel, B.W. and Bush, A.J. (2007) 'Co-morbidity of chronic insomnia with medical problems', *Sleep*, 30 (2): 213-18.

The King's Fund (2012) *From Vision to Action: Making Patient-centred Care a Reality*. Available at: www.kingsfund.org.uk/publications/articles/vision-action-making-patient-centred-care-reality (last accessed 18 March 2013).

The Scottish Government (2009) *Long Term Conditions Collaborative Improving Self Management Support*. Available at: www.scotland.gov.uk/resource/doc/274194/0082012.pdf. (last accessed 20 November 2014).

The Scottish Government (2014) *Self-Directed Support: Practitioner Guidance*. Edinburgh: The Scottish Government.

Tierney, S., Deaton, C., Webb, K., Jones, A. et al. (2008) 'Isolation, motivation and balance: living with type 1 or cystic fibrosis-related diabetes', *Journal of Clinical Nursing*, 17 (7B): 235–43.

Upton, J., Fletcher, M., Madoc-Sutton, H., Sheikh, A., Caress, A-L and Walker, S. (2011) Shared decision making or paternalism in nursing consultations? A qualitative study of primary care asthma nurses' views on sharing decisions with patients regarding inhaler device selection, *Health Expectations*, 14(4): 374–82.

Verbrugge, L.M. and Jette, A.M. (1994) 'The disablement process', *Social Science and Medicine*, 38(1): 1–14.

Verhoeven, F., van Gemert-Pijnen, L., Dijkstra, K., Nijland, N., Seydel, E. and Steehouder, M.I. (2007) 'The contribution of teleconsultation and videoconferencing to diabetes care: a systematic literature review', *Journal of Medical Internet Research*, 9: e37.

Victor, C.R. and Bowling, A. (2012) 'A longitudinal analysis of loneliness among older people in Great Britain', *J. Psychol.*, 146(3): 313–31.

Victor, C.R. and Yang, K. (2012) 'The prevalence of loneliness among adults: a case study of the United Kingdom', *J. Psychol.*, 146(1–2): 85–104.

Vos, T., Flaxman, A., Naghavi, M. et al. (2012) 'Years lived with disability (YLDs) for 1160 sequelae of 289 diseases and injuries 1990–2010: a systematic analysis for the Global Burden of Disease Study 2010', *The Lancet*, 380: 2163–96.

Williams, J., Roth, A., Vatthauer, K. and McCrae, C.S. (2013) 'Cognitive behaviour treatment of insomnia', *Chest*, 143 (2): 554–65.

Willis, E. (2013) 'The making of expert patients: the role of online health communities in arthritis self-management', *J Health Psychol*. Available at: http://hpq.sagepub.com/content/early/2013/08/29/1359105313496446.long (last accessed 2 September 2014).

Wilson, L., Whitehead, L. and Burrell, B. (2011) 'Learning to live well with chronic fatigue: the personal perspective', *Journal of Advanced Nursing*, 67 (10): 2161–9.

Wilson, P.M. and Brooks, F. (2007) 'The Expert Patients Programme: a paradox of patient empowerment and medical dominance', *Health and Social Care in the Community*, 15(5): 426–38.

Wilson, P.M., Kendall, S. and Brooks, F. (2006) 'Nurses' responses to expert patients: the rhetoric and reality of self-management in long-term conditions: a grounded theory study', *International Journal of Nursing Studies*, 43 (7): 803–18.

World Health Organization (2011) *Global Status Report on Non-communicable Disease, 2010*. Geneva: WHO.

World Health Organization (2015) *Chronic Obstructive Pulmonary Disease (COPD)*. Geneva: WHO. Available at: www.who.int/respiratory/copd/en (last accessed 22 February 2015).

Zoffmann, V. and Kirkevold, M. (2005) 'Life versus disease in difficult diabetes care: conflicting perspectives disempower patients and professionals in problem solving', *Qualitative Health Research*, 15, 750–765.

Zoffmann, V. and Kirkevold, M. (2007) 'Relationships and their potential for change developed in difficult type 1 diabetes', *Qualitative Health Research*, 17: 625–38.

Zoffman, V. and Kirkevold, M. (2012) 'Realizing empowerment in difficult diabetes care: a guided self-determination intervention', *Qual Health Res* , 22 (103). Available at: http://qhr.sagepub.com/content/22/1/103 (last accessed 20 November 2014).

11 Caring for the Acutely Ill Adult

PAUL TIERNEY, SAMANTHA FREEMAN AND JULIE GREGORY

All patients, regardless of the setting, have the potential to become acutely and critically unwell. With the general trend of those in hospital being older, sicker and having more complex issues, the need for skills in recognising and responding to the deteriorating patient are becoming increasingly important. Nurses in all clinical areas, and not just those working in critical care environments, should have the knowledge and skills to recognise and respond competently and confidently to the needs of an acutely ill adult.

Caring for a critically unwell adult can also be very challenging, not least because it often involves the use of high tech equipment and monitoring technology which can be a bit worrying to those unfamiliar with such equipment and devices. By exploring the evidence base for the management of severe illness we will provide you with the underpinning knowledge necessary to be able to provide safe and effective care for such patients. The use of patient scenarios and reflective guidance will also help you consider and acknowledge your own limitations, thereby recognising the need to further develop your skills.

After reading this chapter you should be able to:

- Identify the knowledge and skills required to work effectively in acute care settings.
- Critically discuss the comprehensive assessment of an acutely ill adult.
- Recognise and respond to acutely ill adults using appropriate evidence-based strategies.
- Appreciate the importance of using medical devices safely.
- Demonstrate a critical understanding of legal and ethical issues relating to the individual in acute care settings, including consent, confidentiality and best interest principles.

Related NMC competencies

The overarching NMC requirement is that all nurses must:

> be able to recognise and interpret signs of normal and deteriorating mental and physical health and respond promptly to maintain or improve the health and comfort of the service user, acting to keep them and others safe. (NMC 2010a:18)

They must:

> make accurate assessments and start appropriate and timely management of those who are acutely ill, at risk of clinical deterioration, or require emergency care. (DH 2010b:10)

─────────── To achieve entry to the register as an adult ───────────
nurse you should be able to:

- Promote the concept, knowledge and practice of self care with people with acute conditions, using a range of communication skills and strategies.
- Safely use invasive and non-invasive procedures, medical devices, and current techno-logical and pharmacological interventions, where relevant, in medical and surgical nursing practice, providing information and taking account of individual needs and preferences.
- You must be able to evaluate their use, reporting any concerns promptly through appro-priate channels and modifying care where necessary to maintain safety.
- Safely use a range of diagnostic skills, employing appropriate technology, to assess the needs of service users.
- Identify priorities and manage time and resources effectively to ensure that quality of care is maintained or enhanced.

(Adapted from the NMC Standards of Competence for Adult Nursing, 2010a, 2010b.)

Background

The term 'acute care' usually refers to care provided when a patient is suffering from an acute episode of a previously undiagnosed problem (e.g. a stroke or appendicitis), an acute exacerbation of a long-term condition (e.g. a diabetic coma or COPD), or recovering from an accident/trauma or surgery. Acute care environments can be defined as those in which the principal intent is one or more of the following:

- To cure illness or to provide definitive treatment of injury.
- To perform surgery.
- To relieve symptoms of illness or injury (excluding palliative care).
- To reduce the severity of an illness or injury.
- To protect against the exacerbation and/or complication of an illness and/or injury which could threaten life or normal function.
- To perform diagnostic or therapeutic procedures.
- To manage labour (obstetrics).
  (Organisation for Economic Co-operation and Development, 2001)

The reduction in available hospital beds and an increase in inpatient day case activity (National Audit Office, 2012) has resulted in greater demands on many acute care services, leading to the introduction of a variety of emergency and urgent care services across the UK, including Emergency Departments (ED), Minor Injury Units (MIU), Out of Hours Services, Walk-in Centres and NHS 111. Accident and Emergency (A&E) departments may now be classified as Type 1, 2, 3 or 4.

Table 11.1   Accident and Emergency Department types

TYPE	DEPARTMENT
1	Emergency departments are a consultant-led 24-hour service with full resuscitation facilities.
2	Consultant-led mono speciality A&E service (e.g. ophthalmology, dental)
3	Other type of A&E/minor injury which may be doctor-led or nurse-led treating at least minor injuries and illnesses, and can be routinely accessed without appointment
4	NHS walk-in centres

Source: Health and Social Care Information Centre (2014)

Furthermore, A&E attendances in the UK have continued to rise over the decades. Reported A&E attendances in England have rose from nearly 14 million per year in 1987–1988 to over 21 million in 2013–2014 (NHS England, 2014). The need to manage acute hospital admissions safely has therefore led to the introduction of Medical Assessment Units (MAU) and Surgical Assessment Units (SAU) which aim to provide fast-track routes to assessment, diagnosis and subsequent referral to the appropriate speciality.

Adult patients are admitted to hospital for a variety of reasons. Admissions can be planned in advance (i.e. for elective surgery or medical investigations/treatment) or may be as a result of an emergency (i.e. accident or injury, acute sudden illness or exacerbation of a long-term condition). According to the Health and Social Care Information Centre (2013) during 2012–2013, across England there were:

- 5.6 million waiting list admissions (an increase of 1.4% on the previous year and an overall 47% increase over the last 15 years (National Audit Office, 2013);
- 5.3 million emergency admissions (an increase of 1.8% on the previous year);
- 6.1 million day cases.

Whatever the clinical setting, adult nurses must be able to provide timely, safe and effective care which includes an ability to recognise the needs of acutely ill patients, the potential for deterioration in their condition and the ability to respond appropriately. Therefore whilst it is acknowledged that you will need to access other specialist literature in order to develop specific knowledge and understanding relating to the care of adults undergoing specific medical treatments and surgical interventions (see the further suggested reading at the end of this chapter), the main focus for this chapter is upon the systematic assessment and management of an acutely ill patient.

Acute assessment units are often very busy environments and their main aim is to reduce unnecessary hospital admissions, facilitating timely referral to inpatient hospital care within the relevant speciality if necessary. As an adult nurse working in an acute environment you will need to have a good understanding of the altered physiology of illness and the capacity to rapidly observe, assess and monitor patients, interpreting and evaluating your observations and assessments to make sound decisions based upon your clinical judgement. Team working and the ability to communicate effectively with patients and their families as well as other members of the multidisciplinary team will be crucial in order to help to relieve stress and anxiety and to ensure continuity of care. In fact, you will need to draw upon all of the skills and attributes outlined in Part One of this book to fulfil the demands of providing safe, effective and compassionate care to your patients.

> ## ACTIVITY 11.1
>
> Access the following websites and identify the common reasons for hospital admission for adults aged 18 and over (i.e. main specialities, diagnosis and treatment statistics and accidents/external causes):
>
> - England and Wales: Health and Social Care Information Centre website available at www.hscic.gov.uk/
> - Scotland: Information Services Division website available at www.isdscotland.org
> - Northern Ireland: Department of Health, Social Services and Public Safety website available at www.dhsspsni.gov.uk/

Acute medicine

Acute medical emergencies are the most common reason for admission to an acute hospital (Royal College of Physicians, 2007). Acute medicine is now considered a specialism in its own right and many UK hospitals have established Acute Medical Units (AMUs), also known as Medical Assessment Units (MAU), Acute Assessment Units (AAU), and Early Assessment Units (EAU). Scott et al. (2009) suggest that AMUs may reduce inpatient mortality and length of stay, and improve patient and staff satisfaction.

It is recommended that all registered nurses working in such environments should have competences in:

- Immediate Life Support (ILS);
- performing an Early Warning Score (EWS) assessment, its interpretation and escalation as appropriate;
- recording an ECG;
- venepuncture;
- IV drug administration;
- urinary catheterisation (male and female);
- aseptic non-touch technique;
- point of care testing (e.g. use of small bench analysers for blood glucose, blood gases, coagulation tests);
- end of life care;
- handover, transfer and discharge.
  (Adapted from the West Midlands Quality Review Service and the Society for Acute Medicine, 2012)

(Note: Although this list of competencies focuses upon those nurses working in Acute Medical Units you could also argue that they have relevance for adult nurses working in many other clinical settings too.)

STOP AND THINK

How could you ensure that you are able to develop your clinical skills to meet the required competencies highlighted above?

Surgery

There have been significant changes in how surgery is performed in a modern healthcare setting. Just like the medical context, patients are older, sicker, and have more co-morbidity. There has been considerable modifications to management of wound surgical techniques with advances in the use of technology (robotic surgery), microsurgery, and minimally invasive surgical techniques ('keyhole' or laparoscopic surgery). There has also been a significant increase in surgery performed as day cases, following recommendations from the NHS Modernisation Agency (2004) suggesting that day surgery should be considered the norm for elective surgery rather than inpatient surgery. The increased use of day surgery has a number of potential economic benefits, including:

- shorter hospital stays;
- release of facilities for more complex and emergency cases;
- fixed scheduling, reducing cancellations and therefore more efficient theatre use;
- staff reductions (as overnight staffing is usually not necessary);
- a decrease in both the time taken to perform surgical procedures and their cost, taking advantage of advances in surgical and anaesthetic care;
- better use of high-cost operating room apparatus and supplies (WHO, 2007).

The variety of surgical procedures carried out on adults across the UK is vast. However, common surgical procedures include abdominal surgery (e.g. appendicectomy, cholecystectomy, bowel resection), vascular surgery (e.g. varicose vein surgery, aortic repair, insertion of stents), surgical oncology (e.g. resection of tumours), orthopaedic surgery (e.g. joint replacements or fracture repair), and plastic surgery (e.g. skin grafts, surgical repair or reconstruction).

Nursing in a surgical setting involves caring for patients before, during and after surgery and requires the knowledge and skills outlined above in addition to those in the following list:

- Pre-operative, peri-operative and post-operative care.
- Anaesthesia.
- Pain management.
- Infection prevention and control (relevant to every setting but particularly important here).
- Wound care, wound healing, dressings and management of wound drains.

STOP AND THINK

How could you ensure that you are able to develop the knowledge and clinical skills to meet the required competencies highlighted above?

Patients undergoing a planned surgical procedure will often be required to present for a pre-op assessment as an outpatient prior to their admission. Though not all surgery can be planned in advance in this way, whether a patient is undergoing scheduled or emergency surgery adult nurses have a key role in ensuring that patients are not only fully informed about their planned procedure and know what to expect but also that they are fit enough for surgery (though the time available for preparation will differ). If the opportunity is available, it is also a chance to plan for future discharge arrangements. It is argued that this approach can help to reduce patient stress, offers an opportunity to provide reassurance and support, and increases the likelihood of an uneventful recovery and a safer, earlier discharge (NHS Institute for Innovation and Improvement, 2008).

ACTIVITY 11.2

Access the guidelines available below to learn more about pre-op assessment and discharge planning:

- NHS Improving Quality: available at www.nhsiq.nhs.uk
  - o Quality and service improvement tools.
  - o Pre-operative assessment.
  - o Discharge planning.
- National Institute for Health and Care Excellence: available at www.nice.org.uk
- NICE (2003) Preoperative Tests: The Use of Routine Preoperative Tests for Elective Surgery.
- The National Patient Safety Agency: available at www.nrls.npsa.nhs.uk
- WHO (2009) *Patient Safety Checklist: How to do the WHO Surgical Safety Checklist.* Available at: www.nrls.npsa.nhs.uk/patient-safety-videos/how-to-do-the-who-surgical-safety-checklist/
- WHO (2009) *Patient Safety Checklist: How not to do the WHO Surgical Safety Checklist.* Available at: www.nrls.npsa.nhs.uk/patient-safety-videos/five-steps-to-safer-surgery/
- Royal College of Surgeons: available at www.rcseng.ac.uk
- Royal College of Surgeons (2011) *Emergency Surgery: Standards for Unscheduled Surgical Care.*

'Enhanced Recovery' is a comparatively new approach that is being promoted in the NHS. It aims to improve the quality of care by helping patients get better sooner after major surgery and reducing the length of stay in hospital (Enhanced Recovery Partnership Programme, 2010). Enhanced recovery addresses issues in pre-operative, peri-operative and post-operative care. One aim is to ensure that the patient is in the best possible condition for surgery which encompasses the concept of 'prehabilitation' for surgical patients. Elements of the enhanced recovery pathway can be seen in Figure 11.1 overleaf (Enhanced Recovery Partnership Programme, 2010).

Across the NHS, enhanced recovery is being implemented for patients having elective procedures in the four specialities of orthopaedics, colorectal, gynaecological and urological surgery (NHS Improving Quality, 2013). There is a growing body of evidence to support the use of enhanced recovery programmes in patients within these specialities (Aning et al., 2010; Ibrahim et al., 2013; Zhuang et al., 2013; Dwyer et al., 2014). The Enhanced Recovery Partnership now consider that enhanced recovery

The enhanced recovery pathway

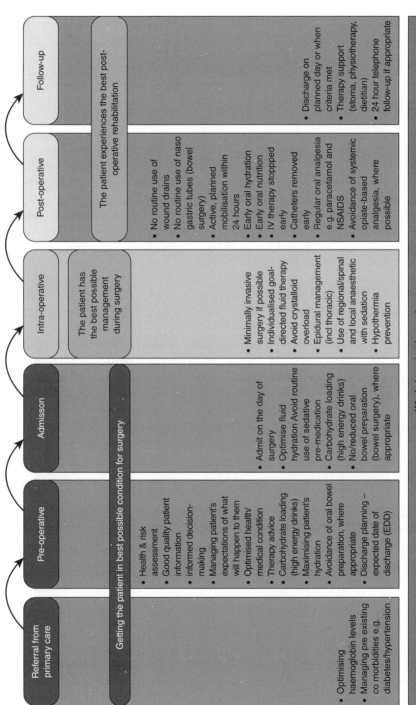

Figure 11.1   The enhanced recovery pathway

Source: Enhanced Recovery Partnership Programme (2010)

should be standard practice for most patients having major surgery, and it has already been implemented in other areas such as emergency surgery and acute medicine (NHS Improving Quality, 2013).

The World Health Organization (2009) advocates the use of the surgical safety checklist in order to promote teamwork and communication in surgery, with an aim to decrease errors and adverse events.

Assessing individuals in an acute care setting

Irrespective of the setting where care takes place, it is imperative that as an adult nurse you are able to accurately assess the needs of your patients. This demands an ability to accurately assess and monitor your patient's condition (on admission and continuously thereafter), check vital signs, develop care plans and safely administer oxygen therapy, IV fluids, medications and pain relief as needed.

So far in this book, we have introduced you to some of the systematic frameworks that can assist you in carefully assessing the needs of your patients. Here we will focus in more depth upon the history-taking and observation element of assessment.

Taking a patient history

The assessment of any individual begins by obtaining a clinical history. History taking in the context of the acutely ill individual may need to be briefer and focused. The scope or depth of the history taking process will need adjusting according to the clinical urgency of the situation. Previously, we have established that history taking is not just simply a fact-finding mission or compiling a list of questions, but is important in the process of establishing a therapeutic relationship. Recognising the need for patients to feel listened to whilst also acknowledging the need for focus, there are a number of mnemonics such as 'OLD CARTS', 'PQRST' or 'SOCRATES' that can be used to guide history taking to elicit more specific information from a patient in relation to a complaint such as pain or any other symptom (e.g. dyspnoea, palpitations, nausea etc.).

> OLD CARTS (Onset, Location, Duration, Character, Aggravating/relieving factors, Radiation, Timing, Severity).
>
> PQRST (Provoking or relieving factors, Quality, Radiation, Severity, Timing).
>
> SOCRATES (Site, Onset, Character, Radiation, Associations, Timing, Exacerbating/relieving factors, Severity).

Table 11.2 gives an example of some of the questions you may need to consider in taking a history of a patient with chest pain using the 'OLD CARTS' mnemonic.

Nurses have long been relied upon to monitor the condition of patients thus ensuring the prompt detection of deterioration or delays in recovery. This demands an ability to be able to recognise and interpret subtle and/or significant changes in the normal physiological parameters of the patient by undertaking specific clinical observations (e.g. blood pressure, pulse and respiratory rate, oxygen saturation, temperature and level of consciousness).

Table 11.2   Example of 'OLD CARTS' mnemonic

Onset

- What brought this on?
- Did it start suddenly or gradually?

Location

- Where exactly is the pain?
- Can you point to where it is?

Duration

- How long has it been there?
- Is it constant or intermittent?

Character

- What is the pain like? Can you describe it to me?
- Consider offering some examples – sharp, dull, aching, stabbing, burning, heavy. It is important however to avoid 'leading' the patient.

Aggravating/relieving factors

- Have you noticed anything that makes it better (e.g. painkillers, other medication such as antacids, positioning)?
- Have you noticed anything that makes it worse (e.g. inspiration, movement, lying down)?

Radiation

- Does the pain radiate to any other location? (To the abdomen, arm, jaw etc.?)

Timing

- When did it start?
- Is it getting better, worse or staying the same?

Severity

- How severe is it?
- Consider using a pain scale (e.g. a 0–10 numeric pain rating).

Other useful questions may ask about associated symptoms, e.g. Do you have any other symptoms with the pain (e.g. dizziness, dyspnoea, nausea)?

---

1. Do you know how to undertake the following clinical observations correctly?

- Blood pressure
- Pulse rate
- Respiratory rate
- Oxygen saturation level
- Blood glucose level
- Temperature
- Level of consciousness.

2. Are you aware of the normal parameters for all of the above?

Many of the clinical observations above can be collated using medical monitoring equipment. Can you think of any risks/disadvantages that can be associated with relying on the use of such equipment?

STOP AND THINK

Whilst we will be exploring some of the frameworks used for detecting patient deterioration later in this chapter, Elliott and Coventry (2012) provide a useful overview of patient monitoring, highlighting the importance of being able to accurately measure and interpret eight vital signs. You may find it useful to access some of the suggested reading at the end of this chapter to ensure that you are able to carry out required clinical observations in the correct manner.

In an emergency setting (e.g. A&E or an Emergency Department) the Manchester Triage System (Mackway-Jones et al., 2013) is used in many settings across the UK. Patients are prioritised into one of five categories (Immediate; Very urgent; Urgent; Standard; Non-urgent). The assessing nurse uses one of a number of flowcharts based on the patient's symptoms and 'discriminators'. Those patients that fall into the Immediate Category need instant treatment; Very Urgent should be treated within 10 minutes; Urgent within one hour; Standard within two hours and Non-urgent within four hours.

Recognising patient deterioration

Admission to hospital can be a disruptive and worrying time for patients and their families. Once in hospital patients ought to feel that they are safe and that they will receive optimum care throughout their stay. However, when suffering from acute illness patients may be unstable and at risk of deterioration due to their altered physiological state. They will often manifest abnormal vital signs, indicating cardiovascular, respiratory or neurological deficits. Unfortunately though there is evidence to suggest that these can go unrecognised by staff, resulting in late treatment, unnecessary admission to critical and intensive care units, and sometimes even death (DH, 2009a). Results from the UK National Cardiac Arrest Audit report the incidence of adult cardiac arrest at 1.6 per 1000 hospital admissions (Nolan et al., 2014). While a significant number of these events occurred in areas such as Coronary Care (CCU) and Intensive Care (ICU) units, over half of cardiac arrests occurred on general wards (Nolan et al., 2014). It is for this reason that all staff – not just those working in acute areas – need to be able to recognise a patient's deterioration and respond quickly and effectively.

In recognition of growing concerns about sub-optimal standards of care within the hospital environment, several clinical guidelines have been published that aim to support healthcare professionals in the assessment and subsequent management of severely ill patients. However, despite regular evidence-based guidelines on resuscitation being produced by the Resuscitation Council UK and significant amounts of time and money being spent on staff training and equipment, survival rates for cardiac arrest remain low. Nolan et al. (2014) reported an overall survival to discharge of 18.4%. While undoubtedly there have been significant advances in resuscitation knowledge and practice over the decades it is not surprising, given the low survival rates, that attention has switched to focusing more on the prevention of cardiac arrest.

STOP AND THINK

Regardless of the setting, nurses need to be aware of the contents of the resuscitation trolley and how to use them:

- Are you prepared to look after a deteriorating patient?
- Do you know about the contents of the resuscitation trolley?
- Would you know how to safely use each piece of equipment?

Track and Trigger systems

Most patients who have a serious adverse event, such as an unplanned ICU admission, cardiac arrest or death, show signs of clinical deterioration in the preceding hours (Schein et al., 1990; Buist et al., 2004). A report from the National Confidential Enquiry into Patient Outcome and Death (NCEPOD) focusing upon patients referred to ICU identified that ward-based recognition of acute illness and its subsequent management was sub-optimal (NCEPOD, 2005). The NCEPOD (2005) report considered that 21% of ICU admissions were avoidable and that sub-optimal care may have been significant enough to have contributed to 33% of deaths.

Subsequently, the National Institute for Health and Clinical Excellence produced the guideline *Acutely Ill Patients in Hospital* (NICE, 2007), addressing the recognition of and response to acute illness in adults in hospital. Similarly, the Scottish Intercollegiate Guidelines Network have also produced the *Care of Deteriorating Patients* guideline (SIGN, 2014). A key priority identified within the NICE (2007:7) guideline is that 'staff caring for patients in acute hospital settings should have competencies in monitoring, measurement, interpretation and prompt response to the acutely ill patient appropriate to the level of care they are providing'.

NICE (2007) also recommended that physiological track and trigger systems should be used to monitor all adult patients in acute hospital settings suggesting that physiological observations should be monitored at least every 12 hours. Track and trigger systems monitor clinical observations ('*Track*') and if predetermined criteria are met a clinical response is activated ('*Trigger*'). Track and trigger systems allow for monitoring patients for signs of clinical deterioration. The signs of clinical deterioration are frequently

Table 11.3   NEWS score

National Early Warning Score (NEWS)*

PHYSIOLOGICAL PARAMETERS	3	2	1	0	1	2	3
Respiration Rate	≤8		9 - 11	12 - 20		21 - 24	≥25
Oxygen Saturations	≤91	92 - 93	94 - 95	≥96			
Any Supplemental Oxygen		Yes		No			
Temperature	≤35.0		35.1 - 36.0	36.1 - 38.0	38.1 - 39.0	≥39.1	
Systolic BP	≤90	91 - 100	101 - 110	111 - 219			≥220
Heart Rate	≤40		41 - 50	51 - 90	91 - 110	111 - 130	≥131
Level of Consciousness				A			V, P, or U

'The NEWS initiative flowed from the Royal College of Physicians' NEWS Development and implementation Group (NEWSDIG) report, and was jointly developed and funded in collabration with the Royal College of Physicians. Royal College of Nursing. National Outreach Forum and NHS Training for Innovation.

Source: Royal College of Physicians (2012)

ss of the cause. NICE (2007) identified six physiological parameters to
track and trigger system:

e.
tions.
3. Temperature.
4. Systolic blood pressure.
5. Heart rate.
6. Level of consciousness (AVPU).

A number of track and trigger systems exist but the Royal College of Physicians (2012)
proposed a 'National Early Warning Score' (NEWS) which would standardise the assessment of the severity of acute illness in the NHS (see Table 11.3). NEWS was not
designed to replace some other scoring systems such as the Glasgow Coma Scale
(Teasdale and Jennett, 1974) but rather to be used in conjunction. The six essential
parameters identified by NICE (2007) in addition to an additional score for patients
requiring oxygen are included in the NEWS. Deviations from normal parameters earn a
score as outlined in Table 11.3. This provides a total NEWS score.

Table 11.4 Outline clinical response to NEWS triggers

NEWS SCORE	FREQUENCY OF MONITORING	CLINICAL RESPONSE
0	Minimum 12 hourly	• Continue routine NEWS monitoring with every set of observations
Total: 1-4	Minimum 4-6 hourly	• Inform registered nurse who must assess the patient • Registered nurse to decide if increased frequency of monitoring and / or escalation of clinical care is required
Total: 5 or more or 3 in one parameter	Increased frequency to a minimum of 1 hourly	• Registered nurse to urgently inform the medical team caring for the patient • urgent assessment by a clinician with core competencies to assess acutely ill patients • Clinical care in an environment with monitoring facilities
Total: 7 or more	Continuous monitoring of vital signs	• Registered nurse to immediately inform the medical team caring for the patient – this should be at least at Specialist Registrar level; • Emergency assessment by a clinical team with critical care competencies, which also includes a practitioner/s with advanced airway skills • Consider transfer of clinical care to a level 2. or 3 care facility, i.e. higher dependency or ITU

Source: Royal College of Physicians (2012)

In addition to the scoring system the Royal College of Physicians (2012) provide an outline of responses to elevated NEWS scores and suggested frequency of monitoring (see Table 11.4). The use of the NEWS can support clinical decision making. It is important to remember that a normal NEWS score does not preclude calling for help when you consider that a patient is unwell. NEWS does not replace clinical judgement. This graded response strategy provides an escalation in response, with higher NEWS scores for those identified as being at risk of clinical deterioration.

ACTIVITY 11.3

The Royal College of Physicians, in conjunction with the Royal College of Nursing and the National Outreach Forum, developed an online training programme in use of the National Early Warning Score (NEWS):

- Access and complete the short training course at the following website: http://tfinews. ocbmedia.com/. This will require that you complete the website registration process.

Calculate the NEWS scores on the patients in the following Case Scenario and write down what action you think should be taken.

Case Scenario

Mariana is a 60-year-old lady who is recovering following a minor operation to remove a skin lesion. Her post-op observations are:

- Respiratory rate 17
- Oxygen saturations 97%
- Temperature 36.2 °C
- Blood pressure 172/84
- Heart rate 74
- Level of consciousness Alert ('A' on the AVPU scale)

Her dressing is intact and there are no signs of discharge or bleeding from her wound.

Rashid is a 62-year-old man admitted with an exacerbation of heart failure. He is complaining of feeling tired and short of breath and has been commenced on supplementary oxygen. He appears drowsy. His current observations are:

- Respiratory rate 22
- Oxygen saturations 96% on supplemental oxygen
- Temperature 37.4 °C
- Blood pressure 96/40
- Heart rate 104
- Level of consciousness Responding to voice ('V' on the AVPU scale)

Mariana has a NEWS total score of 0. The Outline Clinical response suggested by the Royal College of Physicians (2012) would be to continue routine NEWS monitoring. While it is worth noting that Mariana has a raised blood pressure, the Royal College of Physicians acknowledges that this is a risk factor for cardiovascular disease but that a low or falling blood pressure is of more significance in recognising a deteriorating patient.

On the other hand, Rashid has a NEWS total score of 9. The Outline Clinical response suggested by the Royal College of Physicians would be to commence continuous monitoring of vital signs, to inform the medical team caring for the patient, emergency assessment by a clinical team with critical care competencies and to consider a transfer to a level 2 or 3 environment. While each individual component of Rashid's NEWS may not be considered at the extreme, when his condition is considered in its entirety it is evident that he is at considerable risk of clinical deterioration.

STOP AND THINK

- What do you think are the limitations of the track and trigger system outlined above?
- What underpinning knowledge and understanding would you need to be able to interpret the above scores effectively?

Whilst track and trigger systems like NEWS have been widely introduced across the UK, problems in identifying deteriorating patients still exist. Some studies have found that the application of early warning systems varies between organisations, highlighting issues in incomplete or inaccurate recording of required data, an inability to recognise data trends and the timeliness of communication (Donohue and Endacott, 2010; Massey et al. 2010). Coulter-Smith et al. (2013) also argue that systems such as these tend to focus upon the core physiological indicators of severity and that these should be used *in conjunction* with sound clinical judgement based upon experience rather than be seen as a replacement. Therefore the importance of robust clinical assessment and critical reasoning outlined in Chapter 7 (clinical decision making) should not be overlooked.

Critical care

The *Comprehensive Critical Care: A Review of Adult Critical Care Services* report (Department of Health, 2000) provides a classification of the level of critical care that patients need. This report emphasised that critical care services should focus on the level of care that individual patients need rather than on the bed that they may occupy (e.g. a ward bed or ICU bed). The introduction of critical care outreach services developed from this the 'critical care without walls' concept of care based on patient need rather than location. While Ball et al. (2003) suggest that critical care outreach teams may improve patient survival and reduce ICU re-admissions, a review by McGaughey et al. (2007) found the evidence to support this was not clear. However, Pattison and Eastham (2011) acknowledge there can be significant variations in the composition of critical care outreach teams, making research assessing their impact difficult to evaluate. The National Outreach Forum (2012) has produced standards for critical care outreach teams (see Table 11.5).

Table 11.5   Standards for critical care outreach teams

LEVEL	STANDARD
Level 0	Patients whose needs can be met through normal ward care in an acute hospital.
Level 1	Patients at risk of their condition deteriorating, or those recently relocated from higher levels of care, whose needs can be met on an acute ward with additional advice and support from the critical care team.
Level 2	Patients requiring more detailed observation or intervention, including support for a single failing organ system or post-operative care and those 'stepping down' from higher levels of care.
Level 3	Patients requiring advanced respiratory support alone or basic respiratory support together with support of at least two organ systems. This level includes all complex patients requiring support for multi-organ failure.

Source: Department of Health (2000)

Assessment of the critically ill or deteriorating patient using the ABCDE approach

Adult nurses need to be able to perform a comprehensive assessment to identify patient deterioration. The Airway, Breathing, Circulation, Disability, Exposure (ABCDE) approach to the assessment of the critically ill patient is widely advocated (Resuscitation Council UK, 2011; Frost and Wise, 2012).

Thim et al. (2012) suggest that high-quality ABCDE skills among all treating team members can save valuable time and improve team performance. This approach allows for a structured assessment of the patient. The ABCDE approach is beneficial in that it can be used in a variety of settings (pre-hospital and in-hospital) and clinical situations (acute medical and surgical emergencies) with adults and children (Thim et al., 2012). The approach therefore forms the basis of current resuscitation guidelines (Brunker, 2010).

ABCDE principles

The Resuscitation Council UK (2011:12) details some underlying principles to the ABCDE approach as follows:

1. Use the **A**irway, **B**reathing, **C**irculation, **D**isability, **E**xposure approach to assess and treat the patient.
2. Do a complete initial assessment and re-assess regularly.
3. Treat life-threatening problems before moving to the next part of the assessment.
4. Assess the effects of treatment.
5. Recognise that you will need extra help. Call for appropriate help early.
6. Use all members of the team. This enables interventions, e.g. assessment, attaching monitors, intravenous access, to be undertaken simultaneously.
7. Communicate effectively. Use an SBAR (**S**ituation, **B**ackground, **A**ssessment, **R**ecommendation) or RSVP (**R**eason, **S**tory, **V**ital signs, **P**lan) approach.
8. The aim of initial treatment is to keep the patient alive, and achieve some clinical improvement. This will buy time for further treatment and making a diagnosis.

9. Stay calm – remember that it can take a few minutes for treatments to work.
10. The ABCDE approach can be used irrespective of your training and experience in clinical assessment or treatment. The detail of your assessment and what treatments you give will depend on your clinical knowledge and skills. If you recognise a problem or are unsure call for help.

Airway

Walz et al. (2007) recognise that the skill of airway management is important for any healthcare provider caring for critically ill patients. A patient with a compromised airway will quickly deteriorate (Higginson et al., 2011). Problems with decreased levels of consciousness can lead to airway compromise. Sandberg et al. (2013: 20) suggest that 'the awake, alert patient who is able to speak with a normal voice has no immediate threat to the airway'.

Airway obstruction may be partial or complete. With a complete obstruction, a paradoxical respiration pattern may be evident where the chest moves in on inspiration and out on expiration. In the event of airway obstruction Resuscitation Council UK (2011) guidelines for the management of choking may need to be followed:

- Look in the mouth for any potential cause of obstruction such as food, blood, vomit or loose dentures.
- Foreign objects should be removed where possible.
- Suctioning can be used to remove any vomit, blood or secretions from the airway. If the patient has vomited or is at risk of vomiting, you should consider putting them into the recovery position (Frost and Wise, 2012).
- Look for any swelling of the lips or tongue which may be a sign of anaphylaxis. You can assess the ability to cough to clear secretions.
- Listen for additional noises from the airway such as stridor, snoring or gurgling. Stridor is a high pitched sound, which usually occurs on inspiration, which is caused by laryngeal or tracheal obstruction (Moore, 2007). Gurgling may indicate fluids in the airway such as blood, vomit or secretions.

Any significant problems with airway should be treated before moving on to a Breathing assessment. The management of airway compromise may include:

- the use of airway manoeuvres such as head tilt/chin lift or jaw thrust;
- the use of airway adjuncts such as oropharyngeal or nasopharyngeal airways;
- management of choking to appropriate guidelines (back slaps/abdominal thrusts);
- use of suctioning.

Breathing

Moore (2007) states that it is essential that nurses are able to recognise and assess symptoms of respiratory dysfunction to provide early, effective and appropriate interventions. Despite being a sensitive indicator of the deteriorating patient, Ansell et al. (2014) however report that nurses admit circumstances in which they miss observing respiratory rate. Taking and recording a patient's respiratory rate is essential for detecting a patient's condition (Ansell et al., 2014), though the respiratory rate should be counted for a full minute rather than trying to estimate. In addition to the respiratory rate, the depth (shallow, normal or deep) and pattern of breathing (e.g. *Cheyne-stokes* or *Kussmaul*) should be observed.

Look at the effort of breathing – check for the use of accessory muscles such as the sternocleidomastoid and scalene muscles (which help to raise the sternum and first and second ribs) during inspiration and contraction of abdominal muscles during expiration.

Look for 'pursed lip' breathing on expiration and nasal flaring. The patient may be positioned upright to aid chest expansion. Normal breathing is usually quiet.

Listen for additional breathing noises such as wheeze. Olson (2014) warns that if airflow rates are too low a wheeze may not be audible.

Assess the patient's ability to speak in complete sentences. Can they answer your questions easily and fully whilst breathing normally? Observe for signs of cyanosis.

Cyanosis is generally a relatively late finding in the ill patient (McMullen and Patrick, 2013). Moore (2007) notes that central cyanosis usually indicates circulatory or ventilator problems while peripheral cyanosis usually indicates poor circulation. Pulse oximetry is now widely available, and the oxygen saturations should be recorded. 'SpO2' refers to the peripheral oxygen saturation (pulse oximetry) whereas 'SaO2' refers to the arterial oxygen saturation (obtained from an Arterial Blood Gas (ABG) sample).

It is important to acknowledge that oxygen is a treatment for hypoxaemia and not breathlessness. Current clinical guidelines on the use of oxygen should be followed (British Thoracic Society, 2008).

Circulation

An assessment of circulation may start with the fundamental pulse and blood pressure check. While a heart rate may be available from a monitor, a manual pulse check is useful as you can get more information such as the character of the pulse and the rhythm:

- Is the pulse fast and weak which may indicate hypovolaemia?
- Is the pulse regular or irregular?
- Skin temperature can also be assessed while checking the pulse: is the patient cool and clammy or warm to the touch?

Measure the blood pressure. It is advisable to check an abnormal blood pressure reading obtained from a machine with a manual check.

ACTIVITY 11.4

Access and review the MHRA (2013) top ten tips for measuring blood pressure at www.gov.uk (using the search terms 'measuring blood pressure').

IV access is important, particularly if a patient is at risk of hypovolaemia or in need of fluid resuscitation, so it may be necessary to prepare for IV cannulation (NICE, 2013a). Urinary output and fluid balance should also be monitored carefully. A decreased urinary output can be a sign of decreased renal perfusion. NICE (2013) recognise a urinary output of less than 0.5ml/kg/hr as a clinical characteristic of *acute kidney injury*. The capillary refill time (CRT) should also be assessed. A prolonged CRT may indicate reduced skin perfusion, which may indicate poor circulation. However Lewin and Maconochie (2008) warn that while the CRT is a quick and easy bedside test, its results cannot be interpreted with any degree of confidence in the adult population and should not be used in isolation.

If a patient has undergone surgical intervention, wound dressings and drains should be checked regularly and observed for sources of blood loss. In an acutely unwell adult, a 12 lead ECG should also be considered. This is not restricted to only those with a suspected cardiac problem, as a 12 lead ECG can help to identify other clinical problems such as an electrolyte imbalance (e.g. hypo/hyperkalaemia).

Disability

Assess the level of consciousness. This can be done using the AVPU Scale (Figure 11.2) or the Glasgow Coma Scale. Level of consciousness is the earliest and most sensitive indicator of neurological deterioration (Peate, 2013).

- Alert
- Responds to verbal stimuli
- Responds to painful stimuli
- Unresponsive to all stimuli

Figure 11.2   The AVPU Scale

Source: Resuscitation Council UK (2011)

The Glasgow Coma Scale (GCS) can be completed. The best possible score is 15 out of 15 and the worst 3 out of 15. When documenting the GCS it is useful to record not only the total score (i.e. a GCS of 13/15) but also the components of that score (e.g. a of GCS 13/15, i.e. Eyes 3, Verbal 4, Motor 6).

Table 11.6   The Glasgow Coma Scale

Score	Eye opening (E)	Best verbal response (V)	Best motor response (M)
6			Obeys commands
5		Orientated to time and place	Localises to pain
4	Eyes open spontaneously	Confused	Withdrawal from pain
3	Eyes open to speech	Inappropriate words	Flexion to pain
2	Eyes open to pain	Incomprehensible sounds	Extension to pain
1	No eye opening	No verbal response	No motor response

Source: After Teasdale, G. and Jennett, B. (1974) 'Assessment of coma and impaired consciousness: a practical scale', *The Lancet*, 304 (7872): 81–4.

The 'Act FAST' TV campaign in England from Public Health England (2014) aims to improve public awareness of the signs of stroke and the need to call emergency services at the onset of a suspected stroke (Dombrowski et al., 2013). While the Act FAST campaign seeks to raise public awareness, this simple acronym can be used by a nurse as an aid in recognising some of the common signs of a stroke or transient ischaemic attack (TIA). A stroke is a medical emergency that necessitates immediate attention. It is important to recognise the terrible effects of a stroke and the potential consequences of a delayed response (Kavanagh et al., 2011):

- Facial weakness
  - Can the person smile? Has their face fallen on one side?
- Arm weakness
  - Can the person raise both arms and keep them there?
- Speech problems
  - Can the person speak clearly and understand what you say? Is their speech slurred?
- Time to call 999.

  (Public Health England, 2012)

Check the blood glucose level. Approximately one in five in patients with diabetes report having a hypoglycaemic episode whilst in hospital and this rises to two in five in those with Type 1 diabetes (National Diabetes Inpatient Audit, 2013). Diabetes UK advocate the 'make four the floor' rule, signifying a blood glucose reading of 4.0mmol/L as the lowest acceptable level in people with diabetes. The Joint British Diabetes Societies for Inpatient Care guidelines (Walden et al., 2013) outlines treatment strategies for the hospital management of hypoglycaemia in adults with Diabetes Mellitus.

ACTIVITY 11.5

Hypoglycaemia represents a significant clinical problem that all nurses should be able to manage.
  Review the signs/symptoms of hypoglycaemia and consider the management and treatment of hypoglycaemia for the following:

- Adults who are conscious, orientated and able to swallow.
- Adults who are conscious but confused and able to swallow.
- Adults who are unconscious or having seizures.
- Adults who are 'Nil by mouth'.
- Adults requiring enteral feeding.

See the Joint British Diabetes Societies' (JBDS) Hospital Management of Hypoglycaemia in Adults with Diabetes, 2nd edition (Walden et al., 2013). Available at http://www.diabetologists-abcd.org.uk/JBDS/JBDS.htm

Examine the pupils. What size are they? Are they equal? Do they react appropriately to light? You should be aware that some drugs can affect pupil size.

Review the drug chart to assess for any medications that may have caused an altered level of consciousness. It may be necessary to nurse the patient in the recovery position.

Exposure

This is a head to toe check for anything not already discovered on the ABCD check that may suggest a cause for the patient being unwell:

- Check for any rashes, bruising, bleeding or swelling. It is important to maintain the patient's dignity.
- Check temperature.
- Assess if the patient is in any pain.

You should now have some appreciation of how unwell the patient is. Remember, from the principles outlined above that it is important to re-assess regularly.

Evidence-based interventions in acute care
Oxygen therapy

Oxygen therapy is a vital element in the care of an acutely ill adult. Oxygen is widely used in the treatment of a variety of conditions and it is vital that nurses are safe, knowledgeable and competent in its use. It is a drug and should be prescribed for an individual patient depending on their condition. The patient requires a specific dose (concentration) of this drug. Both an inadequate or excessive oxygen dose may be potentially harmful. However, the oxygen dose required varies from patient to patient and indeed within the same patient as their condition changes. It is important to remember that in an emergency situation oxygen can be given immediately and documented later (British Thoracic Society, 2008; National Patient Safety Agency, 2009).

The nurse administering oxygen needs to consider the following:

- Am I aware of the patient's diagnosis and target saturation?
- Does the flow rate need adjusting to achieve that patient's target saturation?
- Am I familiar with the equipment to do this and have I checked this is in working order (e.g. a face mask/nasal cannulae)?
- Have I recorded the oximetry results (saturation levels)?
- Is the tube connected to the right outlet, i.e. oxygen not air?

When using cylinders:

- Have I checked the amount of oxygen in the cylinder before using it?
- Have I calculated how long the oxygen in the cylinder will last?
- Do I make sure empty or near-empty cylinders are replaced immediately?
  (Adapted from the National Patient Safety Agency, 2009)

There are a number of devices available for the delivery of oxygen including nasal cannulae, a simple oxygen mask and a high concentration reservoir mask (a non-rebreathe mask). It is important to acknowledge that the concentration of oxygen that

the patient receives depends not only on the flow rate but also on the type ⌐
the patient's breathing pattern. The British Thoracic Society (2008) produce
for the emergency use of oxygen in adult patients. One essential element o
lines is that oxygen is prescribed according to the target saturation range. Oxygen is
prescribed to a target saturation range of 94–98% for most acutely ill patients and
88–92% for those at risk of hypercapnic respiratory failure. Those administering oxygen
need to monitor the patient and aim to keep saturations within range by adjusting the
oxygen delivery devices or flow rates. Monitoring of saturations and respiratory function
following the administration of supplemental oxygen is essential.

Intravenous therapy

Intravenous (IV) therapy is a common activity that does not always get the attention
it deserves, and takes place in nearly every healthcare setting (Scales, 2008; 2014).
While very commonplace it is easy to become complacent, but a NCEPOD (1999)
report identified that up to 1 in 5 patients receiving IV fluids in hospital could experience complications or morbidity as a result of their inappropriate use.

NICE (2013) has produced guidelines for IV fluid therapy for adults in hospital. The
guidelines suggest that a patient's fluid and electrolyte requirements are identified using the
5Rs: Resuscitation, Routine maintenance, Replacement, Redistribution and Reassessment.
While much of these guidelines is aimed at prescribers, it is important to acknowledge that
managing hydration is a fundamental nursing role (Ugboma and Cowen, 2012). Indicators
that a patient may need urgent fluid resuscitation include the following:

- Systolic blood pressure is less than 100mmHg.
- Heart rate is more than 90 beats per minute.
- Capillary refill time is more than two seconds or peripheries are cold to the touch.
- Respiratory rate is more than 20 breaths per minute.
- National Early Warning Score (NEWS) is 5 or more.
- Passive leg raising suggests fluid responsiveness (NICE, 2013).

JIM

Case Scenario

Jim is 56-year-old gentleman and has had a bowel resection to remove a tumour. The surgery was uneventful, and the surgeons are confident that the entire tumour has been
removed in time, that it has not spread and therefore that this is a curative operation. He
has a urinary catheter, one peripheral cannula in his left forearm and a central line. You are
the nurse who is looking after him that evening, and have just been given handover. On
your initial assessment you find that:

- **A** – he is talking to you.
- **B** – he has a slightly elevated respiratory rate (18) and is receiving 4L/min of oxygen via
nasal specs: his oxygen saturations are 95%.
- **C** – his pulse rate is 92, and manual blood pressure is 135/60: he has no central line monitoring.
- **D** – he is coherent and pain free.

(Continued)

(Continued)

- **E** – there are no obvious rashes, his wound on examination looks clean and dry, and his abdomen looks 'normal'.

An hour later, the patient in the next bed to Jim summons you over, saying that he doesn't think Jim looks well. You re-examine Jim and on examination you find:

- **A** – Jim does answer you.
- **B** – his respiratory rate is now 22, and his oxygen saturations are 92% on 4L/min nasal specs.
- **C** – his pulse rate is now 125, and his manual blood pressure is 90/40: he appears flushed and his temperature is now 38.4°C.
- **D** – his pain score is 8/10.
- **E** – his wound is looking red, there are obvious signs of bleeding and his abdomen looks more distended.
- **What do you think is happening?** Write down in detail the physiological responses and consider what is happening and how this has affected his cardiovascular system, e.g. which component (heart, vessels, blood) is compensating for what?
- What would you do next?

The changes to Jim's cardiovascular and respiratory function are as a result of his body's responses to infection, which rather than his presenting symptoms being local (e.g. at the site of infection) they are systemic and affecting the whole body. He is exhibiting three of the physiological symptoms used as criteria for diagnosing sepsis (e.g. a raised temperature, raised respiratory rate and increased heart rate). Sepsis is the body's response to infection. Although the source of this infection appears to be from his wound site, given the information above, Jim has several potential sites of infection which could be the cause of his sepsis: his surgical procedure, his intravenous access or his urinary catheter. Therefore Jim requires early goal-directed treatment to ensure his sepsis is managed appropriately.

Severe sepsis accounts for approximately one quarter of admissions to general critical care units in the UK (Shahin et al., 2012). Robson and Daniels (2013) consider sepsis a medical emergency and the UK Sepsis Trust (2014) advocate that staff working on all inpatient wards should be aware of the significance of sepsis and have the skills and knowledge to recognise it early and start treatment. Sepsis is defined as 'the presence (probable or documented) of infection together with systemic manifestations of infection', whereas severe sepsis is defined as 'sepsis *plus* sepsis-induced organ dysfunction or tissue hypoperfusion' (Dellinger et al., 2013: 583). Sepsis arises when the body's response to infection injures its own tissues and organs and can lead to shock, organ failure and death if not recognised and treated early (The UK Sepsis Trust, 2014).

The Scottish Intercollegiate Guidelines Network (SIGN) (2014) *Care of Deteriorating Patients'* guideline suggests that any patient whose NEWS score triggers action should be screened for sepsis (and delirium). SIGN recommend that all patients who screen positively for sepsis should be started on the Sepsis Six care bundle, unless their treatment plan dictates otherwise. The Sepsis Six are a set of interventions to be performed in the first hour of suspected sepsis, which can improve survival. These are as follows:

1. Give high flow oxygen.
2. Take blood cultures.
3. Give broad spectrum antibiotics.
4. Give intravenous fluid challenges.
5. Take serum lactate and haemoglobin.
6. Take accurate hourly urine output.

The Sepsis Trust (2012) suggests that a useful way to remember the Sepsis Six is to 'give 3 and take 3'. In other words give oxygen, antibiotics and fluids and take blood cultures, serum lactate and haemoglobin, and urine output.

ACTIVITY 11.6

The UK Sepsis Trust provides a number of online learning resources that are very useful. Access these at the website below and have a look at them in further detail:
http://sepsistrust.org/info-for-professionals/sepsis-learning-resources/

SBAR communication tool

The ABCDE assessment aids in recognising the acutely ill patient. An appropriate response in conjunction with immediate lifesaving interventions (e.g. oxygen administration) is likely to include a call for help. Clear and effective communication between staff is essential to provide effective care and maintain patient safety and the 'SBAR' communication tool can aid this. The SBAR acronym stands for Situation, Background, Assessment and Recommendation. It is a communication tool that can be used to help provide structure to this important conversation on reporting a clinical deterioration in a patient. Originally used by US Navy nuclear submarine personnel, it was adapted for healthcare use by Leonard et al. (2004).

Beliveau (2012) suggests that if SBAR is used consistently not only will the nurse understand how to quickly and concisely gather, organise and report appropriate information but that the recipient can also anticipate how the information will be delivered. SBAR helps to deliver critical information effectively to promote patient safety. A study by DeMeester et al. (2013) found that, following the introduction of SBAR across 16 hospital wards, there was an increased perception of effective communication between nurses and doctors and a reduction in unexpected deaths. It is important to remember the listening skills necessary for the receiver.

ACTIVITY 11.7

Revisit the previous case scenario. How would you report the changes in Jim's condition to the nurse in charge or medical staff? Write down the conversation you would have using the SBAR tool as a guide.

(Continued)

(Continued)

Situation

Identify yourself and where you are calling from. Identify which patient you are calling about and briefly the reason for the call. Leonard et al. (2004) advocate the use of powerful 'critical language' such as 'I'm concerned, this is unsafe', or 'I'm scared' as that will have the effect of gaining the necessary attention of the receiver (e.g. a doctor/senior nurse): 'The reason I am calling is ... '

Background

You need to relay relevant information, including the reason for admission, relevant past medical/surgical history and current management.

Assessment

You need to elaborate what you found on your ABCDE assessment of the patient. You should include the NEWS score and it is helpful to bring relevant information such as the observation chart/notes to the phone when making the call to ensure that you have all the relevant information to hand. You can then state what you think is going on: 'I think that they may be ... '

Recommendation

You should have a clear idea as to what you would like to happen as a result of your call. Are you calling for advice? Do you want an urgent assessment? Or, are you simply providing an update. Do you think that the patient should be transferred to another clinical area such as ICU? You can make suggestions for actions: 'I would like you to ... '

Pain Management

Pain is a very common symptom experienced by people admitted to hospital. The prevalence of pain in hospital settings is estimated to be between 37.5% (Melloti et al., 2005) and 84% (Sawyer et al., 2010). However, despite advances in technology and an increased awareness of the importance of pain management, concerns remain about the management of pain (Wadenstein, 2011). Pain is a subjective individual experience which is affected by many factors: physical, psychological, environmental and social. Some of the factors affecting how people react to pain include the site and nature of the injury, their personality, age, gender, and cultural factors (Godfrey 2005; Strong et al., 2002). As a result of its subjectivity and unique experience, pain is frequently defined by nurses as 'whatever the patient says it is'. Unfortunately though some practitioners do not always appear to believe what their patients say about their pain, though you might ask yourself why would someone either deny or exaggerate this symptom? Uncontrolled pain can have harmful physiological, psychological and emotional effects on an individual (Williams and Salerno, 2012). Pain affects an individual's ability to carry out activities of daily living, for example it affects appetite and the ability to sleep, and it can reduce mobility which in turn can lead to other problems such as chest infection, pressure ulcers, deep veined thrombosis etc. It also causes anxiety, especially if the reason for the pain is not identified, and lowers mood and quality of life. It is therefore important to ensure that you recognise and relieve your patients' pain to prevent unnecessary suffering.

Pain is generally classed into three types: acute, chronic or long-term pain, and malignant pain. Pain associated with a malignancy can be caused by a tumour and/or treatment, such as surgery, radiotherapy and chemotherapy: it can be acute or chronic.

Acute or nociceptive pain is seen as a symptom or warning. It is usually localised, and of short duration when it responds to analgesia and decreases over time as healing progresses. Acute pain is associated with a hospital admission. Some causes of acute pain are myocardial infarction, surgical procedures, acute infections and trauma (Hawthorn and Redmond, 1998).

Chronic pain is defined as having lasted for three months or more, persists after healing would normally be complete and beyond the point where it has value as an indicator of tissue damage (Bond and Simpson, 2006): it has no predicable ending. Back pain is a very common cause of chronic pain in the UK, and arthritis and angina are also common causes of long-term pain problems. The majority of people with chronic non-malignant pain are treated within primary care settings, and when this fails to help they may be referred to a specialist pain management team or unit. Many people admitted to hospital have a long-term pain problem that is unrelated to the reason they have been admitted, but you need to be aware that their pain can result in a prolonged recovery time compared to people without chronic pain.

The treatment modalities and approaches for chronic non-malignant pain are different from and less aggressive than the treatment required for acute pain (McCaffery and Pasero, 1999). Non-pharmacological therapies, including psychological interventions, are frequently used alongside conventional analgesia to help patients cope with this long-term problem. It is important for you to assess how chronic pain has an effect on an individual, their activities of living, its psychological impact, and what the patient understands about their problem.

 YVONNE

Yvonne is a 65-year-old lady who has fallen down stairs at home and been admitted into A&E. She has right-sided chest pain and finds it difficult to breathe. She is suspected to have fractured her ribs as a result of the fall.

On admission her observations are as follows:

- **A** – she can speak to you in full sentences.
- **B** – she has a respiratory rate of 28, her respirations are shallow and her oxygen saturations are 95% with no oxygen being supplied.
- **C** – her pulse is 112, strong and regular, and her blood pressure is 185/90.
- **D** – she is coherent but very distressed and her pain score is 9/10.
- **E** – she is very pale and sweaty, has bruising to her right arm and her right ankle is swollen.

What do you think is Yvonne's main problem?
What might happen if this is not resolved?

The A&E doctor has requested an x-ray of her chest and ankle and as the nurse responsible for her care:

- Would you be happy to send her straight to radiology?
- What care would be appropriate prior to transfer?

(Continued)

Case Scenario

(Continued)

Yvonne is prescribed the following analgesia:

- Morphine IV, 10mgs PRN.
- Morphine orally, 10–20mgs 2–4 hourly.
- Paracetamol 1gram, orally or IV, QDS.

What do you feel is the most appropriate analgesia, and by which route would you administer it?

List your observations of Yvonne: how frequently should they be conducted?

What other possible side effects would you monitor?

Is there any other analgesia that may help?

Once Yvonne's pain is controlled, how would you expect her A–E observations to alter?

What non-pharmacological interventions could be administered by you and may help reduce Yvonne's pain?

The assessment and measurement of pain are fundamental to the diagnosis of the cause of pain, selecting an appropriate analgesia therapy, use of other therapies, and evaluating and then modifying that therapy (Australian and New Zealand College of Anaesthetists, 2010). In other words, the management of pain develops from pain assessment and it is the first step in the decision-making process.

The patient's report of pain is the most reliable indicator of pain and it is essential to listen and believe that individual (Schofield and Dunham, 2003). Pain scales or tools provide a standard means of assessing pain – they are used to measure or establish the level of pain. Patients can be encouraged to use them to communicate their pain experience and they help to evaluate the effect of treatment and indicate when a review of pain therapy is required (Williamson and Hoggart, 2005; Ruder, 2010). There are a number of pain assessment scales that ask patients to rate their pain, and these have been found to be easy to use and highly valid and reliable. The successful use of these pain scales depends on a patient's ability to use the scales and careful interpretation of the scores by healthcare professionals (Williamson and Hoggart, 2005). The Visual Analogue Scale, Numerical Rating Scale and Verbal Descriptor Scale are examples of patient rating scales.

The *Visual Analogue Scale* (VAS) consists of a 10cm line with anchor words at each end of the line, from 'no pain' to 'worst pain imaginable'. A mark is made on the line by the patient with a pen or pencil and is measured on the line (Schofield and Dunham, 2003). Alternatively a plastic or metal slide-ruler may be used as an alternative to paper (Mohan et al., 2013). This tool has limited practical use in acute care settings but can be used in outpatient clinics.

The *Numerical Rating Scale* (NRS) asks the patient to verbally rate their pain as a number (0–10), with 0 indicating no pain and 10 the worse pain imaginable (Wood, 2004; Mohan et al., 2013). It is quick and easy to use in patients who can communicate effectively (Ruder, 2010; Mohan et al., 2013). Some patients do have difficulty converting their experience into a number and its use is limited when communication is a problem.

The *Verbal Descriptor Scale* (VDS) asks the patient to indicate which word describes their pain. Examples of descriptors are No Pain, Mild Pain, Moderate Pain and Severe

Pain. It is quick and easy to use and it is valid and fits with the WHO's analgesic ladder (Wood, 2004). There is limited range to assess changes in pain intensity and the ratings are subject to a patient's interpretation of the words used. Numbers have been adopted to help document VDS, for example no pain = 0, mild pain = 1, moderate = 2, and severe pain = 3.

However, the assessment scales above only rate the intensity of pain and a more comprehensive assessment would include how pain affects the activities of daily living. For example, you could use one of the mnemonics described earlier, such as OLD CARTS or SOCRATES, to explore this in more depth.

When a patient is unable to communicate and describe their pain, for example someone in ICU or following a CVA or with cognitive impairment, including dementia, pain can be assessed through observing behaviours. A number of behavioural pain assessment tools have been devised, for example the Critical Care Pain Observation Tool (CPOT) (Gelmas et al., 2006) and the Abbey Scale and Pain Assessment IN Advanced Dementia (PAINAD) (Warden et al., 2003; Abbey et al., 2004) for people with dementia. The critical care tool relies on physiological changes to help identify pain in addition to observing facial expression and agitation. The tools devised for people with dementia includes verbalisation, facial expression, body movements, changes in interaction, changes in activities of living and mental status changes. The Abbey Tool also includes physiological changes and any physical damage that may be causing pain.

- How is pain assessed in your current placement area?
- Have you observed the use of observational pain assessment tools?
- How effective are the tools in identifying and assessing pain?

STOP AND THINK

Pain management interventions

Once pain has been identified and assessed it is managed using pharmacological and non-pharmacological interventions, often in combination. It is important that adult nurses have an understanding of the pain management options available. It has already been established that pain is an individual experience and as such the effectiveness of interventions can vary between individuals, with wide differences in the reaction to interventions, i.e. both pharmacological and non-pharmacological pain measures.

Pharmacological pain management

There is a choice of analgesic drugs available depending on the nature and severity and the individual patient's reaction to medication. It is important that you advise patients of the benefits of reducing their pain and to stress that analgesia is taken regularly to prevent pain, rather than waiting for pain and to then take analgesia. This is because waiting for pain leads to the individual 'chasing the pain' rather than managing or controlling it. The effectiveness of analgesia has been studied and systematic reviews of randomised controlled trials produced (these studies can be found at the Oxford Pain Site available at www.medicine.ox.ac.uk/bandolier/Extraforbando/APain.pdf).

The World Health Organization's analgesic ladder (1986)

Despite being the object of debate and critsim, The WHO (1986) analgesic ladder offers a useful 'step-by-step' approach to pain management. There are three main classes of analgesia: Paracetamol (simple analgesia), Non-Steroidal Anti-Inflammatory Drugs (NSAID) and Opioids. These are well established and are incorporated into the ladder.

This analgesic ladder relates to the intensity of pain:

Step 1 = Mild pain, Paracetamol and NSAID

Step 2 = Moderate pain, Paracetamol, NSAID and mild opiate

Step 3 = Severe pain, Paracetamol, NSAID and strong opiate

It can be applied to all types of pain (e.g. acute, chronic or malignant). In acute severe pain the patient would start at step 3 of the ladder and as the pain reduces move towards step 1.

Simple analgesia

Paracetamol can be taken orally as tablets, capsules, syrup or soluble preparations, though it should be avoided in active liver disease. The daily maximum dose of 4 grams should never be exceeded as it can cause liver damage and/or failure. It is important to stress this aspect and to check that patients are not taking any other medication that may contain Paracetamol (e.g. cough and flu remedies or combination analgesia, such as Co-dydramol).

Non-Steroidal Anti-Inflammatory Drugs (NSAID)

NSAID can be taken orally or applied as a gel for mild to moderate muscular skeletal pain. They act by blocking the prostaglandins responsible for some of the inflammatory response to tissue damage (Bond and Simpson, 2006). Systematic reviews of randomised controlled trials of NSAID have found them to be very effective for the mild to moderate pain associated with dysmenorrhea, joint and muscle pain, post-surgical pain, toothache etc. They can reduce swelling and pain at site and improve mobility (McQuay and Moore, 1998). Some patients find that one NSAID is more effective than others (Bond and Simpson, 2006).

Opioid analgesia

Opioid analgesia is derived from the opium poppy and is regulated under the *Misuse of Drugs Act* (1971). Strong opioids are classed as Controlled Drugs (CD). A prescription is therefore always required for opioid analgesia. Opiates are agonist-type drugs that combine with opiate receptors found mainly in the periphery, spinal cord and brain

(Bond and Simpson, 2006). They interfere with the transmission of the pain signal within the spinal cord and change an individual's perception of the pain (Williams and Salerno, 2012). Systematic reviews have found opioids to be more effective when used in combination with Paracetamol and NSAID (Doherty et al., 2011).

When caring for a patient using opioid analgesia it is important to consider possible side effects and carefully monitor their reaction to the medication. Anticipate constipation and inform the patient of the problem by advising them how to prevent constipation with adequate fluids etc. Laxatives may be required. Anti-emetics may be required initially and anti-histamines can also help with itchiness and any rash – both of these symptoms will become less of a problem after a few days. Many healthcare professionals and members of the public fear addiction and will avoid using opioid analgesia as a result. However, addiction is rare when analgesia is required and the importance of good pain control should always be emphasised (Gregory, 2014).

Morphine is considered the cornerstone of pain relief for severe pain. It is relatively cheap and available in many forms, orally and parentally. The dose of morphine required for individuals varies in its ability to provide similar pain relief; therefore this needs to be adjusted according to a patient reaction (Bond and Simpson, 2006). Patient Controlled Analgesia (PCA) is a system commonly used following surgery, which aims to overcome some of this individual variation. PCA is a device (usually electronic) that enables the patient to deliver a small pre-determined dose of morphine IV (usually 1–2 mgs) via a demand button or handset. There is a 'lockout' safety feature that means the patient does not receive morphine more than every five minutes.

Nitrous Oxide 50% and Oxygen 50% (Entonox) is a medical gas indicated for procedural pain. It has been traditionally used in maternity and emergency departments, and increasingly in hospital wards and departments for painful procedures such as wound care. It is quickly effective, within a few deep breaths, easy to use, and provides the patient with an element of control and distraction from the procedure. It has few side effects (mainly nausea), can be used with other analgesics, and is considered safe for all age groups (Gregory, 2008).

Non-pharmacological pain interventions

Pain is not just a physical event and responds to a variety of treatments and often a combination of strategies. Some of the non-pharmacological and less invasive interventions that can be used alongside analgesia to help pain include the following.

Psychological interventions help people to cope with their pain. Also known as cognitive-behavioural therapies they can be relatively simple or complex interventions. The aim of these interventions is to decrease or change the individual's perception of pain (Hawthorn and Redmond, 1998). Some of the strategies include the use of distraction, music therapy, meditation, guided imagery and relaxation.

Distraction is easily applied and aims to take the patient's mind off the pain. If the individual focuses their attention on the painful stimulus it becomes more intense. It is a useful strategy that is frequently used during procedures such as a dressing change. Focusing the mind on other stimulus is thought to reduce the pain intensity. Mental distraction involves carrying out a mental activity, such as counting, reciting a poem or prayer, and behavioural task distraction, for example reading a book, or listening to the radio, watching TV, playing a computer game (Hawthorn and Redmond, 1998). The ability to distract an individual from the pain does not indicate that the pain is not real; believing the patient during the assessment and encouraging the use of distraction are therapeutic. Music has also been found to be effective in reducing pain by distraction, relaxation, reducing anxiety and allowing increased feelings of control (Hawthorn and Redmond, 1998). The choice of music is important and should be suitable to ensure it helps the patient relax. Pain, muscle tension and anxiety are closely linked and helping an individual reduces muscle tension, anxiety and therefore the pain intensity. A simple technique is deep breathing exercises, as they are a form of distraction and help patients to relax (Hawthorn and Redmond, 1998).

Evaluation or re-assessment of pain to establish the effectiveness of interventions is as important as the initial assessment. Monitoring side effects, such as gastric irritation and constipation, to ensure patients continue with their medication may be necessary. Alternative medications may be required or titration of the dose considered to provide adequate pain relief with lower side effects. The use of non-pharmacological interventions can be suggested and encouraged once the pain is tolerable. For many patients an increase or improvement in activity may be as important as the reduction of pain intensity and should be included in the evaluation of pain management interventions.

Caring for a patient with an artificial airway

Many patients in need of critical care will have a temporary tracheostomy sited. They may require this to remain in situ when discharged from ICU to the ward. In fact, some patients with a tracheostomy are nursed in other clinical environments such as community settings (Freeman, 2011). As an adult nurse you will need to be aware of the additional equipment required, any potential risks, and how to manage these.

A tracheostomy is a surgically created opening in the wall of the trachea below the cricoid cartilage. The indications for a temporary tracheostomy to be sited are:

- to protect the airway;
- to aid the removal of excessive secretions;
- to aid weaning from mechanical ventilation (Intensive Care Society, 2008).

You can find further useful information at the following website: www.tracheostomy. org.uk

Case Scenario

JAN

Jan is 42 and has a temporary tracheostomy in place following an ICU admission. She was admitted with respiratory failure following a long stay in hospital as a result of her chronic renal failure. She is no longer requiring ventilation and is breathing unsupported via her tracheostomy with 35% humidified oxygen. She is due to be transferred to your ward.

- What additional equipment do you think you will need at Jan's bedside?
- In relation to this, what are the nursing implications of caring for someone with a temporary tracheostomy?
- What are the potential complications?

According to the Intensive Care Society (2008), when caring for a patient with a temporary tracheostomy it is important that nursing staff are familiar with and able to use the following additional equipment which should be immediately available:

- An operational suction unit (which should be checked at least daily) with suction tubing attached and a Yankeur sucker.
- Appropriately sized suction catheters.
- Non-powdered latex free gloves, aprons and eye protection.
- Spare tracheostomy tubes of the same type as inserted: one the same size and one a size smaller.
- Tracheal dilators.
- Rebreathing bag and tubing.
- Catheter mount or connection tracheostomy disconnection wedge.
- Tracheostomy tube holder and dressing.
- 10ml syringe (if tube cuffed).
- Artery forceps.
- Resuscitation equipment.

The potential complications of a temporary tracheostomy are listed below:

- Airway occlusion.
- Displaced tubes.
- Blocked tubes.
- Air leaks.
- Impaired cough.
- Surgical emphysema.
- Infection-wound/chest.
- Haemorrhage.
- Tracheal stenosis.
- Ulcerartion or tissue damage.
- Altered body image (Intensive Care Society, 2008).

Note: there are some differences in resuscitation approaches for individuals who have a temporary tracheostomy. If effective ventilation can be provided with a bag/valve then continual chest compressions should be carried out and ventilate the patient with approximately 10 breaths per minute.

If not then ask the following:

- Is the tube patent?
- Can a suction catheter be passed down?
- Can you change the inner cannula?
- Remove and cover stoma and ventilate via the patient's mouth (The Resuscitation Council, 2010).

Medical technology

Medical technology and devices are widely used in current healthcare settings and are likely to play a greater part in future nursing practice. The increased use of medical technology is evident in the treatment of a variety of patient groups and clinical settings. However, the use of medical technology can significantly increase overall healthcare costs and therefore effective use of this technology is essential. Moreover, whilst medical technology can be used to support and complement, it can never replace good nursing care.

ACTIVITY 11.8

- How many medical devices have you already used in clinical practice?
- Do you know how to use them safely?

Now access the MHRA (2014) checklist:
Medicines and Healthcare Products Regulatory Agency (MHRA) (2014) *Devices in Practice: Checklists for Using Medical Devices.* Available at http://www.mhra.gov.uk

- If there was an incident involving a patient in your care, based on your knowledge, understanding and documentation, could the care you provided be challenged? (e.g. How detailed or accurate is your documentation?)

Adult nurses are responsible for ensuring that all the medical devices/equipment they are likely to use are checked regularly to ensure that everything is in working order. You will also need to be aware of the potential pitfalls of using medical devices and the impact that these can have on patient safety. The Medicines and Healthcare Products Regulatory Agency (MHRA) is responsible for regulating all medicines and medical devices in the UK. Vincent et al. (2001) estimated that approximately 10% of patients in NHS hospitals experienced a patient safety incident, with about half of those considered preventable with ordinary standards of care. Most incidents that are reported to the Reporting and Learning System (RLS) relate to acute care. The issue of patient safety has been recognised as a priority for the NHS in documents such as *Building a Safer NHS for Patients* (Department of Health, 2001), *Seven Steps to Patient Safety* (NPSA, 2004) and *Safety First* (Department of Health, 2006).

Patient safety is the responsibility of all health professionals (Rylance, 2014). It is important to understand potential threats to patient safety and nurses need to be aware of the potential problems if they are to improve. This responsibility applies equally to near-misses as to actual incidents. If a near-miss happened to you or your patient it could happen to others. By reporting a near-miss you have the potential to prevent an incident from happening to others.

Legal and ethical considerations in acute care

Nurses working in acute care environments may be faced with a number of situations or decisions that have ethical or legal considerations. The nurse must approach these situations with due care and deliberation.

Consent

Consent should be obtained prior to any examination, treatment or care provided to a patient. 'Consent' is the patient's agreement or permission for the examination, treatment or care to occur. It is based on the fundamental principle of autonomy, whereby the patient has the right to choose what happens to their own body.

The Department of Health (2009b: 9) guidance on consent considers that 'For consent to be valid, it must be given voluntarily by an appropriately informed person who has capacity to consent to the intervention in question (this will be the patient or someone with parental responsibility for a patient under the age of 18, someone authorised to do so under a Lasting Power of Attorney (LPA) or someone who has the authority to make treatment decisions as a court appointed deputy'. Considering this statement, three key questions need to be considered:

- Does the person have capacity?
- Is the consent given voluntarily?
- Has the person received sufficient information?

Each of these elements will now be considered.

Does the person have capacity?

The assessment of a person's capacity to give or withhold consent is considered in rela-tion to a specific decision. While the individual may not have capacity to make some decisions they may still retain capacity for other decisions. For example a patient may not have capacity to make a decision regarding a surgical procedure but could retain capacity to consent (or not) to having their clinical observations (e.g. blood pressure) checked.

The *Mental Capacity Act* (2005) provides guidance on the issue of capacity and has five key principles:

1. Every adult has the right to make his or her own decisions and must be assumed to have capacity to make them unless it is proved otherwise.
2. A person must be given all practicable help before anyone treats them as not being able to make their own decisions.

3. Just because an individual makes what might be seen as an unwise decision, they should not be treated as lacking capacity to make that decision.
4. Anything done or any decision made on behalf of a person who lacks capacity must be done in their best interests.
5. Anything done for or on behalf of a person who lacks capacity should be the least restrictive of their basic rights and freedoms. (Office of the Public Guardian, 2014)

If the patient lacks capacity a decision may be made in the patient's best interests. The *Mental Capacity Act* 2005 Code of Practice (2007) provides guidance on how best to establish a patient's best interests. This will include trying to establish the patient's previous wishes and feelings and may involve consulting carers, family or friends.

Is the consent given voluntarily?

Consent should be obtained voluntarily without coercion. Healthcare providers can be considered to be in a position of power, while patients may be in a vulnerable or stressed state. Likewise family members can place undue pressure on a patient regarding decision making and this needs to be considered. Ideally, the patient should not feel pressurised into making a decision quickly, without having had adequate time to consider their options. The patient has the right to withdraw consent at any time.

Has the person received sufficient information?

Information should be provided to a patient in a way that they can readily understand. The use of highly technical or medical jargon should be avoided. Information should be balanced, outlining potential benefits and the risks along with potential alternatives (if any). The use of interpreting services should be considered when appropriate.

In the emergency situation consent should still be sought from competent patients, but if this is not possible (e.g. unconscious patient) care can be provided that is in the patient's best interests i.e. that which is lifesaving or aimed at preventing serious deterioration.

Case Scenario

 JACK

Jack is 65 he is in Type II respiratory failure and his condition is deteriorating. He has had a previous admission to the ICU and is refusing artificial ventilation. However some colleagues believe the patient to be delirious which is affecting his decision making.

What are your thoughts about this case in relation to the following:

- Complexity in care delivery.
- Complexity in care management.
- Complexity in ethical decision making.

Do you know the difference between Type I and Type II respiratory failure?

Jack has Type II respiratory failure which refers to poor carbon dioxide excretion from the lungs. Type I respiratory failure relates to low oxygen levels passing through the lungs into the bloodstream. Type I is referred to as *hypoxaemia* and Type II *hypercapnia* but patients can have both. Jack will require increased observation, and as noted earlier due to the potential for need of advanced respiratory support may need to be moved to a higher level of care. His wish not to be artificially ventilated may be due to impaired decision making as a result of his deteriorating respiratory function or may be due to his past ICU experience. This will need to be assessed carefully to establish if Jack does have the capacity to make an informed decision. The team will need to support and advocate for a patient in situations such as this and the involvement of family members is also key to ensuring treatment and care are in the best interests of the patient.

Delirium is a very common problem in the acute setting with Ryan et al. (2013) estimating that it may affect one in five of general hospital inpatients. It is defined by Maldonado (2008) as an acute change in cognition, inattention and a disturbance of consciousness. Delirium can develop over a short period of hours or days and fluctuate over time (Griffiths and Jones, 2007). NICE (2010) guidelines for delirium identify those at risk as:

- aged 65 years or older;
- having cognitive impairment (past or present) and/or dementia;
- having a current hip fracture;
- having a severe illness.

Additionally, Ely et al. (2001) noted that patients needing intensive care have a high probability of developing delirium due to multi-system illness, their co-morbidities, the use of psychoactive medications and age. Delirium is the most common neurological diagnosis amongst adult patient within the ICU (Guenther et al., 2012) and yet is often missed by staff. This is possibly due to each patient with delirium displaying different clinical symptoms. Patients can be restless, agitated and aggressive, possibly trying to remove a line and catheters, often referred to as *hyperactive* delirium (NICE, 2010). These patients are easily identified, however a group that are often missed are those patients experiencing *hypoactive* delirium. These patients become quiet, withdrawn and sleepy (NICE, 2010). It is vital that this patient group is adequately assessed, diagnosed and treated. A study carried out by Micek et al. (2005) explored the relationship with the assessment of delirium using the validated Confusion Assessment Method for ICU (CAM-ICU) and the use of physical restraint and continual sedation infusions. They found that patients experiencing delirium (as established by the CAM-ICU tool) were more likely to be physcially restrained and sedated. The CAM-ICU tool is one of the most common tools for identifying delirium in the ICU which can be used by nursing staff and has been found to be a valid and reliable measure (Krahne et al., 2005).

Decisions regarding CPR

Where do people die? While most people would prefer to die in their 'own home' (whether this be their own residence, a nursing home or old people's home), currently most people who die in the UK die in hospital. The National End of Life Care Intelligence Network (NEoLCIN) (2010) reported than in England 58% of the population die in hospital and only around 19% of people die in their own residence.

In acknowledging this there are issues regarding decision making at the end of life including those encompassing CPR, The British Medical Association (BMA), Resuscitation Council UK and the Royal College of Nursing (2014) *Decisions Relating to Cardiopulmonary Resuscitation* document provides some guidance. Some of the main points are as follows:

- 'Where no explicit decision about CPR has been considered and recorded in advance, there should be an initial presumption in favour of CPR'.
- 'Every decision about CPR must be made on the basis of a careful assessment of each individual's situation'.
- 'Clear and full documentation of decisions about CPR, the reasons for them, and the discussions that informed those decisions are an essential part of high-quality care'.
- 'Each decision about CPR should be subject to review based on the person's individual circumstances.'
- 'Any decision about CPR should be communicated clearly to all those involved in the patient's care'.
- 'A DNACPR (Do Not Attempt CPR) decision does not override clinical judgement in the unlikely event of a reversible cause of the person's respiratory or cardiac arrest that does not match the circumstances envisaged when that decision was made and recorded. Examples of such reversible causes include but are not restricted to: choking, a displaced tracheal tube or a blocked tracheostomy tube'.
- 'Making a decision not to attempt CPR that has no realistic prospect of success does not require the consent of the patient or of those close to the patient. However there is a presumption in favour of informing a patient of such a decision'.

ACTIVITY 11.9

1. Access the following website to read the above documents related to CPR: www.resus.org.uk/pages/DecisionsRelatingToCPR.pdf
2. Access and read the following British Psychological Society document: Joyce, T. (2007) *Best Interests Guidance on Determining the Best Interests of Adults who Lack the Capacity to Make a Decision (or Decisions) for Themselves (England and Wales)*. Leicester: The British Psychological Society.

STOP AND THINK

How could you use the guidance above to inform the decision-making process when considering Jack's 'best interests'?

Caring for a group of patients

A survey of nine European countries by Aiken et al. (2014) assessed the link between nurse staffing, training and patient mortality. While the main finding of the survey was that higher levels of nurse staffing and training were associated with lower patient mortality, it also revealed significant variations in nurse-to-patient staffing levels across Europe. The survey reported an average patient-to-nurse ratio of 8.8:1 (a 5.5–11.5 range). The National Institute for Health and Clinical Excellence (2014) has produced guidance for safe nurse staffing levels for adult inpatient wards in acute hospitals. While much of the guidance provides information relevant from an organisational perspective there are recommendations for nurses in charge of shifts to assess if the nursing staff available on the day are able to meet patients' nursing needs.

Aston et al. (2010: 108) identify a series of items that the nurse needs to consider when caring for a group of patients:

- How you utilise information that has been handed over to you by previous staff.
- Deciding if you need more information.
- Assessing or reassessing patients.
- Prioritising care.
- Planning care.
- Deciding what to delegate and who you can delegate to.
- How to manage time efficiently.
- How to respond to changes/incidents/issues that arise.
- Adapting your initial plans.

There are a number of factors to consider in prioritising care for a group of patients or indeed one patient. Time management and prioritising care are interlinked. While you should have a patient-centred approach to care and avoid considering patient care as simply 'tasks to be done', a 'to do list' can help you focus. Making a list can also make it easier to prioritise and delegate. This prioritisation can lead to a plan of care. As you are no doubt aware, it is important to acknowledge that this plan of care is devised in collaboration with the patient, as what the patient considers most important may vary from your perspective on what is important. **It is the individual and not the tasks that are the priority.** It is important that this plan of care is not considered a fixed or permanent schedule, as patient priorities can and do change.

In thinking about how to manage time effectively you should consider if there is the potential for multitasking. It is important that you use the best evidence available to support your decision making. Priority setting is based on assessment. The nurse needs to be flexible and able to adapt to changing priorities and demands. You should remember that you are providing care as part of a team and consider decision making as part of a team. Effective teamwork can impact on patient outcomes. A nurse needs to be able to work in a collaborative manner as part of a team to ensure patient safety.

Acute hospital care of the older person

While the UK population is ageing, it is those aged over 85 who are showing the fastest population increase (Office for National Statistics, 2012). Conroy and Cooper (2010) recognise that 'the acute clinical problems and needs of older patients are often substantially different from those of younger patients'. The Kings Fund (2014: 27) report, *Making Our Health and Care Systems fit for an Ageing Population*, emphasises that '.. acute hospital care must meet the needs of older patients with complex co-morbidities, frailty and dementia'. Acknowledging that almost 50% of the ICU population are over 65 years of age, McCormack (2014) stresses the importance of critical care nurses acknowledging their role as gerontological nurses.

The older adult may be considered at higher risk while in the acute setting. While the National Patient Safety Agency (2010) reports an average of 5.6 falls per 1,000 bed days in acute hospitals, over 80% of reported falls happened in those aged over 65 years, with those aged over 85 at highest risk.

The Alzheimer's Society (2009) report provides some interesting statistics:

- 97% of nursing staff and nurse managers reported that they always or sometimes care for someone with dementia.
- 47% of carer respondents said that being in hospital had a significant negative effect on the general physical health of the person with dementia, which wasn't a direct result of the medical condition.
- Over a third of people with dementia who go into hospital from living in their own homes are discharged to a care home setting.
- 77% of carer respondents were dissatisfied with the overall quality of dementia care provided.
- 89% of nursing staff respondents identified working with people with dementia as very or quite challenging.

The report also identified key areas of dissatisfaction identified by carer respondents: nurses not recognising or understanding dementia; a lack of person-centred care; not being helped to eat and drink; a lack of opportunity for social interaction; not as much involvement in decision making as wished for (for both the person with dementia and carer); and the person with dementia being treated with a lack of dignity and respect. Key areas of concern as identified by nursing staff respondents were: managing difficult/unpredictable behaviour; communicating; not having enough time to spend with patients and provide one-to-one care; wandering/keeping people on the ward; and ensuring patient safety.

Bridges et al. (2010) warn that 'older patients in hospital may feel worthless, fearful or not in control of what happens, especially if they have impaired cognition or communication difficulties'. The Royal College of Nursing (2011) provides five principles to supporting good dementia care in the hospital setting:

1. Staff who are skilled and have time to care.
2. Partnership working with carers.
3. Assessment and early identification.
4. Care that is individualised.
5. Environments that are dementia friendly.

Supporting the families of acutely ill patients

When a person is acutely unwell the psychological distress within family members is an inherent factor that a nurse needs to be mindful of and they should do their utmost to provide appropriate support. Informing an individual that their loved one has become acutely unwell and is possibly moving to a department such as an ICU can result in a number of different responses and behaviours. The ability to calm feelings of panic and distress felt by patients, family and friends is an important aspect of care that cannot be overlooked, and will place significant demands upon your communication skills and ability to demonstrate empathy, compassion and understanding. For example, the society we currently live in is diverse and as a nurse you will encounter very different types of 'family'. In fact, due to this the term 'significant other' is often used. A lot of high care areas such as ICUs have very strict visiting rules related to family only, and yet as adults we have significant others who may want to visit and offer support to the acutely unwell person. These restrictions can put increased strain on an already stressed individual trying to visit. Additionally, families may be left waiting whilst interventions are carried out, such as a line insertion or x-rays. Nursing staff must remain vigilant in updating families and visitors about the reasons why they have been asked to wait.

The families of those admitted to an ICU are often in a highly anxious state and are also confronted with a highly technical environment with their loved one at the centre attached to a myriad of different devices: therefore it is vital they are adequately supported. Families can also provide a crucial contribution to the person's care. Many patients following acute illness requiring an ICU stay have problems recalling elements of their illness and care; families can provide this insight into the experience (Paule and Rattey, 2008). More importantly families can provide reassurance and support. A study conducted by Kean and Mitchell (2013), which explored how ICU nurses perceived families, found that families made a notable contribution to patient care, however the nursing staff felt they needed to remain in control of that involvement.

- What factors would influence your decision to limit visiting to close family members?
- Reflect on the placements you have already experienced: what sort of reception do families and visitors get?
- How do you feel about families witnessing resuscitation? Find out what the policy is in your placement area in relation to families witnessing resuscitation.

You may want to read the guidance from the Resuscitation Council UK at www.resus.org.uk

STOP AND THINK

ACTIVITY 11.10

Access and read the Intensive Care Society's (1998) *Guidelines for Bereavement Care in Intensive Care Units.*

Enhancing the patient experience

Within the NHS there has been some progression in the way that the 'quality' of the care being provided is assessed. While traditional measures looking at clinical effectiveness (e.g. Standardised Mortality Ratios) and safety have unquestionable significance, the importance of the patient experience is now recognised.

A number of studies have explored the link between an ICU admission and the occurrence of Post-Traumatic Stress Disorder (PTSD) and have noted a link between the risk of developing PTSD and the acuity of illness, the pharmacological agent used, co-morbities, age and psychological problems pre-admission (Scragg et al., 2001; Cuthbertson et al., 2004; Jones et al., 2007; Girard et al., 2007). Those patients experiencing PTSD following ICU re-experience their ordeal in the form of flashbacks. It is possible that there are adverse effects on a person's emotional well-being long after they are discharged from the ICU, and patients and their families may need to be aware of this as many patients leave with some physical changes which may initially be the focus of their recovery.

The National Institute for Health and Care Excellence (2012a, 2012b) has produced clinical guidance and a set of quality standards on improving the experience of care for people using adult NHS services. These documents contain some key themes, including providing an individualised service, family and carer involvement, getting the basics right and clear communication.

STOP AND THINK

- As an adult nurse working in a critical/intensive care setting, what could you do to try to enhance the experience of the patients you care for?

ACTIVITY   11.11

Access and review the following NICE guidelines: NICE (2009) 'Rehabilitation after critical illness' (CG83). Manchester: NICE.
Make a note of all of the areas where you as an adult nurse could positively influence the patient experience.

There has been significant improvement in the immediate follow-up of ICU patients with the development of outreach or follow-up teams which include a clinical psychology input. There has also been a move towards maintaining patient diaries to aid recall and document the patient journey through an ICU when their awareness was impeded. Completing diaries for ICU patients has been developed and researched in many Scandinavian countries, however uptake of this method across UK ICUs has been slow, with increased workload often cited as a barrier to implementation.

Summary

Nurses have a central role in ensuring safe patient care. This chapter has discussed the knowledge, skills and attributes needed by adult nurses working in an acute care setting. We have also focused upon the knowledge and skills needed in the assessment and recognition of the acutely ill adult. The signs of clinical deterioration can happen many hours before a cardiac arrest. Early detection of patient deterioration gives an opportunity to improve patient outcomes by providing timely and appropriate care. National Early Warning Scores are a valuable tool in achieving this, but it is important to remember that if you are concerned about a patient's safety and are not sure what to do you should call for help. A comprehensive assessment using the ABCDE approach and use of the SBAR communication tool can help you in these situations.

Medical technology is part of the modern healthcare environment and is not limited to critical care areas. While the 'technical' aspects of nursing may be appealing to nurses working in acute care, these cannot and must not be promoted at the expense of providing compassionate nursing care. A nurse should use appropriate technology for the benefit of patients but also be aware of the potential of over-reliance. For example, a nurse should not have to rely on pulse oximetry to be able to identify that a patient with an increased respiratory rate, who is cyanotic, using accessory muscles and unable to talk in complete sentences with an audible wheeze, is unwell.

The profile of patients in the acute care setting and the way that care is provided are changing. Patients who have a greater level of acuity tend to be older and have more co-morbidity. Acute care environments need to adapt to these changes. It is important to remember that the acute care environment can be a scary place for patients and their families.

Suggested further reading

Bickley, L.S. (2013) *Bates' Guide to Physical Examination and History Taking*, 11th edition. Philadelphia: Lippincott, Williams & Wilkins.

British Geriatric Society (2012) *Quality Care for Older People with Urgent Care Needs* (The 'Silver Book'). Available at: www.bgs.org.uk/index.php/bgscampaigns-715/silverbook (last accessed 18 March 2015).

Brooker, C. and Nichol, M. (2011) *Alexander's Nursing Practice*, 4th edition. London: Churchill Livingstone.

O'Driscoll, B.R., Howard, L.S. and Davison, A.G. on behalf of the British Thoracic Society (2008) 'Guideline for the emergency oxygen use in adult patients', *Thorax*, 63, Supp VI.

Page, K. and McKinney, A. (2012) *Nursing The Acutely Ill Adult*. London: Sage.

Resuscitation Council UK (2011) *Immediate Life Support Manual*, 3rd edition. London: Resucitation Council.

References

Abbey, J.A., Piller, N., DeBellis, A., Esterman, A., Parker, D., Giles, L. and Lowcay, B. (2004) 'The Abbey Pain Scale. a 1-minute numerical indicator for people with late-stage dementia', *International Journal of Palliative Nursing*, 10(1): 6–13.

Aiken, L., Sloane, D., Bruyneel, L., Van de Heede, K., et al. for the RN4CAST Consortium (2014) 'Nurse staffing and education and hospital mortality in nine European countries: a retrospective observational study', *The Lancet*, 383(9931): 1824–30.

Alzheimers Society (2009) *Counting the Cost: Caring for People with Dementia on Hospital Wards*. London: Alzheimers Society.

Aning, J., Neal, D., Driver, A. and McGrath, J. (2010) 'Enhanced recovery: from principles to practice in urology', *BJU Int*; 105 (9): 1199–201.

Ansell, H., Meyer, A. and Thompson, S. (2014) 'Why don't nurses consistently take patient respiratory rates?', *British Journal of Nursing*, 23(8): 414–18.

Appleby, J. (2013) 'Are accident and emergency attendance increasing?' The King's Fund Blog. Available at: www.kingsfund.org.uk/blog/2013/04/are-accident-and-emergency-attendances-increasing (last accessed 17 October 2014).

Aston, L., Wakefield, J. and McGown, R. (eds) (2010) *The Student Nurse Guide to Decision Making in Practice*. Maidenhead: Open University Press.

Australian and New Zealand College of Anaesthetists (2010) *Acute Pain Management: Scientific Evidence*, 3rd edition. Melbourne: Australian and New Zealand College of Anaesthetists.

Baillie, L. (2009) 'Patient dignity in an acute hospital setting: a case study', *International Journal of Nursing Studies*, 46 (1): 23–37.

Ball, C., Kirby, M. and Williams, S. (2003) 'Effect of the critical care outreach team on survival to discharge from hospital and readmission to critical care: non-randomised population based study', *British Medical Journal*, 327: 1014.

Beliveau, E. (2012) Cited in Buttaro, T.M. and Barba, K.M. (eds) *Nursing Care of the Hospitalized Older Patient*. Oxford: Wiley-Blackwell.

Bond, M.R. and Simpson, K.H. (2006) *Pain: Its Nature and Treatment*. Edinburgh: Churchill Livingstone.

Bridges, J., Flatley, M. and Meyer, J. (2010) 'Older people's and relatives' experiences in acute care settings: systematic review and synthesis of qualitative studies', *International Journal of Nursing Studies*, 47: 89–107.

British Medical Association, the Resuscitation Council UK and the Royal College of Nursing (2014) *Decisions Relating to Cardiopulmonary Resuscitation*, 3rd edition. Guidance from the British Medical Association, the Resuscitation Council UK and the Royal College of Nursing (previously known as the 'Joint Statement'). Available at: http://resus.org.uk/pages/dnacpr.htm (last accessed 17 October 2014).

British Thoracic Society (2008) 'Guideline for the emergency oxygen use in adult patients', *Thorax,* 63: Supp VI.

Brunker, C. (2010) 'A brief history of resuscitation and beyond: as easy as ABCDE', *British Journal of Neuroscience Nursing*, 6(5): 232–5.

Buist, M., Bernard, S., Nguyen, T., Moore, G. and Anderson, J. (2004) 'Association between clinically abnormal observations and subsequent in-hospital mortality: a prospective study', *Resuscitation,* 62: 137–41.

Conroy, S. and Cooper, N. (2010) *Acute Medical Care of Elderly People*. British Geriatric Society. Available at: www.bgs.org.uk/index.php/topresources/publicationfind/goodpractice (last accessed 18 March 2015).

Coulter-Smith, M.A., Smith, P. and Crow, R. (2013) 'Critical review: a combined conceptual framework of severity of illness and clinical judgement for analysing diagnostic judgement in critical illness', *Journal of Clinical Nursing*, 23: 784–98.

Cuthberson, B.H., Hull, A., Stachen, M. and Scott, J. (2004) 'Post Traumatic Stress Disorder after critical illness requiring General Intensive Care', *Intensive Care Medicine*, 30 (4): 450–5.

Dellinger, R., Levy, M. et al. and the Surviving Sepsis Campaign Committee including the Pediatric Subgroup (2013) 'Surviving Sepsis Campaign: international guidelines for the management of severe sepsis and septic shock: 2012', *Critical Care Medicine*, 41(2): 580–637.

DeMeester, K., Verspuy, M., Monsieurs, K.G. and Van Bogaert, P. (2013) 'SBAR improves nurse-physician communication and reduces unexpected death: a pre and post intervention study', *Resuscitation,* 84: 1192–6.

Department of Health (2000) *Comprehensive Critical Care: A Review of Adult Critical Care Services*. Available at: http://webarchive.nationalarchives.gov.uk/20130107105354/http://www.dh.gov.uk/prod_consum_dh/groups/dh_digitalassets/@dh/@en/documents/digitalasset/dh_4082872.pdf (last accessed 17 October 2014).

Department of Health (2001) *Building a Safer NHS for Patients: Improving Medication Safety*. London: DH.

Department of Health (2006) *Safety First: A Report for Patients, Clinicians and Healthcare Managers*. London: DH.

Department of Health (2009a) *Competencies for Recognising and Responding to Acutely Ill Patients in Hospital*. Leeds: DH.

Department of Health (2009b) *Reference Guide to Consent for Examination or Treatment*, 2nd edition. London: DH.

Department of Health (2013) *The Mid Staffordshire NHS Foundation Trust*. Public inquiry chaired by Robert Francis QC (The Francis Report). London: The Stationery Office.

Diabetes UK (2013) *Inpatient Care for People with Diabetes*. Available at: www.diabetes.org.uk/About_us/What-we-say/Improving-diabetes-healthcare/Inpatients-care-for-people-with-diabetes/ (last accessed 17 October 2014).

Doherty, M., Hawkey, C., Goulder, M., et al. (2011) 'A randomised controlled trial of ibuprofen, paracetamol or a combination tablet of ibuprofen/paracetamol in community-derived people with knee pain', *Ann Rheum Dis*, 70: 1534–41.

Dombrowski, S.U., Mackintosh, J., Sniehotta, F., Arajo-Soares, V., Rodgers, H., Thomson, R., Murtagh, M., Ford, G., Eccles, M. and White, M. (2013) 'The impact of the UK "Act FAST" stroke awareness campaign: content analysis of patients, witness and primary care clinicians' perceptions', *BMC Public Health*, 13: 915.

Donohue, L.A and Endacott, R. (2010) 'Track, trigger and teamwork: communication of deterioration in acute medical and surgical wards', *Intensive Crit Care Nurs.*, 26 (1):10–7.

Dowdy, D., Eid, M., Sedrakyan, A., Mendez-Tellez, P., Pronovist, P., Herridge, M. and Needham, D. (2005) 'Quality of life in adult survivors of critical illness: a systematic review of the literature', *Intensive Care Medicine*, (32): 1115–24

Dwyer, A.J., Thomas, W., Humphry, S. and Porter, P. (2014) 'Enhanced recovery programme for total knee replacement to reduce the length of hospital stay', *J Orthop Surg (Hong Kong)*, 22 (2): 150–4.

Elliott , M and Coventry, A (2012) 'Critical Care: The eight vital signs of patient monitoring', *British Journal of Nursing*, 21 (10), 621–5

Ely, E.W., Inouye, S.K., Bernard, G.R., Francis, J., May, L., Truman, B., Speroff, T., Gautam, S., Margolin, R., Hart, R.P. and Dittus, R. (2001) 'Delirium in mechanically ventilated patients: validity and reliability of the Confusion Assessment Method for the Intensive Care Unit (CAM-ICU)', *Journal of the American Medical Association*, 286: 2703–10.

Enhanced Recovery Partnership Programme (2010) *Delivering Enhanced Recovery: Helping Patients to Get Better Sooner After Surgery*. Available at: http://webarchive.nationalarchives.gov.uk/20130107105354/http://www.dh.gov.uk/prod_consum_dh/groups/dh_digitalassets/@dh/@en/@ps/documents/digitalasset/dh_115156.pdf (last accessed 17 October 2014).

Freeman, S. (2011) 'Care of adult patients with a temporary tracheostomy', *Nursing Standard*, 26 (2): 49–56.

Frost, P. and Wise, M. (2012) 'Early management of acutely ill ward patients', *British Medical Journal*, 345.

Gelmas, C., Fillian, L., Puntillo, K., Viens, and Fortier, M. (2006) 'Validation of a critical care pain observational tool in adults', *American Journal of Critical Care*, 15 (4): 421.

Girard, T.D., Shintani, A.K. and Jackson, J.C. (2007) 'Risk factors for post-traumatic stress disorder symptoms following critical illness requiring mechanical ventilation', *Critical Care Medicine*, 11: R28.

Godfrey, H. (2005) 'Understanding pain part 1: pain management', *British Journal of Nursing*, 14 (17): 846–52.

Gregory, J. (2008) 'Using nitrous oxide and oxygen to control pain in primary care', *Nursing Times*, 104(37): 24–6.

Gregory, J. (2014) 'Dealing with acute and chronic pain: part one – assessment', *Journal of Community Nursing*, 28(5): 83–6 .

Griffiths, R.D. and Jones, C. (2007) 'Deliriums, cognitive dysfunction and Posttraumatic Stress Disorder', *Current Opinion in Anaesthesiology*, 20 (2): 124–9.

Grissinger, M. (2010) 'Reducing errors with injectable medications', *Pharmacy and Therapeutics*, 35(8): 428–51.

Guenther, U., Weykam, J., Andorfer, U., Theuerkauf, N., Poop, J., Ely, W. and Putensen, C. (2012) 'Implications of objective vs subjective delirium assessment in surgical intensive care patients', *American Journal of Critical Care*, 21(1): 12–20.

Hanson, R.M. (2014) 'Is elderly care affected by nurse attitudes? A systematic review', *British Journal of Nursing*, 23(4): 225–9.

Hawthorn, J. and Redmond, K. (1998) *Pain: Causes and Management*. Oxford: Blackwell Sciences Ltd.

Health and Social Care Information Centre (2013) *Hospital Episode Statistics: Admitted Patient Care 2012–13*. Available at: www.hscic.gov.uk (last accessed 16 October 2014).

Health and Social Care Information Centre (2014) *Accident and Emergency Department Types*. Available at: www.datadictionary.nhs.uk/data_dictionary/attributes/a/acc/accident_and_emergency_department_type_de.asp?shownav=1 (last accessed 17 October 2014).

Health Foundation (2013) *Patient Safety*. Available at: www.health.org.uk/areas-of-work/topics/patient-safety/patient-safety/ (last accessed 17 October 2014).

Higginson, R., Jones, B. and Davies, K. (2011) 'Emergency and intensive care: assessing and managing the airway', *British Journal of Nursing*, 20(16): 973–7.

Ibrahim, M.S., Alazzawi, S., Nizam, I. and Haddad, F.S. (2013) 'An evidence-based review of enhanced recovery interventions in knee replacement surgery', *Ann R Coll Surg Engl.* 95 (6): 386–9.

Intensive Care Society (2008) *Standards for the Care of Adult Patients with a Temporary Tracheostomy*. London: The Intensive Care Society.

Intensive Care Society (2009) *Levels of Critical Care for Adult Patients. Standards and Guidelines*. London: The Intensive Care Society.

Jones, C., Backman, C., Capuzzo, M., Flaatten, C., Rylander, R. and Griffiths, D. (2007) 'Precipitation of Post-Traumatic Stress Disorder following intensive care: a hypothesis generating study of diversity in care', *Intensive Care Medicine*, 33 (6): 978–85.

Kavanagh, S., Cambell, J. and Rudd, A. (2011) 'Impact of the FAST campaign', *British Journal of Neuroscience Nursing*, 7 (5): 626.

Kean, S. (2014) 'How do intensive care nurses perceive families in intensive care? Insights from the United Kingdom and Australia', *Journal of Clinical Nursing*, 23 (5–6): 663–72.

Kean, S. and Mitchell, M. (2014) 'How do ICU nurses perceive families in intensive care? Insights from the United Kingdom and Australia', *Journal of Clinical Nursing*, 23(5–6): 633–672.

Keogh, B. (2013) *Review into the Quality of Care and Treatment Provided by 14 Hospital Trusts in England: Overview Report*. Available at: www.nhs.uk/NHSEngland/bruce-keogh-review/Documents/outcomes/keogh-review-final-report.pdf (last accessed 17 October 2014).

Krahne, D., Heymann, A. and Spies, C. (2006) 'How to monitor delirium in the ICU and why it is important', *Clinical Effectiveness in Nursing*, 269–79.

Leonard, M., Graham, S. and Bonacum, S. (2004) 'The human factor: the critical importance of effective teamwork and communication in providing safe care', *Qual Saf Healthcare*, 13 Supp.

Lewin, J. and Maconochie, I. (2008) 'Capillary refill time in adults', *Emerg Med J.*, 25: 325–6.

Mackway-Jones, K., Marsden, J. and Windle, J. (2013) *Emergency Triage: Manchester Triage Group*, 3rd edition. Chichester: Wiley.

Maldonado, J.R. (2008) 'Delirium in the Acute Care setting: characteristics, diagnosis and treatment', *Critical Care Clinics*, 24: 657–722.

Massey, D., Aitken, L.M. and Chaboyer, W. (2010) 'Literature review: do rapid response systems reduce the incidence of major adverse events in the deteriorating ward patient?', *Journal of Clinical Nursing*, 19: 3260–73.

McCaffery, P. and Pasero, C. (1999) *PAIN: Clinical Manual*, 2nd edn. St Louis: Mosby.

McCormack, B. (2014) 'Critical care nursing and the older people – is there an issue?', *Nursing in Critical Care*, 19(4): 164–5.

McFarland, J., Tighe, S., O'Sullivan, K., Trzepacz, P., Meagher, D. and Timmons, S. (2013) 'Delirium in an adult acute hospital population: predictors, prevalence and detection', *BMJ Open*, 3: e001772.doi:10.1136/bmjopen-2012-001772

McGauhey, J., Alderdice, F., Fowler, R., Kapila, A., Mayhew, A. and Moutray, M. (2007) 'Outreach and early warning systems (EWS) for the prevention of intensive care admission and death of critically ill adult patients on general wards', *Cochrane Database of Systematic Reviews 2007,* Issue 3, Art. No.: CD005529. doi: 10.1002/14651858.CD005529.pub2.

McMullen, S.M. and Patrick, W. (2013) 'Cyanosis', *American Journal of Medicine,* 126(3): 210–212.

McMullen, S. and Ward, P. (2013) 'Cyanosis', *The American Journal of Medicine,* 126 (10): 211–12.

McQuay, H. and Moore, A. (1998) *An Evidence- based Resource for Pain Relief.* Oxford: Oxford University Press.

Medicines and Healthcare Products Regulatory Agency (MHRA) (2014) *Devices in Practice. Checklists for Using Medical Devices.* Available at: www.mhra.gov.uk/home/groups/dts-bs/documents/publication/con007424.pdf (last accessed 17 October 2014).

Melotti, R.M., Samolsky-Dekel, B.G., Ricchi, E., et al. (2005) 'Pain prevalence and predictors among inpatients in a major Italian teaching hospital. A baseline survey towards a pain free hospital', *European Journal of Pain,* 9(5):485–95.

Micek, S.T., Anand, N.J., Laible, B.R., Shannon, W.D. and Kollef, M.H. (2005) 'Delirium as detected by the CAM-ICU predicts restraint use among mechanically ventilated medical patients', *Critical Care Medicine,* 33 (6): 1260–65.

Mohan, H., Ryan, J., Whelan, B. and Wakai, A. (2013) 'The end of the line? The Visual Analogue Scale and Verbal Numerical Rating Scale as pain assessment tools in the emergency department', *Emergency Medicine* 27: 372–75.

Moore, T. (2007) 'Respiratory assessment in adults', *Nursing Standard,* 21 (49): 48–56.

National Audit Office (2012) *Healthcare Across the UK: A Comparison of the NHS in England, Scotland, Wales and Northern Ireland.* Available at: www.nao.org.uk/wp-content/uploads/2012/06/1213192.pdf (last accessed 17 October 2014).

National Audit Office (2013) *Emergency Admissions to Hospital: Managing the Demand,* HC 739 Session 2013–14 31 October. London: NAO.

National Confidential Enquiry into Patient Outcome and Death (NCEPOD)(1999) *Extremes of Age.* Available at: www.ncepod.org.uk/1999ea.htm (last accessed 17 October 2014).

National Confidential Enquiry into Patient Outcome and Death (NCEPOD) (2005) *An Acute Problem?* Available at: www.ncepod.org.uk/2005report/summary.pdf (last accessed 17 October 2014).

National Diabetes Inpatient Audit (2013) *National Diabetes Inpatient Audit. National Summary.* Available at: www.hscic.gov.uk/catalogue/PUB13662/nati-diab-inp-audi-13-nat-rep.pdf (last accessed 17 October 2014).

National End of Life Care Intelligence Network (NEoLCIN) (2010) *Variations in Place of Death in England: Inequalities or Appropriate Consequences of Age, Gender and Cause of Death.* Available at: www.endoflifecare-intelligence.org.uk/home (last accessed 17 October 2014).

National Institute for Health and Clinical Excellence (2007) *Acutely Ill Patients in Hospital: Recognition of and Response to Acute Illness in Adults in Hospital, NICE Clinical Guideline 50.* London: NICE.

National Institute for Health and Clinical Excellence (2009) *Rehabilitation after Critical Illness. NICE Clinical Guideline 83.* London: NICE.

National Institute for Health and Clinical Excellence (2010) *Delirium: Diagnosis, Prevention and Management.* London: NICE.

National Institute for Health and Clinical Excellence (2011) *Diabetes in Adults. Quality Standard (QS6).* London: NICE.

National Institute for Health and Care Excellence (2012a) *Patient Experience in Adult NHS Services: Improving the Experience of Care for People using Adult NHS Services. NICE Clinical Guidance 138.* London: NICE.

National Institute for Health and Care Excellence (2012b) *Quality Standard for Patient Experience in Adult NHS Services. NICE Quality Standards* (QS15). London: NICE.

National Institute for Health and Care Excellence (2013) *Acute Kidney Injury: Prevention, Detection and Management of Acute Kidney Injury Up to the Point of Renal Replacement.* NICE Clinical Guideline 169. London: NICE.

National Outreach Forum (2012) *Operational Standards and Competencies for Critical Care Outreach Services.* Available at: www.norf.org.uk/ (last accessed 2 December 2014).

National Patient Safety Agency (2004) *Seven Steps to Patient Safety.* Available at: www.nrls.npsa.nhs.uk/resources/collections/seven-steps-to-patient-safety/ (last accessed 17 October 2014).

National Patient Safety Agency (2007a) *Recognising and Responding Appropriately to Early Signs of Deterioration in Hospitalised Patients.* London: NHS/NPSA.

National Patient Safety Agency (2007b) *Patient Safety Alert: Promoting Safer Use of Injectable Medicines.* Available at: www.nrls.npsa.nhs.uk/resources/?entryid45=59812 (last accessed 17 October 2014).

National Patient Safety Agency (2009) *Rapid Response Report: Oxygen Safety in Hospitals.* Available at: www.nrls.npsa.nhs.uk/resources/type/alerts/?entryid45=62811&p=2 (last accessed 17 October 2014).

National Patient Safety Agency (2010) *Slips, Trips and Falls Data Update June 2010.* Available at: www.nrls.npsa.nhs.uk/resources/patient-safety-topics/patient-accidents-falls/ (last accessed 17 October 2014).

NHS England (2014) *A&E Annual Activity Statistics, NHS and Independent Sector Organisations in England.* Available at: www.england.nhs.uk/statistics/statistical-work-areas/ae-waiting-times-and-activity/weekly-ae-sitreps-2014-15/ (last accessed 17 October 2014).

NHS Improving Quality (2013) *Enhanced Recovery Care Pathway: A Better Journey for Patients Seven Days a Week and a Better Deal for the NHS.* Progress review (2012/2013) and level of ambition (2014/2015). London: NHS.

NHS Institute for Innovation and Improvement (2008) *Enhanced Recovery Programme.* Available at: www.institute.nhs.uk/quality_and_service_improvement_tools/quality_and_service_improvement_tools/enhanced_recovery_programme.html (last accessed 2 December 2014).

NHS Modernisation Agency (2004) *10 High Impact Changes for Service Improvement and Delivery: A Guide for NHS Leaders.* Available at: www.nursingleadership.org.uk/publications/HIC.pdf (last accessed 17 October 2014).

NMC (2010a) *Standards for Pre-registration Nursing Education.* Available at: http://standards.nmc-uk.org (last accessed 19 November 2014).

NMC (2010b) *Standards for Competence for Registered Nurses.* Available at: www.nmc-uk.org/Documents/Standards/Standards%20for%20competence.pdf. (last accessed 19 November 2014).

Nolan, J., Soar, J., Smith, G., Gwinnutt, C., Parrott, F., Power, S., Harrison, D., Nixon, E. and Rowan, K. on behalf of the National Cardiac Arrest Audit (2014) 'Incidence and outcome of in-hospital cardiac arrest in the United Kingdom National Cardiac Arrest', *Resuscitation,* 85: 987–92.

Office for National Statistics (2012) *Population Ageing in the United Kingdom, its Constituent Countries and the European Union.* Available at: www.ons.gov.uk/ons/rel/mortality-ageing/focus-on-older-people/population-ageing-in-the-united-kingdom-and-europe/rpt-age-uk-eu.html (last accessed 17 October 2014).

Office of the Public Guardian (2014) *How to Make Decisions under the Mental Capacity Act 2005.* Available at: www.gov.uk/government/collections/mental-capacity-act-making-decisions (last accessed 10 March 2015).

O'Driscoll, B.R., Howard, L.S. and Davison, A.G. on behalf of the British Thoracic Society (2008) 'BTS guideline for emergency oxygen use in adult patients', *Thorax,* 63: Supp VI.

Olson, K. (2014) *Oxford Handbook of Cardiac Nursing,* 2nd edition. Oxford: Oxford University Press.

Organisation for Economic Co-operation and Development (OECD) *Health Data 2001: A Comparative Analysis of 30 Countries, OECD, Paris, 2001, Data Sources, Definitions and Methods.* Available at: http://stats.oecd.org/glossary/detail.asp?ID=4 (last accessed 17 October 2014).

Pattison, N. and Eastham, E. (2011) 'Critical care outreach referrals: a mixed-method investigative study of outcomes and experiences', *Nursing in Critical Care*, 17(2): 71–82.

Paul, F. and Rattey, J. (2008) 'Short and long term impact of critical illness on relatives: literature review', *Journal of Advanced Nursing*, 62: 276–92.

Peate, I. (2013) *The Student Nurse Toolkit: An Essential Guide for Surviving Your Course.* Chichester: Wiley-Blackwell.

Public Health England (2012) *Act FAST*. Available at:http://campaigns.dh.gov.uk/category/act-fast/ (last accessed 27 January 2015).

Public Health England (2014) *Act FAST* TV Campaign. Available at:http://www.gov.uk/government/news/act-fast-campaign/ (last accessed 17 January 2015).

Resuscitation Council UK (2011) *Immediate Life Support Manual*, 3rd edition. London: Resuscitation Council UK.

Robson, W. and Daniels, R. (2013) 'Diagnosis and management of sepsis in adults', *Nurse Prescribing*, 11(2): 76–82.

Royal College of Nursing (2011) *Dementia: Commitment to the Care of People with Dementia in Hospital Settings*. Available at: www.rcn.org.uk/development/practice/dementia/commitment_to_the_care_of_people_with_dementia_in_general_hospitals (last accessed 2 December 2014).

Royal College of Physicians (2007) *Acute Medical Care: The Right Person, in the Right Setting, First Time*. Available at: www.rcplondon.ac.uk/sites/default/files/documents/acute_medical_care_final_for_web.pdf (last accessed 17 October 2014).

Royal College of Physicians (2012) *National Early Warning Score (NEWS): Standardising the Assessment of Acute-illness Severity in the NHS*. Available at: www.rcplondon.ac.uk/sites/default/files/documents/national-early-warning-score-standardising-assessment-acute-illness-severity-nhs.pdf (last accessed 17 October 2014).

Ruder, S. (2010) '7 tools to assist hospice and home care clinicians in pain management at end of life', *Home Healthcare Nurse*, 28 (8): 458–68.

Ryan, D.J., O'Regan, N.A., o Caoimh, R., Clare, J., O'Connor, M., Leonard, M., (2012) 'Delirium in an adult acute hospital population: predictors, prevalence and detection', *British Medical Journal Open*, 2:e001772.

Rylance, P.B. (2014) 'Improving patient safety and avoiding incidents in renal units', *Journal of Renal Nursing*, 6 (1): 24–8.

Sandberg, M., Nakstad, A., Berlac, P., Hyldmo, P.K. and Boylan, M. (2013) 'Airway assessment and management'. In T. Nutbeam and M. Boylan (eds), *ABC of Prehospital Emergency Medicine*. London: BMJ.

Sawyer, J., Haslem, L., Daines, P. and Stilo, K. (2010) 'Pain prevalence study in a large teaching hospital in Canada. Round 2: lessons learnt?', *Pain Management Nursing*, 11 (1): 45–55.

Scales, K. (2008) Intravenous therapy: a guide to good practice, *British Journal of Nursing*, 17 (19) Supp.

Scales, K. (2014) 'IV fluid therapy', *Nursing Standard*, 28(23): 19.

Schein, R.M., Hazday, N., Pena, M., Ruben, B.H. and Sprung, C.L. (1990) 'Clinical antecedents to in-hospital cardiopulmonary arrest', *Chest*, 98 (6): 1388–92.

Schofield, P. and Dunham, M. (2003) 'Pain assessment: how far have we come in listening to our patients?', *Professional Nurse*, 18 (5): 276–9.

Scott, I., Vaughan, L. and Bell, D. (2009) 'Effectiveness of acute medical units in hospitals: a systematic review', *International Journal for Quality in Healthcare*, 21(6): 397–407.

Scottish Intercollegiate Guidelines Network (SIGN) (2014) *Care of Deteriorating Patients*. Available at: www.sign.ac.uk/guidelines/fulltext/139/index.html (last accessed 17 October 2014).

Scragg, P., Jones, A. and Fauvel, N. (2001) 'Physiological problems following ICU treatment', *Anaesthesia*, 56 (9): 9–14.

Sepsis Trust (2012) *The Sepsis Six*. Available at: http://survivesepsis.org/the-sepsis-six/ (last accessed 2 December 2014).

Shahin, J., Harrison, D. and Rowan, K. (2012) 'Relation between volume and outcome for patients with severe sepsis in United Kingdom: retrospective cohort study', *British Medical Journal*, 344: e3394.

Strong, J., Unruh, A.M., Wright, A. and Baxter, D.G. (2002) *Pain: A Textbook for Therapists*. Edinburgh: Churchill Livingstone.

Teasdale, G. and Jennett, B. (1974) 'Assessment of coma and impaired consciousness: a practical guide', *The Lancet*, 304 (7872): 81–4.

The King's Fund (2014) *Making Our Helath and Care System Fit for an Ageing Population*. Available at: www.kingsfund.org.uk/publications/making-our-health-and-care-systems-fit-ageing-population (last accessed 2 December 2014).

Thim, T., Krarup, T., Grove, E., Rohde, C. and Lofgren, B. (2012) 'Initial assessment and treatment with the Airway, Breathing, Circulation, Disability, Exposure (ABCDE) approach', *International Journal of General Medicine*, 5: 117–21.

Ugboma, D. and Cowen, M. (2012) 'Managing hydration'. In I. Bullock, J. Clark and J. Rycroft-Malone (eds), *Adult Nursing Practice: Using Evidence in Care*. Oxford: Oxford University Press.

UK Sepsis Trust (2014) *General Ward Toolkit*. Available at: http://sepsistrust.org/info-for-professionals/clinical-toolkits/ (last accessed 17 October 2014).

Vincent, C., Neale, G. and Woloshynowych, M. (2001) 'Adverse events in British hospitals: preliminary retrospective record review', *British Medical Journal*, 322: 517–19.

Wadensten, B., Frojd, C., Swenne, C., Gordh, T. and Gunningburg, L. (2011) 'Why is pain still not being assessed adequately? Results of a pain prevalence study in a university hospital in Sweden', *Journal of Clinical Nursing*, 20: 624–34.

Walden, E., Stanisstreet, D., Jones, C., Graveling, A. on behalf of the Joint British Diabetes Societies for Inpatient Care (2013) *The Hospital Management of Hypoglycaemia in Adults with Diabetes Mellitus*. Available at: www.diabetologists-abcd.org.uk/JBDS/JBDS.htm (last accessed 17 October 2014).

Walz, J.M., Zayaruuzny, M. and Heard, S.O. (2007) 'Airway management in critical illness', *Chest*, 131 (2): 608–20.

Warden, V., Hurley, A.C., Volicer, L. (2003) 'Development and psychometric evaluation of the Pain Assessment in Advanced Dementia (PAINAD) Scale', *Journal of the American Medical Directors*, (Jan/Feb): 9–15.

West Midlands Quality Review Service and the Society for Acute Medicine (SAM) (2012) *Quality Standards for Acute Medical Units (AMUs)*. Available at: www.acutemedicine.org.uk/resources/quality-standards/ (last accessed 17 October 2014).

Williams, C. and Salerno, S. (2012) 'The patient in pain'. In D. Tait, D. Barton, J. James and C. Williams (eds), *Acute and Critical Care in Adult Nursing*. London: Sage.

Williamson, A. and Hoggart, B. (2005) 'Pain: a review of three commonly used pain rating scales', *Journal of Clinical Nursing*, 14: 798–804.

Wood, S. (2004) 'Factors influencing the selection of an appropriate pain assessment tools', *Nursing Times*, 100 (35) 42–7.

World Health Organization (1986) *Cancer Pain Relief*. Geneva: WHO.

World Health Organization (2007) Policy Brief. *Day Surgery: Making it Happen*. Available at: www.euro.who.int/__data/assets/pdf_file/0011/108965/E90295.pdf (last accessed 17 October 2014).

World Health Organization (2009) *WHO Guidelines for Safe Surgery: Safe Surgery Saves Lives*. Available at: http://whqlibdoc.who.int/publications/2009/9789241598552_eng.pdf?ua=1(last accessed 17 October 2014).

Zhuang, C.L., Ye, X.Z., Zhang, X.D., Chen, B.C. and Yu, Z. (2013) 'Enhanced recovery after surgery programs versus traditional care for colorectal surgery: a meta-analysis of randomised controlled trials', *Dis Colon Rectum*, 56 (5): 667–78.

12 Caring for the Older Person

EMMA STANMORE AND CHRISTINE BROWN WILSON

This chapter will provide an opportunity for you to consider how care of the older person is delivered from an individual perspective and how we might promote the principles of *person-centred care* when caring for an older person in everyday practice.

It will explore how the principles of health promotion (with particular reference to physical activity and falls prevention) can be applied to promote independence and improve the quality of life for older people. It shall also address other key topics such as dignity in care, empowerment and choice in relation to the care of older people, including persons with dementia or 'frailty'. A key aim will be for you to begin to question your own perceptions of older people using examples of myths and stereotypes that can often influence how we value and view ageing in our society. The chapter hopes to promote an understanding of the principles of anti-discriminatory practice with reference to age and consider how this is applied in practice. Most importantly, we also hope to demonstrate the necessity of using biography throughout the assessment process, appreciating the experience, skills and wisdom of older people both to enrich our nursing practice and enhance person-centred care.

After reading this chapter you should be able to:

- Understand the current challenges around planning and delivering high-quality care to frail older people in a variety of settings.
- Consider the principles of anti-discriminatory practice through examining myths and stereotypes that may detrimentally influence the care of older people, including those with dementia.
- Identify how dignity and compassion might be promoted for older people in everyday practice.
- Evaluate the role of the nurse in establishing the needs and preferences of older people and their carers through the use of person-centred and biographical care planning.
- Understand the importance of preventative care and health promotion for older people with particular reference to physical activity and falls prevention.
- Explore the principles of independence, empowerment and choice for the delivery of care and the role of technology in supporting these principles.

Related NMC competencies

The overarching NMC requirements are that all nurses must:

adapt their practice to meet the changing needs of people, groups, communities and populations and ... practice in a holistic, non-judgmental, caring and sensitive manner that avoids assumptions, supports social inclusion; recognises and respects individual choice; maintains dignity and human rights and acknowledges diversity. Where necessary, they must challenge inequality, discrimination and exclusion from access to care. (NMC, 2015)

―――――――――― To achieve entry to the register as an adult ――――――――――
nurse you should be able to:

- Promote the rights, choices and wishes of all adults, paying particular attention to equality, diversity, and the needs of an ageing population.
- Understand and apply current legislation to all service users, paying special attention to the protection of vulnerable people, including those with complex needs arising from ageing, cognitive impairment, and those approaching the end of life.
- Support and promote the health and well-being of people, including those affected by ill-health, disability and ageing.
- Work in partnership with service users, carers, families, groups, communities and organi-sations. You must manage risk, and promote health and well-being, while aiming to empower choices that promote self-care and safety.
- Build partnerships and therapeutic relationships through safe, effective and non-discriminatory communication. You must take account of individual differences, capabilities and needs.
- Take every opportunity to encourage health-promoting behaviour through education, role modelling and effective communication.

(Adapted from the NMC Standards of Competence for Adult Nursing, 2010a, 2010b.)

Background

It is a cause for celebration that people in the United Kingdom are living longer and on the whole healthier lives than ever before. This reflects our advancement in areas such as healthcare technologies, pharmacology, education, better living conditions and reduced childhood mortality. For the first time in history we have more people over the age of 60 than those under the age of 18 (ONS, 2011), with the 'oldest old' (over the age of 85) being the fastest growing demographic. It is for this very reason that all adult nurses need to be adequately prepared to care for older people to ensure that their individual needs are met. It would be logical to think that as older people are the core users of the NHS this would lead to more expertise within this field of care in nursing and healthcare. Yet this does not appear to be the case, with recent reports repeatedly highlighting a picture of poor or variable care for older people (Cornwell, 2012; RCP, 2012; Francis, 2013), and you will be aware that we are currently in the aftermath of the publication of Francis's public inquiry into the serious failings at Mid Staffordshire NHS Foundation Trust that highlighted the need for the delivery of compassionate care for older people. We think it important to re-iterate again that the report revealed a negative culture of disengagement, low morale, tolerance of poor care and long-term understaffing that led to high mortality rates, undignified care and shocking levels of patient and staff complaints that had been unaddressed by those in authority. There are lessons to be learned here for all healthcare providers.

The positive side of these perturbing reports is that they have resulted in an opportunity to transform services for older people, in which nurses will have a key role. As older people account for the majority of patients, all adult nurses should receive adequate preparation, including developing the skills needed to work with patients who are cognitively impaired (e.g. those with dementia) or frail. Indeed, one of the key recommendations in the Francis Report (2013) is that the specialist requirements of caring for older people should be recognised by the introduction of a new status of a registered older person's nurse.

There have been a number of other government actions to help put care of older people at the centre of healthcare that include an improved publicly available ratings system for the inspection of healthcare organisations with a greater emphasis on compassionate care. Tailored education, training and support are to be offered to nursing staff to promote the values of compassion, dignity and respect, and there is to be a reduction in unnecessary bureaucracy by streamlining inspections, information sharing and the improved use of technology amongst frontline staff to give more time and a greater emphasis on caring. There has also been a governmental push to recruit people into the care workforce who demonstrate a desire and ability to care for others (DH, 2013). Therefore, as a result of these policies, we may see some important leadership changes in the care of older people, with a greater recognition of the skills required for competent and compassionate care, and nurses need to seize these opportunities to make a difference.

Identify the key nursing skills required to effectively care for older people to overcome the shortcomings of the Francis Report.

- How might you demonstrate these skills in everyday practice?
- Provide one or two examples where you might implement these skills.

STOP AND THINK

Dispelling myths and stereotypes

Before discussing the challenges of caring for a growing population of older people further it is important to recognise the value and importance of older people as individuals with beneficial societal roles and influences. Ageing should not just signify decline and disease. Many older adults continue to perform at exceptionally high levels and learn new skills, as well as coping with major life changes such as retirement and bereavement. With age comes a wealth of experience, wisdom and skills that are a rich resource for all generations. The state pension age will be increasing gradually between 2010 and 2020, many men women will retire at different ages. The last women to retire at 60 have already done so. Between now and 2016 the retirement age for women will rise to around 63. Then between 2016 and 2018 it will rise to 65. According to a recent survey, 76% of older people believed that the country fails to make good use of the skills and talents of older people (Age UK, 2009). However, we know that older people can be as productive as younger generations and we perhaps need to discard any stereotypes regarding what we think it means to be 'old' (Bowers et al., 2013). Older people should not be seen as an homogeneous group with burdensome needs, but as diverse individuals with the ability to contribute to society and the same right to dignified, personalised care as any other generation.

Myths can be described as stories propagated within a society, often as a means of educating people with regard to the values and morals of society. In the global society in which we currently live, myths now emerge from advertising through a range of media. In terms of ageing, such myths either portray old age as a sign of decline and increasing decrepitude, or as a heroic point in life, where older adults overcome the adverse effects of ageing to do things that would be expected of younger members of society (e.g. running marathons). Neither of these views are particularly helpful for older people as they do not recognise the individual nature of ageing or the context in which people live in their later years (Minkler, 1996). These views have been perpetuated by early sociological research, resulting in the disengagement and activity theories and more latterly the theory of successful ageing (for further discussion of these theories, please refer to the suggested Further Reading at the end of this chapter).

We stereotype people by placing them in a group with others whom we believe all have similar traits and so will behave in similar ways, and this is often used as a mechanism to mentally organise workload. Additionally, by stereotyping people in this way we risk seeing them as 'different' and so can justify treating them differently. For older people, this may mean treating them with less dignity than other groups of people in our care. The language we use often refers to the stereotypes we subscribe to (Fiske et al., 2002). For example, referring to older people as 'the elderly' suggests we believe that all older people have a limited capacity for development as they are in a period of decline. This may be used to justify nursing older people in bed for longer periods, because they already have limited mobility and a limited capacity to recover. However, when we consider the personal nature of ageing we cannot assume that all older people approach their ageing in the same way (Bond et al., 2007). Therefore, we might conclude that the myths and stereotypes of ageing in our society may have an adverse impact on older people when they present to healthcare environments. For example, nurses in busy environments may unknowingly use stereotypes to make quick decisions when faced by an increasing workload. Some nursing students, for example, have recounted how qualified staff nurses see older people being admitted to wards and make assumptions based on these stereotypes, such as the expectation that an older person will suffer from incontinence or dementia (Brown Wilson et al., 2013). These decisions may then have an adverse impact on the care of older people, as nurses are often the gatekeepers for referrals to other healthcare professionals/ services.

STOP AND THINK

Consider two older people you know or have cared for who are of similar ages.

- What influences their approach to ageing?
- Are there any similarities or differences?
- What do you attribute these to?
- Do you think your views have an impact on how you might care for older people?

No-one will be immune from societal stereotypes, but an awareness of when myths or stereotypes are being used to make judgements about the older person and their care is the first step in minimising the potential harm these may cause. In addition, adopting an approach to care that focuses on the person and enables the practitioner to see the condition in context to the person will also lessen the impact negative stereotypes may have. As nurses we must challenge the stereotype of ageing as a period of decline, and support older people in maintaining and enhancing their quality of life by improving their health in ways that are meaningful to them.

The challenges of caring for older people

Older people are the main users of health services in both hospitals and the community and this trend is likely to continue. Increasing age brings with it the risk of living with one or more long-term medical conditions and hospitals are struggling to cope with fewer beds and increasing numbers of emergency admissions, largely due to the increase in older patients (RCP, 2012). The growing number of older people will bring new challenges to those nurses responsible for the care of older people, as well as new opportunities to ensure high-quality care is experienced and maintained for older people and their carers.

Traditionally, care of the older person has been seen as a less attractive career pathway in comparison to other specialist areas of adult nursing, but in reality it is a rewarding and challenging field of nursing that is ripe for further development and innovation. There are opportunities for nurses to pioneer and transform services designed to support older people to live longer in their own homes, using assistive technologies, and to deliver better preventative care or specialist inpatient care that incorporates their needs and preferences.

Technologies, such as telehealth (see Chapter 10, p. 298), are currently expanding due to their potential to enable more older people to receive care under the supervision of a healthcare team, reducing costly home visits and improving quality of care as well as preventing accidents and crises. Early findings from the large Whole System Demonstrator trial in the UK found that telehealth is associated with lower mortality and emergency admission rates (Steventon et al., 2013). There are also growing numbers of 'Smart homes' with embedded health devices such as movement and fall sensors, programmes to manage complex medication regimes and microprocessors in appliances, furniture and clothing that collect health monitoring data.

Despite these technological advances that aim to enable people to remain active at home for longer, the benefits achieved to date still require further research (Greenhalgh et al., 2012). The process of developing and implementing telehealth technologies requires co-ordination and commitment between numerous professions and organisations. However, nurses are in a key position to support, implement and evaluate new technologies to ensure that these are introduced using the best evidence, with joined-up service provision, and most importantly, what older people want.

Consider an older person that you know:

- What technology do they use in everyday life?
- How might this or a similar technology be used to enhance their health or maintain their independence as they age?

STOP AND THINK

The care of older people can be emotionally demanding and requires qualities such as compassion, empathy and patience alongside specialist *gerontological* education and training to ensure that nurses are equipped to meet their complex care needs using a person-centred approach. Caring for older people also requires an understanding of the physiological changes that take place as we age, with in-depth knowledge of long-term conditions such as diabetes, depression, arthritis, cardiovascular disease, respiratory conditions and dementia, to name but a few.

We know that older people, given the right help and support, would prefer to live in their familiar homes and communities for as long as possible (Age UK, 2009). However, Smith et al. (2011) argue that many of the current undergraduate nurse education programmes focus on acute hospital care for patients with single organ or infectious diseases, in contrast to many older people who have complex care needs or multiple co-morbidities and predominantly use primary care services as well as hospitals. Indeed, the current model of acute care is geared towards treatment and cure and is not well suited to older patients living with complex needs. There is also the consideration of the complexities of poly-pharmacy and the interaction between multiple medications and their side effects, and the need to give preventative care to enable older people to stay independent and disease-free. As an adult nurse caring for older people, you will need to build upon and develop the knowledge and understanding you should have already gained from reading the previous chapters in this book in order to be able to support those with complex, often interrelated co-morbidities, the frail 'oldest old' and the growing number of people with dementia in an already over-stretched health service. This may require you to undertake additional gerontological courses in the future to gain the skills required for the care of older people. Developing the specialised skills and knowledge to care for older people and a positive attitude to ageing at an individual as well as organisational level should drive a sustainable improvement in service provision and improve dignity in care for older people.

Maintaining dignity for the older person

Dignity in care refers to the care and support in any setting that promotes and maintains a person's self-respect, whatever their circumstances, health, age or any other such difference. The Social Care Institute for Excellence (n.d.) defines dignity as '... a state, quality or manner worthy of esteem or respect; and (by extension) self respect', and although you could argue 'dignity' often means different things to different people, it is clear to an older person when they have not received dignified care which can result in feelings of embarrassment and humiliation. From the perspective of an older person in hospital, a nurse helping to maintain their dignity means taking the time to find out about their usual routines, needs and preferences rather than expecting individuals to conform to standardised hospital routines; a small action that nevertheless can make on older person feel valued. Being thoughtful, polite and caring not only enriches the care that is delivered but can also reduce the person's anxiety and increase their confidence. For example, simply reading an excerpt from a book that is of interest to a patient who is blind shows that you are trying to do what really matters to the patient and applying this to your practice.

Nordenfelt and Edgar (2005) describe four ways of understanding dignity (Figure 12.1): dignity we earn by our actions (*Dignity of Merit*) and the person we are in society (*Dignity of Identity*), dignity we feel within ourselves (*Dignity of Moral Status*) and dignity we deserve because we are human (*Menschenwürde*). These are interrelated concepts with Dignity of Merit and Identity conferred on us by others. If people treat us with dignity because they feel our position in society warrants it, this then this will support our own sense of worth leading to self-respect. Each of these notions is under-pinned by the respect we should show to all people because they are human beings. However, if respect is not shown then our sense of dignity becomes eroded, which then impacts adversely on our self-respect (Nordenfelt and Edgar, 2005).

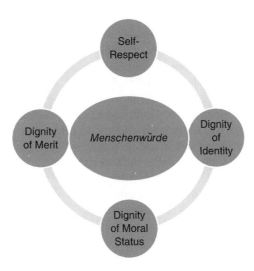

Figure 12.1

Source: Adapted from Nordenfelt and Edgar (2005)

This conceptual definition of dignity was defined as part of a wide European study conducted by Bayer et al. (2005) which examined how older people themselves experi-enced dignity. Older people gave examples of how their dignity was compromised when their views were not respected by healthcare professionals, they were not addressed directly, or their opinion was not sought. Such actions imply a lack of respect. A report for Help the Aged (Levenson, 2007) also identified a number of principles in how dig-nity might be enhanced (see the Dignity box overleaf). These included the importance of staff respecting older people and ensuring facilities were well maintained and clean. Autonomy was considered to be a key issue and included supporting older people to maintain independence wherever possible, ascertaining how people wish to be involved in their care and then including them in the decision-making process (Magee et al., 2008). Overall, maintaining dignity is about treating people as people and not objects. This demonstrates respect for the individual and builds trust between the professional and the person receiving care.

Dignity

Dignity in care is inseparable from the wider context of dignity as a whole.

Dignity is about treating people as individuals.

Dignity is not just about physical care.

Dignity thrives in the context of equal power relationships.

Dignity must be actively promoted.

Dignity is more than the sum of its parts.

(Adapted from Levenson, 2007.)

The previous chapter highlighted some issues related to the provision of care for older people in acute settings. We will now explore this a little further. When older people are admitted to hospital, they will ignore assaults on their dignity whilst they are unwell as the key focus is their recovering (Jacelon, 2003). However, as they progress from the acute phase of their illness they become more aware of such assaults. In her observational study, Jacelon (2003) found that many older people attempted to address this by interacting with staff and developing reciprocal relationships. One interpretation of this study might be that healthcare professionals become so focused on one approach to care that they don't always realise the impact their actions can have on a person's dignity. If we return to the four notions of Dignity (Figure 12.1), we might understand such actions as an effort by the older person to enhance their dignity of moral status (because they were trying to help staff) as the dignity conferred by others was not forthcoming.

Furthermore, people with dementia are more likely to suffer assaults on their dignity as they may not be able to communicate in a way that is understandable to busy healthcare professionals. This is often compounded by their being in a unfamiliar environment and having their usual routines disrupted. Moreover, many people with dementia may be admitted to a healthcare environment with an underlying medical problem such as an infection that is not recognised due to the overlying symptoms of dementia, which then results in poor consequences for the person (All-Party Parliamentary Group on Dementia, 2011).

Case Scenario

 ## MRS CROSS

Consider the needs of Mrs Cross, a 70-year-old lady with impaired hearing and poor eyesight, who has been admitted to hospital for treatment due to viral pneumonia.

- Make a list of the practical ways in which nursing and hospital staff could work to maintain Mrs Cross's dignity in the example above.
- Consider simple methods such as keeping her informed and being polite. For instance, how would you communicate effectively, considering her needs and preferences?
- What would you have to consider in order to be able to assist her with her personal hygiene needs?
- What difficulties might you face in a busy hospital ward?

Write down your thoughts and reflections.

(There are some websites listed at the end of this chapter that contain useful information when considering dignity and the care of older people.)

Compassion, choice and empowerment in healthcare

Previous chapters have highlighted the value of compassion, patient choice and empowerment in healthcare provision. However, we feel this is important enough to re-iterate it again here in relation to caring for the older person.

Compassionate and effective care in this context requires nurses to be able to respond in an ever-changing environment and place the care of the older person and their individual needs at its forefront. We need to be able to focus on the things that matter to older patients and their families and not just base our decisions on medical protocols or guidelines.

The Care Quality Commission (CQC) regularly inspects hospitals, care homes and primary care centres in the UK to ensure that services are effective, safe and compassionate. They publish their findings from these inspections and encourage services to make improvements where shortfalls in care are identified. In terms of the care of older people, the CQC have made recommendations in a number of NHS services that included the recruitment of specialist care of the older person nurses, more consultant geriatricians, increasing staffing levels, and the introduction of a 'Compassionate Care Training Programme' for all staff working with older people.

However, it is often difficult from these reports to identify what is meant by terms such as 'caring' or 'compassion'. One example of care that lacks compassion would be that of nurses telling older people to use an incontinence aid rather than being taken to the toilet (Abrahams, 2011). Similarly, research reports comparable issues such as nurses or caregivers making the assumption an older person is not hungry rather than finding out the underlying reason for why they are not eating (Tadd et al., 2011). These reports describe everyday occurrences observed in busy ward environments that imply a lack of compassion, dignity and respect. These terms are considered integral to modern-day healthcare but may be difficult for nurses to see how it applies to their everyday care, allowing practices such as those described above to creep into the workplace culture. Such practices may occur when we fail to consider the impact of our approach to care when we look after older people.

Think about how you might improve the care you deliver to older people across each of the 6Cs and consider how any improvements that you introduce could be measured to demonstrate change.

(Note: the measurement of compassion may be difficult as compassion is not always visible. Think about novel ideas, such as collecting patient case studies where compassion was demonstrated or introducing short patient feedback forms in your work setting that could be used to recognise good examples of care or areas that need further improvement.)

STOP AND THINK

The responsibility for improving the quality of older people's care needs to be taken at an individual level as well as by nurses in leadership positions. As nurses lead by example, the culture and environment of undervaluing older people can be changed to one of empowerment of older people and putting their perspective first. Many older patients

n support from family caregivers, and it's generally these caregivers who
ns and complaints about the quality of care, as acknowledged in the Francis
rt (Francis, 2013).

One recent study exploring the views of older people in their choice of care for intermediate care services (involving care at home, and a short admission to a care home or
an intermediate care unit) reported mixed views from patients on whether they received
choice about their care and also about how much they wanted to be involved in the
decisions about this (Stanmore, 2011). Pickard and Glendinning (2002) recommend
that older carers should receive real choice about the extent of their involvement in care
giving, and that healthcare professionals should anticipate the needs of older carers and
provide a more proactive service when offering help. This is even more vital for those
of us caring for people with dementia. Critical points where more support is required
by carers include the diagnosis of dementia, when taking on an active caring role, and
when the capacity of the person with dementia declines (Newbronner et al., 2013).
These are important opportunities for health professionals to support family caregivers
with advice and signposting. For example, counselling and peer support groups have
been found to be helpful for family caregivers in the early stages of the dementia
(Sorensen et al., 2008).

As an adult nurse, you will need to be proactive in involving older people in their care
decisions from the onset: giving explanations, managing expectations, and involving
families in decision making and discharge planning. The implementation of this advice
would ensure that older carers would also feel more supported and valued. However, as
highlighted above, some older people may not initially appear to be particularly interested in being involved in the choice and decision making for their care. Amongst older
people the attitude of 'whatever the doctor thinks is best', rather than voicing their own
preferences or opinions, may still reflect a medical model of healthcare. In addition, not
all older patients are in a fit state to make decisions when they are acutely ill. Nevertheless,
a solution to whether or not to involve the patient in choice and decision making is to
ensure that this is offered at the initial assessment, but with the opportunity of allowing
the patient to opt out if they feel more comfortable with a chosen advocate making the
decisions for them. They could later on become more involved in their healthcare decisions as they recover. Person-centred care does not stop at assessment and should be
incorporated throughout a patient's care. Patients are entitled to be involved in their
healthcare decisions, even with a diagnosis of dementia, and as you are already aware
the involvement of patients should be embedded in the structures of all aspects of NHS
healthcare (DH, 2001).

Biographical approach to care

So how can we ensure that older people receive the person-centred care they deserve?
It is by valuing the older person for who they are, understanding what is important
and ensuring significant routines are maintained in their care that we deliver person-
centred care. We start this by developing an understanding of the biography of the
older person that supports us in valuing them as a person first and then considering
their needs as a patient or client in this context. This is even more crucial when a
person has dementia, as the disruption to their everyday routines can cause anxiety
and upset which may result in behaviours that challenge staff. Involving the older
person's caregiver at the assessment stage can support staff in providing appropriate
care that values the person by implementing usual routines that make the person feel

more comfortable in unfamiliar surroundings (see the box below on a biographical approach to care planning).

A Biographical Approach to Care Planning

- Encourage the client (and their carers) to talk about how they approach their life.
- Try to develop a rapport with your patient by talking about everyday events and people during care routines.
- Use belongings, photos etc. as triggers for discussion.
- Recognise the unique assets and characteristics of each person and build on these when planning care.
- Build on lifelong interests shared by patients and their families to offer them the opportunity to experience new things and interests in the context of their care.

We may think we do this already, but as busy healthcare professionals we will often focus on the condition the person presents with first, with the needs of the older person a secondary consideration. It is when focusing on the condition rather than the person becomes established practice that we begin to see examples of poor care as described by the Ombudsman (Abrahams, 2011) and Francis (2013). Nurses are often in the frontline as regards patient care and as such it is our care that comes under close scrutiny. These reports repeatedly provide examples of poor care related to older people and/or people with dementia that could be addressed by recognising what is important to the older person and their family. Families often provide biographical information to nurses but when nurses do not recognise the value of this information, they may appear not to have sufficient time to care or be seen as losing their compassion. Families will then subsequently make judgements on the quality of care and will tend to be more critical when they perceive this information is not being listened to or acted upon (Jurgens et al., 2012; Clissett et al., 2013).

Promoting person-centred care with older people and those with dementia

Person-centred care has been identified as a way of improving the care of older people (McCormack and McCance, 2006) and those with dementia (Brooker, 2004). Of course, not all older people will have dementia, but the risk of some dementias, such as Alzheimer's disease, multiplies with age. This suggests that increased longevity may also increase the amount of people diagnosed with a dementia. The aim of person-centred care is to focus professionals' attention on the person rather than the condition. Kitwood (1997) believes that considering the emotional needs of the person alongside their physical needs will enhance the care of people with dementia. Brooker (2004) has developed these principles further into the VIPS Model:

- Valuing the person with dementia.
- Providing Individualised care.
- Recognising the Perspective of the person with dementia.
- And examining the Social environment in which the person is located (Røsvik et al., 2011). We will focus on the case of a person with dementia again in more detail later in the Chapter.

Recognising that our patient is a person first is now considered a guiding principle across all models of healthcare. For example, the Institute of Medicine's (IOM, 2001) definition of patient-centred care includes respecting needs, values and preferences, as well as providing for emotional as well as physical support. However, many of these models lack specific guidance as to how these might be put into practice (Dewing, 2004), with Goodrich and Cornwell (2008) finding that few healthcare professionals in the UK could describe what was meant by patient-centred care.

STOP AND THINK

Draw a time-line of your life and consider how some of the events that have been significant have shaped how you approach your life today.

- Consider an older person you know in your personal life: how have events in their life shaped how they make decisions about their health?
- For this older person, what are the significant routines in their life that might be disrupted if they require health and social care support?
- How might you, as a concerned relative, try to influence their care?

The approach that nurses should use with all older people is characterised by understanding the biography of the person and seeing beyond the immediate context of illness (McCormack and McCance, 2006). A systematic review of patient experience in acute hospitals suggests that older people and their families want staff to recognise who they are and what is important to them, to involve them in decision making and support them in maintaining links with their community whilst in hospital (Bridges et al., 2010). Dewar (2011) found that asking patients a series of questions about what was important to the person and any fears they had made patients and families feel more involved in their care.

Brown Wilson (2013) develops the use of biography to consider what is significant in a person's life, including day-to-day routines that give the older person's life meaning, or for the person with dementia, provide an understandable structure to their day. Nurses are often able to develop insights into this biographical information through the daily contact they have with patients in providing care, such as giving out medication, bathing, dressing, and supporting people at mealtimes. This information may not be shared as a routine because it might not be considered relevant to the nursing care of this person (Brown Wilson, 2013). The challenge for nurses is the need to consider how to document information such as this so it becomes part of accepted practice when caring for the older person rather than it depending upon who is on shift at that time.

Implementing person-centred care

This chapter has suggested a number of ways by which the principles of person-centred care can be implemented as a mechanism by which to promote dignity when working with and caring for older people. However, it is recognised that the environment in which care is delivered and organised also has an impact on the implementation of approaches such as person-centred care (McCormack and McCance, 2010; Brown Wilson et al., 2013).

McCormack and McCance (2010) identified that the care environment is a key feature of their model of person-centred nursing, suggesting that a range of factors such as organisational systems, physical environment, skill mix and staff relationships needs to be taken into consideration. Each of these will make a contribution or act as a barrier to the implementation of person-centred care. Often person-centred care may be considered something additional as some of these factors may require additional work and sometimes be beyond the control of ward-based staff. Brown Wilson (2009) offers a number of factors based on smaller organisations that may be of value in supporting ward-based staff and students in implementing a person-centred approach by integrating these into their current practice:

- Leadership.
- Staff motivation.
- Teamwork.
- A consistent approach to care.
- Continuity of care.

Leadership that is approachable, able to generate trust, supportive of staff in resolving conflict, and promotes an exchange of information to support staff in their decision making, is more likely to develop positive relationships in the workplace (Anderson et al., 2003). Brown Wilson (2009) suggests that this style of leadership can also come from those delivering day-to-day care in ways such as role modelling good practice.

To get to know a person and then implement significant changes to their care plan requires a continuity of staff who will adopt a person-centred approach. Initially, sharing biographical knowledge may be dependent upon developing relationships with specific members of staff, but once this information is disseminated continuity can be promoted, even when the same nursing staff are on duty, through a consistent approach to care. This is possible even when the staffing levels and skill mix may be sub-optimal.

The personal philosophy of staff members, their beliefs and values, will be integral to a person-centred approach (McCormack and McCance, 2006; Brown Wilson and Davies, 2009). This is represented in Figure 12.2, as staff who are motivated by a 'do unto others' philosophy are more likely to create a focus on the person. This means that these nurses are able to take into account what the older person considers important in their care and then seek to implement care in this way. Brown Wilson (2009) found that a critical mass of staff working with the same philosophy was more likely to result in a focus on the person. Therefore, this implies that developing a culture in the work environment where an older person is listened to and their needs are acted on is more likely to deliver a person-centred approach to care.

Older people and families will often seek to make a direct contribution to, or influence their care, through the development of relationships with staff (Jacelon, 2003; Brown Wilson, 2009; Clissett et al., 2013). Adopting a biographical approach to care planning is one way of recognising and valuing this contribution. This may highlight the reasons behind different behaviours, supporting staff in making sense of these given their workload.

Looking back at the Case Scenario in Chapter 10 (p. 217), how might a person-centred ward philosophy have changed the way care was delivered on Lucy's ward?

STOP AND THINK

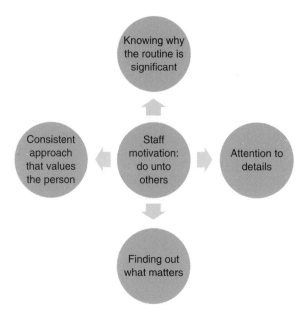

Figure 12.2

Source: Brown Wilson (2013)

For older people, finding out what is important in their life is the first step in implementing person-centred care.

MR SMITH

Mr Smith's pain had been attributed to his age. He was being treated for depression as he appeared withdrawn. On speaking with Mr Smith, the nurse found that he had always been an active and outgoing man and enjoyed volunteering at the local hospital. However, he was now unable to continue to do this due the pain in his knees, which restricted his mobility. Finding out what was significant to Mr Smith was then transferred into action by referring to other members of the multidisciplinary team to investigate the cause of the pain. In the meantime, the nurse arranged for transport for Mr Smith to attend a day centre which he enjoyed.

Understanding frailty in the older person

One of the key challenges for supporting people as they age is their increasing level of frailty. *Frailty* is a much-used term that remains poorly defined, with no consensus on its definition (Mitniski et al., 2004). Some have defined it as a collection of deficits, namely the more people have wrong with them, the frailer they are (Mitnitski et al., 2005), with others suggesting it is a specific syndrome represented by weight loss, exhaustion, low physical activity and slowness (Fried et al., 2004). Despite these various definitions there is increasing recognition that frailty is a physiological syndrome that causes an older person to be more vulnerable to adverse health outcomes (Ferrucci et al., 2004). This is due mainly to a decline in physiological function across multiple systems, often due to co-morbid conditions. This results in the older person's system having limited ability to respond to internal stressors internally, such as viruses or environmental stressors such as changes in temperature for example. This approach suggests that frailty is not simply a result of the ageing process and so should not be defined by chronological age but by how the older person's body responds to different stressors.

Rockwood et al. (2006) undertook a large-scale study testing the hypothesis that, at a given age, frailty can be defined in relation to how many deficits an older person has, such as problems with mobility, nutrition, and the ability to undertake Activities of Daily Living (ADL) (Roper et al., 2000). This accumulation of deficits is important as it may tip the balance between an older person being able to live independently in the community or requiring institutional care (Rockwood et al., 1994). A Frailty Index, developed to summarise a person's health status by counting the number of deficits, is then used to infer the relative frailty of an individual (Mitnitski et al., 2005). The work undertaken by Rockwood et al. (2006) suggests that it is the accumulation of these deficits that is important for health outcomes, rather than the individual nature of each deficit. This understanding is vital for nurses in healthcare, as we will often focus on the nature of a deficit.

It is very tempting to think about frailty as a fixed condition, i.e. 'once you become frail there is no going back'. However, this work should challenge us to consider how older people may be supported to reduce their deficits rather than accepting these are a result of age. Rockwood et al. (1994) consider frailty as a balance (see Figure 12.3). For older people who are well, the scales are tipped towards *assets* (medical and social). Increasing frailty then brings the scales into alignment until one additional problem may tip the scales in favour of *deficits*. However, the nature of those deficits may be amenable to treatment to enable the balance between assets and deficits to change. For example, if a deficit is related to walking, then simple exercises can improve that deficit.

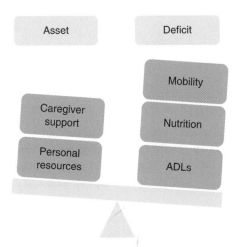

Figure 12.3   Interpretation of Frailty Balance based on Rockwood et al., 1994

There is substantial evidence that older people with frailty benefit from assessment and intervention that is whole-person-centred, multidisciplinary, iterative and case-managed; this is also known as the Comprehensive Geriatric Assessment (CGA) (Ellis et al., 2011). Physiological function, the reactions of the body to pharmaceutical treatments, and responses to health challenges and injury, all change with age. The syndromes frequently presenting in older patients (e.g. cognitive impairment, stroke, fragility fractures, falls, syncope and incontinence) are different from those seen in younger populations.

When using the CGA to assess frailty (see the box on the following page) the more deficits the older person has, then the greater is their risk of poor outcomes.

However, when nurses consider these domains, they tend to consider each issue as an isolated problem. Considering issues of nutrition, mobility and continence for example as indicators of frailty may promote a more holistic assessment of the person. In any assessment it is vital that we understand the significance of the presenting issues to the older person themselves. So we need to consider the clinical significance of these issues from that person's perspective, i.e. what is most important to that person and what intervention is required to support that person in achieving their personal goal. By doing this, we place an older person at the centre of the assessment process and provide an opportunity to learn more about that individual, their current situation and desires for the future.

———— Assessing frailty using CGA domains based ———— on Jones et al. (2004)

Cognitive status (no cognitive impairment=no problem; cognitive impairment/no dementia=mild problem; delirium or dementia=severe problem).

Mood and motivation.

Communication (vision, hearing, speech).

Mobility, balance (scored at the highest level of independence with aids where used).

Bowel function.

Bladder function.

IADLs and ADLs (rated as no impairment=no problem, IADL impairment=mild problem, ADL impairment=major problem).

Nutrition.

Social resources (scored as a problem if there was need for additional help).

Note: For a Frailty Index, score problems in each domain were scored as 0 (no problem), 1 (a minor problem), or 2 (a major problem). For evaluating the contribution of each domain, the mode of the three ratings determined the value for each subject.

Case Scenario

 ### MR JONES

Mr Jones has been admitted to your ward. He is generally a well 88-year-old man but was unable to get out of bed this morning. The community nurses could not find a specific problem with him but were unable to move him from the bed and so he was admitted.

On assessment Mr Jones states he is eating regularly but admits he has lost weight over the past three months as his trousers now feel loose. He is eating light meals that can be prepared in a microwave as he has lost interest in cooking. He walks his dog once a day but only covers a short distance. He has a slow walking speed and tends to shuffle his feet when he walks. He is struggling to do his housework and needs help with the garden. He wishes to remain in his own home.

Using the domains of the Comprehensive Geriatric Assessment identify how frail you think Mr Jones is and why. What are the risks for him if these deficits are not addressed? What nursing actions do you think would benefit him and how would these enable him to retain his independence?

Promoting the health of older people

Caring for older people is not just about treating them during illness, it is also about keeping them well and educating them about how to stay healthy and active for as long as possible. Although it is widely understood that health promotion for older people may encompass activities such as blood pressure control, flu immunisation or smoking cessation, it should be recognised that every contact with an older person may present an opportunity to promote healthy behaviour and lifestyle.

Opportunities for nurses to promote health may be related to screening for the early detection of conditions, or identifying whether the older person would benefit from preventative advice or assessment for asymptomatic disease such as hypertension or osteoporosis. Early identification of dementia is also important to ensure that treatment, support and follow-up can be put into place so that the sufferer and their families can receive ongoing care and review. Likewise, recognising through assessment the need for screening for cancers such as breast, prostate and colon (that are increasingly remediable to surgery or chemotherapy) can lead to much improved outcomes when these diseases are identified early on in their natural history. Similarly, being on the lookout for signs of depression (another common condition in older people) can lead to early diagnosis and treatment that can greatly improve quality of life in older people.

Simple health-promoting measures, such as checking when an older person last had their vision or hearing ability checked and referring to appropriate services, can improve their general health and well-being and assist in them maintaining their ability to remain independent. Similarly, establishing whether an older person is experiencing difficulties with urinary incontinence can lead to effective prevention and treatment that will also impact positively on a person's self-esteem. Although urinary incontinence is treatable, fewer than half of patients with urinary incontinence report their symptoms to a physician and suffer in silence (Orrell et al., 2013). This is usually because they are too embarrassed, they consider their problem a normal part of ageing, absorbent devices are readily available, or they have low expectations of treatment or fear surgery. Developing positive, therapeutic relationships with older people may enable them to more readily disclose symptoms that may be a source of embarrassment (Fultz and Herzog, 2000), leading to diagnosis and treatment.

Educating older people to optimally manage chronic conditions such as arthritis or diabetes is also a key part of the adult nurse's health-promoting role. For instance, reinforcing healthy dietary advice or encouraging physical activity will not only improve the condition but also reduce the likelihood of developing other co-morbid diseases. Diet and lifestyle influences can have a considerable impact on health during the life course (WHO, 2002). In a study of dietary patterns and lifestyle among individuals aged 70 to 90 years, adherence to a Mediterranean diet and healthy lifestyle was associated with a more than 50% lower rate of all causes and cause-specific mortality (Knoops et al., 2004).

377

r activities may also encompass a reassessment or review of a patient's
ng ongoing needs or their understanding of safe administration and
for older people taking four or more medicines (known as poly-
al to their GP or pharmacist for a medication review has been shown to
ficial in reducing medication-related complications. These increase with the
of medications consumed, both prescribed and over the counter. Medication
management studies in older people have shown that they are more likely to experience
adverse consequences and have a lower tolerance of drug side effects; to be at greater risk
of inappropriate prescribing; are more likely to be uncertain about physician instructions;
are more likely to have greater difficulties ordering and collecting their medicines; and are
prone to have difficulties administering their medicines because of cognitive, sensory, or
physical impairment (Rogers et al., 2014). Therefore, taking the time to assess patients'
needs in managing their medication, and teaching about the safe administration and possible
side effects, could save much distress, reduce hospital admissions, and be potentially life saving.

Case Scenario

MRS FIELDS

Mrs Fields, a 78-year-old woman with coronary heart disease, congestive heart failure and
hypertension, lives at home with her spouse. She decided to stop taking her diuretics due
to continence problems and was admitted to hospital with worsening heart failure. The
nursing assessment revealed that a number of general practitioners had visited Mrs Fields
and adjusted her medication to improve control of her heart failure. One of the community
nurses was also visiting to assess and manage continence problems, but neither the doctors
nor the nurse were aware of each other's visits.

What nursing and health-promoting actions do you think would benefit Mrs Fields? How
would these actions enable her to safely return home and effectively manage her medication? What could be done to improve multidisciplinary communication to prevent incidents
like this case from occurring again?

What additional training would you find useful in enabling you to support older people
to manage their medicines effectively?

Promoting physical activity in older people

For many older people, an inactive life can lead to poor mental health and feeling dissatisfied, depressed and socially isolated. Participation in meaningful activity is important for maintaining relationships and feelings of purpose, as well as improving physical
and mental health (NICE, 2008). Research over the last twenty-five years has shown
that physically active older people experience a better quality of life, less social isolation
and maintain their function and independence, compared to those who remain sedentary (Wilmoth et al., 2013).

Current evidence suggests that as adult nurses we should be encouraging older people
to remain active and independent, rather than disempowering them or overly increasing
their reliance on health professionals.

There are a number of important reasons for encouraging physical activity or exercise in older people: it can be health promoting for instance, as resistance exercises

(those that incorporate strength training) can maintain or improve bone health to prevent osteoporosis. Exercise can also be disease preventing: for example, it can lower blood pressure and cholesterol, prevent heart disease and diabetes, and has also been associated with preventing certain types of cancer (CDC, 1996; WHO, 2007; BHF, 2010).

There are further myths and stereotypes about older people being unable to remain physically fit and active. Those working in exercise science could inform us that older people are capable of functioning at exceptionally high levels and that decline occurs on an individual basis, dependant on factors such as lifestyle and genetics. We know from research studies that older people, even those in their nineties, are able to reverse the effects of ageing through regular muscle strengthening and balance exercises (Fiatarone et al., 1990). Therefore it is important for nurses to encourage activity and exercise with older people, whatever their ability, and to assist them to find local facilities or give advice on home-based exercises that will maintain and improve their physical function.

Some of the benefits that can be used to encourage older people to become more active and remain active are listed in Table 12.1. Possibly the most important points listed here are the benefits in maintaining independence and a social network, as losing these abilities are some of the biggest fears for older people. When talking to patients about staying active and not sitting for longer than an hour they may not be not be highly motivated to do so, but if it is explained that this could be the difference in staying independent at home for longer they may be much more motivated to increase their physical activity.

Table 12.1 Advantages of physical activity and risks associated with sedentary behaviour

Physically active behaviour	Sedentary behaviour
Increased ability to maintain social network	Reduced postural stability
Reduced fatigue	Decreased function and independence
Improved ability to maintain a stable weight	Decreased quality of life
Better quality of life	Increased risk of pressure ulcers
Possible improved survival	Significantly decreased bone density and increased risk of osteoporosis
Improved bone density and lowered risk of osteoporosis	
Improved muscle strength and balance	Can negatively affect mental health
Quicker reaction time	Increased risk of obesity and associated morbidities (e.g. cardiovascular disease, Type 2 diabetes, cancer)
Improved *proprioception*	
Improved mental health and cognitive function	

Source: CMO (2011); Sherrington et al. (2008)

As a nation we are becoming increasingly sedentary and there have been many recent governmental campaigns aimed at getting people to be more active to target obesity and social isolation and to encourage longer working lives (DH, 2009). Sedentary behaviour accelerates the loss of performance and older people already lose 1–2% of functional ability each year. Just one week of bed rest reduces a person's strength by approx 20% and spine bone density by 1% (LeBlanc et al., 1987). If you consider how much time older people in care homes spend either sitting down or in bed you can understand their increased risk of fractures and falls. All older adults should minimise the amount of time spent being sedentary (sitting) for extended periods and nurses can educate and encourage older people to be as active as possible.

So how active should older people be? This very much depends on the individual, taking into consideration their current health and how active they already are. In 2011, the first ever UK-wide published guidelines (CMO, 2011) outlined the amount of physical activity that older adults (65 years and over) should be doing to benefit their health:

- Older adults who participate in any amount of physical activity gain some health benefits, including the maintenance of good physical and cognitive function.
- Some physical activity is better than none, and more physical activity provides greater health benefits.
- Older adults should also undertake physical activity to improve muscle strength on at least two days a week.
- Older adults at risk of falls should incorporate physical activity to improve balance and co-ordination on at least two days a week.(CMO, 2011)

However, research suggests that there are many barriers (actual and perceived) for older people to overcome to be able to effectively participate in physical activity. Some patients are just too unwell, yet others may think that exercise is not good due to their condition but in actual fact their health would greatly benefit if they did increase their physical activity, for example patients needing cardiac rehab or those with rheumatoid arthritis (Stanmore, 2013a). Some patients try exercise but don't see any immediate observed positive effects – this is because some of the benefits are not immediately obvious and the person may need to become a little fitter before they experience any improvements in their health. Other people may not like the social contact in classes or find they get too fatigued or feel pain, whilst others struggle with motivation or feel they have other more important priorities in their life. Furthermore there may be practical difficulties such as getting to an available class. These barriers can be overcome with help and an individualised approach, so when encouraging an older person to exercise involve them in developing a programme and help them to find a class or sport that they can take part in. Remember, there is something for everyone. Skelton et al. (2005) demonstrated in their strength and balance training study of older people that in three months 65–90 year olds were able to rejuvenate twenty years of lost strength.

Exercise should incorporate some kind of aerobic or endurance tasks, some flexibility and resistance exercises (e.g. weight bearing), in particular the lower limbs, and some functional task training that is individualised according to the needs and preferences of the person. There is even research being published about the benefits of Wii Fit, Xbox Kinect and other virtual reality gaming systems for exercise that are proving to be beneficial for older people in the home or care home environment (van Diest et al., 2013).

ACTIVITY   12.1

Consider the types of exercise facilities, classes or services that are suitable for older people in your local community:

- What do you think might be the barriers for the attendance of older people for each of these activities?
- How might these barriers be overcome using an individualised approach and considering the person's significant routines?

Visit your library or search the internet for facilities local to you that are suitable for older people–remember the importance of finding out what is the older person's interests and needs to tailor this to their preferences. There are also some websites listed at the end of this chapter that contain useful information when considering physical activity and older people.

Falls prevention for older people

A common myth or stereotype of older people is that falling is often accepted as a natural part of the ageing process. Looking at the research we can see that as many as 40% of falls can be predicted and prevented (Gillespie et al., 2012), but this message needs to reach older people (and some health professionals) who continue to think that falls are inevitable.

The National Council on Ageing (2013) produced a list of the ten most common misconceptions about falls in older adults, such as, 'It won't happen to me', 'It's just a normal part of growing older', 'If I limit my activity, I won't fall', 'As long as I stay at home, I can avoid falling', 'Muscle strength and flexibility can't be regained', and 'Taking medication doesn't increase my risk of falling'. So we can conclude that older people also need re-educating about these misconceptions and that as nurses we should be re-iterating the positive message that falls can be prevented with support.

It is true, however, that falls are common in older people, yet many older people are unaware of their risk of falling. Around one in three people aged over 65, and half of those aged over 80, fall at least once a year, and this rate increases with age and for those living in care homes (AGS/BGS, 2010). Approximately 10% of falls will result in fractures, and most concerning is that falls resulting in hip fractures commonly lead to death or institutional care within a year. Fear of falling is also a key concern that can restrict social activity and lead to older adults becoming more sedentary and isolated. The risk of falls is then exacerbated due to the resulting muscle weakness and balance difficulties. Therefore, it is imperative that nurses raise awareness of the importance of falls risk screening and assessment of older people with other health professionals, older people and their carers/relatives.

We can easily identify those who are most at risk of a fall by asking questions related to the most notable risk factors. Fall risk factors for older people can be categorised as biological, behavioural, and psychosocial (see Figure 12.4).

A history of a previous fall is the best predictor of a future fall, and any older person who responds positively to this question should receive support on preventing further falls. For some older people, reduced physical activity causes their balance and muscle strength to deteriorate and their reaction time and gait speed slow, so the ability to remain steady and upright becomes much more challenging. We know that older people are generally more sedentary and this can increase the likelihood of a fall.

Having poor strength and balance, gait problems and a fear of falling along with some diseases such as Parkinson's, stroke, rheumatoid arthritis and dementia increase the likelihood of falls, as does having poor vision, foot pain and incontinence (WHO, 2007; Stanmore et al., 2013b). We know that taking more than four types of medicine and

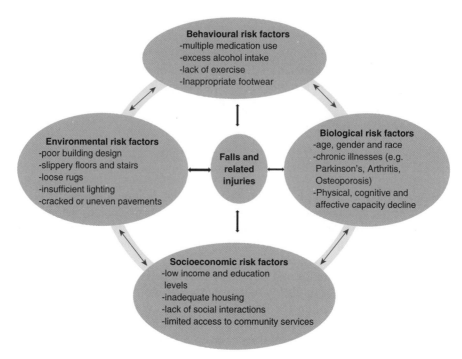

Figure 12.4   Risk factors associated with an increased risk of falls

(NICE, 2013; WHO, 2007)

certain types of medicine (e.g. antidepressants, diuretics, analgesics and antipsychotic medicines) also increases a person's fall risk. In addition, a person's environment can also increase the likelihood of falls too, for example tripping hazards or uneven surfaces in the home (NICE, 2013).

Over the last three decades, researchers have conducted falls prevention trials with older people by modifying either a single risk factor or multiple risk factors. Both strategies have been shown to be effective in reducing the rate of falling. One Cochrane systematic review (Gillespie et al., 2012) assessed the effects of interventions to reduce the incidence of falls in older people living in the community and included 159 clinical trials. The researchers concluded that group and home-based exercise programmes, incorporating balance and strength training exercises, effectively reduced falls, as did Tai Chi. Overall, these exercise programmes reduced fractures. Home safety interventions were found to be effective, especially in people at a higher risk of falling and when carried out by occupational therapists. The review concluded that falls prevention strategies can be cost saving. This evidence could be used by nurses to reduce the risk of falling and improve the quality of life for older people.

A first line approach for adult nurses (in the hospital, home and in care homes) to identify older individuals at high risk of falls would be to ask if the patient has fallen in the last year, and if so the frequency, injuries and circumstances of the fall(s). How older people and health professionals classify a fall can differ. A stumble or trip where the person is able to respond and recover is not a fall. The following wording is recommended when asking older people about falls: 'In the past month, have you had any fall including a slip or trip in which you lost your balance and landed on the floor or ground or lower level?' (Lamb et al., 2005). A positive history of falls should trigger an in-depth assessment to identify modifiable risk factors that can be dealt with by the health professional (Figure 12.5).

To target those who are at a high risk of falls but who have not yet fallen, a short assessment of the individual's functional and physical ability may be carried out using:

- The FICSIT Four Test Balance Scale (Rossiter-Fornoff et al., 1995).
- The Timed Up and Go Test (Podsiadlo and Richardson 1991).

The FICSIT Four Test Balance Scale is a short balance test that includes four timed static balance tasks of increasing difficulty using different positioning of the participants' feet and has also been extensively tested for validity and reliability (Rossiter-Fornoff et al., 1995). The validated Timed Up and Go Test measures the time it takes for an individual to rise from a chair, walk three metres at a normal pace with their usual assistive device, turn, return to the chair and sit down. A time of 12 or more seconds indicates an increased risk of falling (Podsiadlo and Richardson, 1991). These physical checks have been safely performed on thousands of older people (Robertson et al., 2002) and there are videos available on the internet that can teach health professionals to perform them correctly with older people (for example www.cdc.gov/homeandrecreationalsafety/Falls/steadi/videos.html).

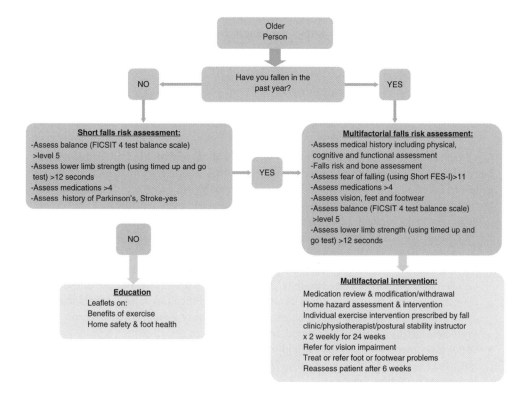

Figure 12.5 Algorithm of falls risk screening tool (based on Stanmore, 2013b; AGS/BGS, 2010; Nandy et al., 2004)

Strength and balance exercises are particularly good at reducing the risk of falls, increase bone health (therefore reducing the risk of fractures), and can have other beneficial properties such as improving mood and social contact.

ACTIVITY 12.2

Find out more about trained postural stability instructors or therapists that deliver strength and balance exercises for older people by contacting local community physiotherapy departments or visit the website of Later Life Training.
(For a directory of trained staff within local regions see www.laterlifetraining.co.uk

We know that group and home-based exercise programmes delivered by trained professionals can be effective in reducing falls and improving function. In terms of prescribing, the optimum dose and timing of exercise programmes for reducing falls, and the criterion for a minimal effective exercise dose equates to a twice-weekly programme over 24 weeks (Sherrington et al., 2008). *Tai chi* is a type of exercise that many older people enjoy due to its relaxing properties and it is known to reduce the risk of falls. Many local leisure centres and libraries can give further details about available classes. Referrals to physiotherapists, specialist falls services, occupational therapists, postural stability instructors and GPs (for a medication review) could be carried out by nurses to ensure that evidence-based practice is carried out for older people. A home assessment by an occupational therapist or community nurse would also be invaluable to highlight any fall hazards that may be present on the person's home environment (see the case scenario below).

Case Scenario

MRS BIRCH

Mrs Birch is a 79-year-old independent lady who lives at home with her frail husband who has Parkinson's disease. She has been having difficulties sleeping and has recently had a couple of falls during the night, resulting in some minor bruising and a small laceration to her right shin. The community nurse is requested to visit and assess Mrs Birch.

How would you conduct a bio-psychosocial assessment with Mrs Birch, thinking about her individual needs and care? What is normal for Mrs Birch? What has changed?

- *Physical assessment*: past medical history, current health status, co-morbidities; nocturia: detailed falls assessment (see Figure 12.5); medications – prescribed and use of over the counter, type and frequency; sleep duration, quality, difficulties falling asleep/staying asleep/un-refreshing sleep/daytime sleepiness, sleep apnoea; wound assessment.
- *Psychological assessment*: assess mood, anxiety, cognition.
- *Social assessment*: lifestyle; formal and informal support; environment; exercise levels; husband's needs; what is important to Mrs Birch and her husband, their interests, past occupations, hobbies, family etc

How could you ensure a biographical approach is incorporated into your assessment?

Ensuring that older people receive regular eyesight checks and treatment for visual problems (e.g. cataract surgery) can be helpful in preventing falls, as can wearing well-fitting, anti-slip shoes. As many older people can be taking a number of different types of medicines it is important that they receive a regular review of their medication (in particular the review of psychotropic medicines) so that this can be modified if necessary.

Fear of falling can negatively affect individuals and their ability to maintain social networks and maintain independence. A simple measure of fear of falling, such as the validated Short Falls Efficacy Scale-International (Kempen et al., 2008) can be undertaken to identify those with low levels of confidence. People who recurrently fall would benefit from a more detailed multi-factorial assessment and an individual falls prevention programme from a trained clinician or at a falls prevention clinic.

Dementia and delirium

More than 800,000 people are living with dementia in the UK alone, a figure expected to rise to over a million by 2021 (Alzheimer's Disease Society, 2012). Dementia is not one condition but a syndrome characterised by a decline of mental and physical abilities including communication. There are many types of dementia, the most common being Alzheimer's disease (AD), Vascular Dementia (VD), fronto-lobal dementia and dementia with Lewy bodies. Although the majority of people affected by dementia are over 65, approximately 17,000 people under this age are also affected by early onset of the disease (Alzheimer's Society, 2012).

AD is characterised by a progressive deterioration of brain function, whereas people with a diagnosis of VD may experience a rapid decline in function followed by a period of no decline before the next rapid decline (for further details of the aetiology of dementia, see the SCIE resources at the end of this chapter). The most important issue for nurses is to understand that the behaviour exhibited by people living with dementia will be dictated by the type of dementia they have and the area of the brain most affected. It is widely accepted that dementia is a journey for the person living with the condition *and* the caregivers supporting them (Newbronner et al., 2013). The deterioration of abilities will also vary from person to person which further instils the need for individualised person-centred care (Social Care Institute for Excellence, 2013). Equally, family caregivers will have different needs (Newbronner et al., 2013) so it is important that nurses don't adopt a 'one size fits all' approach to supporting families. Often the person with dementia may present to services at a point of crisis and so families may be stressed and tired and require additional support from staff (Jurgens et al., 2012).

Memory function, reasoning and communication are generally the common factors most affected by the onset of dementia. This presents challenges for staff in acute and busy environments as people with dementia are not able to communicate in the same way as older people without dementia. This may result in outbursts of aggressive or challenging behaviour caused by frustration. Family caregivers are able to share knowledge about the person's daily routines that may help to reduce frustration and subsequent behaviours. In addition the person will be exposed to the confusing effects of moving between departments and/or wards and seeing a number of different people, when they may only be used to seeing one or two people per day. Equally, they may be experiencing pain or feeling ill and being bombarded with information from multiple sources, which may cause additional stress resulting in different psychological responses (see Table 12.2).

Admissions often cause disruption for the caregiver as well as the person with dementia, and caregivers often seek to work in partnership with staff to minimise this disruption (Clissett et al., 2013). However, nurses do not always recognise this and may ignore the support being offered. This can have a negative effect by making families more critical of the care being provided (Jurgens et al., 2012). It is important that nurses recognise the needs of caregivers to be involved, and listen to the information they provide about the needs of the person with dementia (Clissett et al., 2013).

Table 12.2   Common responses for people with dementia to hospital

Psychological	Physical
• Stress	• Disturbance in relation to activities of living
• Fear	e.g.
• Agitation and/or aggression	• Sleep patterns
• Vocalisations	• Nutrition
• Wandering or excessive walking	• Hydration
• Searching	• Elimination
• Wanting to go home	• Mobility

Clarke et al. (2003) undertook a pilot investigation into supporting care staff undertake life history work with people living with dementia to improve person-centred care in an acute context. By encouraging older people to talk about their life experiences staff are able to gain a fuller appreciation of people's needs, concerns and aspirations (Clarke et al., 2003). Life story work is being used more widely across dementia care and usually involves the construction of a life story book (McKeown et al., 2006), although it is recognised that in acute care this can take more time than is available to staff (Clarke et al., 2003). However, a practice development project undertaken with staff in a dementia environment suggests that the focused use of biographical information can also promote person-centred practice and is a helpful mechanism to involve families (Brown Wilson et al., 2013).

It is important that nurses do not make assumptions about the behaviour of people living with dementia attributing it solely to their dementia; changes in behaviour may also be a result of underlying physical issues such as pain or the onset of infection. Family caregivers can provide important information on the changes they may have observed immediately prior to admission. For example, a Urinary Tract Infection (UTI) continues to be a reason for older people being admitted to hospital. Using questionnaires to document the cues an older person might exhibit to suggest a change in their condition has been found to be acceptable to both nurses and patients in acute services (Hill, 2012). Infection in older people may result in delirium, which often presents with cognitive confusion and may be misdiagnosed as dementia. The key difference between the two conditions is that the cognitive confusion that presents with delirium is acute in onset and improves with appropriate treatment. Busy staff may confuse delirium with dementia but often families can provide accurate information about the older person's cognition before the admission. Involving family caregivers in the assessment process may facilitate important diagnoses such as delirium.

Delirium is a little understood condition that when experienced by older patients often results in increased length of stay and poorer outcomes as older people may have less resources to cope with illness and/or the ill effects caused by hospitalisation. This situation may be further compounded if nurses subscribe to the myth that all older people are likely to be confused because of their age, rather than a result of underlying and treatable conditions. Delirium is different from dementia as it is acute in onset, often with families telling healthcare staff that their family member is not generally confused. There are a number of risk factors associated with delirium, for example age, fever, co-morbidities, malnutrition, dehydration and low serum albumin (Siddiqi et al., 2007). There are few effective known interventions, but there is a recognition that following a comprehensive assessment, a multi-factorial approach is required to treat the underlying causes (Siddiqi et al., 2007).

In one practice development project, nurses were able to identify and treat the early onset of delirium when patients and relatives identified early behavioural or cognitive changes that might go unrecognised by staff (Hill, 2012).

 ## MR BANKS

Mr Banks has been sent by his general practitioner to the emergency department due to second degree burns on his right leg from his electric fire. On initial assessment he appears unkempt, wearing soiled clothes, in a confused state, and disorientated to time and place. The emergency doctors request an urgent care home placement, prescribe painkillers and non adhesive, antimicrobial wound care dressings. You are asked to assist the social worker to set up the care home package and to contact the family. On contacting the family you discover that Mr Banks is usually self caring but since his wife died six weeks ago he has not been coping at home, has not been eating and drinking, and has stopped going out bowling with his friends.

What further assessments need to be carried out in order to gain a comprehensive, systematic and comprehensive nursing assessment of Mr Banks' needs? What acute problems or illnesses could have led to his delirium? What nursing actions do you think would benefit Mr Banks and how would these enable him to return home and maintain his independence?

Case Scenario

Chapter summary

As an adult nurse, you must be aware of the myths and stereotypes of ageing and ensure these are not influencing key decisions in how you support older people. Subscribing to the myths of ageing or stereotyping older people may precipitate decisions leading to a lack of dignity in care giving. Seeing the person not the condition is essential to ensure the dignity of older people, including those living with dementia, is maintained.

Person-centred care delivery in any setting challenges a nurse to see the person rather than the condition, and is a further mechanism whereby dignity can be enhanced in caregiving. Adopting a biographical approach to care planning is a first step in identifying what is important to the older person and how this might be integrated into their care. For people living with dementia, knowing their usual routines and working to ensure these are maintained in unfamiliar environments will enable staff to understand their responses.

Healthy lifestyles are as influential as genetic factors in helping older people avoid the decline traditionally associated with ageing. Many chronic diseases can also be prevented by maintaining a healthy and active lifestyle throughout the life course. As an adult nurse, you will be well placed to advise on health promotion factors such as physical activity, healthy diets, smoking cessation, immunisation uptake and optimum management of chronic diseases to prevent a deterioration in health. Regular physical activity has been shown to contribute to improvements in both physical and psychological function, including a reduction of depressive symptoms. It contributes to a healthier independent life style by significantly improving the functional capacity and quality of life for older people. Older people also need to be aware of the high risk of falls and should be encouraged to undertake strength and balance exercises to try and reduce falls and fall-related fractures and injuries, as well as improve their functioning. Older people with a history of falls should be referred to a fall prevention clinic or a trained therapist for a comprehensive assessment of risk factors and a tailored programme to prevent further falls.

Not all older people are frail, but the risk of frailty increases with age and sometimes a small loss of function may precipitate a crisis with a risk of poor outcomes. Frailty is a physiological syndrome characterised by multiple deficits in system functioning. Some of the manifestations, such as reduced walking speed or gait problems, are reversible even at an advanced age.

Adult nurses may be the first contact when a patient struggles with memory problems or may be the one that families discuss their concerns with when a relative is not coping. They need to be aware of the support available and encourage patients with early signs of dementia to seek a diagnosis recognising the impact on the person and family when a diagnosis of dementia is made. Adult nurses also need to have an understanding of the differences between acute delirium and dementia, and act as advocates for older people to ensure that they receive a comprehensive assessment and person-centred care. The behaviour exhibited by people living with dementia will vary from person to person and so personalised care needs to be given to ensure individual needs are met.

In summary, there is still much to explore about caring effectively for older people but we hope that this chapter will encourage you to use approaches that value the older person and achieve positive changes that will affect us all as we grow old.

Suggested further reading

Bond, J., Peace, S.M., Dittmann-Kohli, F. and Westerhof, G. (2007) *Ageing in Society: European Perspectives on Gerontology*. London: Sage.

Brown Wilson, C. (2013) *Caring for Older People: A Shared Approach*. London: Sage.

Cornwell, J. (2012) *The Care of Frail Older People with Complex Needs: Time for a Revolution*. London: The King's Fund. Available at: www.kingsfund.org.uk/publications/care-frail-older-people-complex-needs-time-revolution (last accessed 16 September 2014).

McCormack, B. and McCance, T. (2010) *Person Centred Nursing: Theory and Practice*. Oxford: Wiley Blackwell.

Melzer, D., Tavakoly, B., Winder, R., Richards, S., Gericke, C. and Lang, I. (2012) 'Healthcare quality for an active later life: improving quality of prevention and treatment through information: England 2005 to 2012'. Peninsula College of Medicine and Dentistry, Ageing Research Group. Available at: www.exeter.ac.uk/media/universityofexeter/medicalschool/pdfs/Health_Care_Quality_for_an_Active_Later_Life_2012.pdf (last accessed 16 September 2014).

NHS Wales (2013) *Integrated Assessment, Planning and Review Arrangements for Older People: Guidance for Professionals in Supporting the Health, Care and Well-being of Older People*. Cardiff: Welsh Assembly Government.

Reed, J., Clarke, C. and McFarlane, A. (2011) *Nursing Older People: A Textbook for Nurses*. Buckinghamshire: Open University Press.

The Scottish Government (2013) *Scotland's National Dementia Strategy: 2013-16*. Edinburgh: The Scottish Government.

The Scottish Government (2014) *The Prevention and Management of Falls in the Community: A Framework for Action for Scotland 2014/2015* (Consultation Document). Edinburgh: The Scottish Government.

Tolson, D., Booth, J. and Schofield, I. (eds) (2011) *Evidence Informed Nursing with Older People*. Oxford: Blackwell.

Welsh Government (2014) *Declaration of Rights for Older People in Wales*. Cardiff: Welsh Assembly Government.

For more information about the biology of ageing, see Arking, R. (2006) *The Biology of Ageing: Observations and Principles,* 3rd edition. Oxford: Oxford University Press.

For more information about long-term conditions in older people, see Goodwin, N., Curry, N., Naylor, C., Ross, S. and Duldig, W. (2010) *Managing People with Long-term Conditions: An Inquiry into the Quality of General Practice in England*. London: The King's Fund. Available at: www.kingsfund.org.uk/document.rm?id=8757 (last accessed 19 August 2014).

Additional resources

There are a number of good websites that can be readily accessed to help increase your knowledge about health promotion, dignity, dementia, and exercise for older people, access accredited courses, and gain access to validated tools to screen and assess individuals at risk of falls:

Age UK: website for information on health and well-being for older people at: www.ageuk.org. uk

Baillie, L., Gallagher, A. and Wainwright, P. (2008) *Defending Dignity: Challenges and Opportunities*. London: RCN.

Bridges, J., Flatley, M., Meyer, J. and Brown Wilson, C. (2009) *Best Practice for Older People in Acute Care Settings (BPOP): Guidance for Nurses*. Available at: http://nursingstandard. rcnpublishing.co.uk/shared/media/multimedia/index.htm (last accessed 10 March 2015).

British Geriatric Society resources on the diagnosis and treatment of delirium are available at: www.bgs.org.uk (last accessed 10 March 2015).

Dignified Revolution: www.dignifiedrevolution.org.uk

Elvish, R., Burrow, S., Cawley, R., et al. (2013) '"Getting to Know Me": the development and evaluation of a training programme for enhancing skills in the care of people with dementia in general hospital settings', *Ageing Ment Health*, 18(4).

Healthcare Quality Strategies for more information about the issues of medication and falls. Available at: www.hqsi.org

The King's Fund Project on Dementia at: www.kingsfund.org.uk

Later Life Training website for online support and audio files on specific exercises and training programmes for falls prevention. Available at: www.laterlifetraining.co.uk (last accessed 10 March 2015).

Prevention of Falls Network for Dissemination website for resources, updates and an online forum for advice and discussion. Available at: http://profound.eu.com (last accessed 10 March 2015).

Royal College of Nursing's dignity campaign. Available at: www.rcn.org.uk

Royal College of Nursing's dementia resources. Available at: www.rcn.org.uk

Social Care Institute for Excellence's dementia resources. Available at: www.scie.org.uk/ publications/dementia/index.asp (last accessed 10 March 2015).

References

Abrahams, A. (2011) *Care and Compassion? Report of the Health Service Ombudsman on Ten Investigations into NHS Care of Older People.* London: HMSO.

Age UK (Age Concern and Help the Aged) (2009) *One Voice: Shaping our Ageing Society.* London: Age Concern.

All-Party Parliamentary Group on Dementia (2011) *The £20 Billion Question: An Inquiry into Improving Lives through Cost-effective Dementia Services.* Available at: www.alzheimers.org.uk/site/scripts/download_info.php?fileID=1207 (last accessed 19 August 2014).

Alzheimer's Society (2012) *Dementia 2012.* London: Alzheimer's Society.

American Geriatrics Society, British Geriatrics Society, and American Academy of Orthopaedic Surgeons Panel on Falls Prevention (AGS/BGS) (2010) 'Clinical Practice guideline: Prevention of falls in older persons', *J Am Geriatr Soc.* Available at: www.americangeriatrics.org/files/documents/health_care_pros/JAGS.Falls.Guidelines.pdf (last accessed 19 August 2014).

Anderson, R.A., Issel, L.M. and McDaniel Jr., R.R. (2003) 'Nursing homes as complex adaptive systems: relationship between management practice and resident outcomes', *Nursing Research,* 52(1): 12–21.

Arking, R. (2006) *The Biology of Ageing: Observations and Principles.* New York: OUP.

Bayer, T., Tadd, W. and Krajcik, S. (2005) 'Dignity: the voice of older people', *Quality in Ageing,* 6 (1): 22–9.

Bond, J., Peace, S.M., Dittmann-Kohli, F. and Westerhof, G. (2007) *Ageing in Society: European Perspectives on Gerontology.* London: Sage.

Bowers, H., Lockwood, S., Eley, A., Catley, A., Runnicles, D., Mordey, M., Barker, S., Thomas, N., Jones, C. and Dalziel, S. (2013) *Widening Choices for Older People with High Support Needs.* York: Joseph Rowntree Foundation.

Bridges, J., Flatley, M. and Meyer, J. (2010) 'Older people's and relatives' experiences in acute care settings: systematic review and synthesis of qualitative studies', *International Journal of Nursing Studies,* 47: 89–107.

British Heart Foundation (BHF) (2010) *A Toolkit For the Design, Implementation and Evaluation of Exercise Referral Schemes,* BHF National Centre, Loughborough University.

Brooker, D. (2004) 'What is person centred care in dementia?', *Reviews in Clinical Gerontology,* 13: 215–22.

Brown Wilson, C. (2009) 'Developing community in care homes through a relationship-centred approach', *Health and Social Care in the Community,* 17(2): 177–86.

Brown Wilson, C. (2013) *Caring for Older People: A Shared Approach.* London: Sage.

Brown Wilson, C. and Davies, S. (2009) 'Using relationships in care homes to develop relationship centred care: the contribution of staff', *Journal of Clinical Nursing,* 18: 1746–55.

Brown Wilson, C., Swarbrick, C., Pilling, M. and Keady, J. (2013) 'The senses in practice: enhancing the quality of care for residents with dementia in care homes', *Journal of Advanced Nursing,* 69(1): 77–90.

Centers for Disease Control and Prevention (1996) *Physical Activity and Health: A Report of the Surgeon General Executive (Summary).* Washington, DC: US Department Of Health And Human Services.

Chief Medical Officer (2011) *Public Health Guidelines on Physical Activity for Older Adults.* London: Department of Health.

Clarke, A., Hanson, E.J. and Ross, H. (2003) 'Seeing the person behind the patient: enhancing the care of older people using a biographical approach', *Journal of Clinical Nursing,* 12: 697.

Clissett, P., Porrock, D., Harwood, R. and Gladman, J. (2013) 'Experiences of family carers of older people with mental health problems in an acute general hospital: a qualitative study', *Journal of Advanced Nursing,* 69(12): 2707–16.

Cornwell, J. (2012) *The Care of Frail Older People with Complex Needs: Time for a Revolution.* London: The King's Fund/The Sir Roger Bannister Health Summit, Leeds Castle.

Department of Health (2001) *Involving Patients and the Public in Healthcare: A Discussion Document*. London: DH.

Department of Health (2009) *Be Active, Be Healthy: A Plan for Getting the Nation Moving*. London: DH.

Department of Health (2012) *Compassion in Practice: Nursing, Midwifery and Care Staff, Our Vision and Strategy*. London: DH.

Department of Health (2013) *Patients First and Foremost: The Initial Government Response to the Report of The Mid Staffordshire NHS Foundation Trust Public Inquiry*. London: DH.

Dewar, B. (2011) 'Caring about Caring: An Appreciative Inquiry about Compassionate Relationship-Centred Care'. Unpublished PhD thesis, Edinburgh Napier University. Available at: http://researchrepository.napier.ac.uk/4845/ (last accessed 19 August 2014).

Dewing, J. (2004) 'Concerns relating to the application of frameworks to promote person-centredness in nursing older people', *International Journal of Older People Nursing*, 13(3a): 39–44.

Ellis, G., Whitehead, M.A., O'Neill, D., Langhorne, P. and Robinson, D. (2011) 'Comprehensive geriatric assessment for older adults admitted to hospital', *Cochrane Database of Systematic Reviews*, Issue 7. Art. No.: CD006211. doi: 10.1002/14651858.CD006211.pub2.

Ferrucci, L., Guralnik, J.M., Studenski, S., et al. (2004) 'Interventions on Frailty Working Group: designing randomized, controlled trials aimed at preventing or delaying functional decline and disability in frail, older persons: a consensus report', *J Am Geriatr Soc*; 52: 625–34.

Fiatarone, M.A., Marks, E.C., Ryan, D.T., Meredith, C.N., Lewis, A., Lipsitz, M.D. and Evans, W.J. (1990) 'High-intensity strength training in nonagenarians', *Journal of the American Medical Association*, 263 (22): 3029–34.

Fiske, S.T., Cuddy, A.J., Glick, P.C. and Xu, J. (2002) 'A model of (often mixed) stereotype content: competence and warmth respectively follow from perceived status and competition', *Journal of Personality and Social Psychology*, 82(6): 878–902.

Francis, R. (2011) *The Mid-Staffordshire NHS Foundation Trust Public Enquiry* Available at: www.midstaffspublicinquiry.com/news/2011/12/transcript- thursday-1–december-2011 (last accessed 18 March 2015).

Francis, R. (2013) *Report of the Mid Staffordshire NHS Foundation Trust Public Enquiry*. London: DH.

Fried, L.P., Ferrucci, L., Darer, J. et al. (2004) 'Untangling the concepts of disability, frailty, and co-morbidity: implications for improved targeting and care', *J Gerontol A Biol Sci Med Sci*; 59A: M255–M263.

Fultz, N.H.A. and Regula Herzog, A.R. (2000) 'Prevalence of urinary incontinence in middle-aged and older women: a survey-based methodological experiment', *J Ageing Health*, 12: 459–69.

Gillespie, L.D., Robertson, M.C., Gillespie, W.J., Sherrington, C., Gates, S., Clemson, L.M. and Lamb, S.E. (2012) 'Interventions for preventing falls in older people living in the community', *Cochrane Database of Systematic Reviews*, Issue 9. Art. No.: CD007146. doi: 10.1002/14651858.CD007146.pub3.

Goodrich, J. and Cornwell, J. (2008) *Seeing the Person in the Patient: The Point of Care Review Paper*. London: The King's Fund.

Goodwin, N., Curry, N., Naylor, C., Ross, S. and Duldig, W. (2010) *Managing People with Long-term Conditions: An Inquiry into the Quality of General Practice in England*. London: The King's Fund. Available at: www.kingsfund.org.uk/document.rm?id=8757 (last accessed 19 August 2014).

Greenhalgh, T., Procter, R., Wherton, J., Sugarhood, P. and Shaw, S. (2012) 'The organising vision for telehealth and telecare: discourse analysis', *BMJ Open*, 2: 4.

Hill, K. (2012) 'Critical to care: improving the care to the acutely ill and deteriorating patient', Foundation of Nursing Studies Project Report. Available at: http://fons.org/library/report-details.aspx?nstid=18132 (last accessed 19 August 2014).

Institute of Medicine (IOM) (2001) *Crossing the Quality Chasm: A New Health System for the 21st Century*. Washington, DC: National Academy Press.

Jacelon, C. (2003) 'The dignity of elders in acute care hospital', *Qualitative Health Research*, 13 (4): 543–56.

Jones, D., Song, X. and Rockwood, K. (2004) 'Operationalizing a frailty index from a standardized comprehensive geriatric assessment', *J AmGeriatr Soc*, 52: 1929–33.

Jurgens, F., Clissett, P., Gladman, J. and Harwood, R. (2012) 'Why are family carers of people with dementia dissatisfied with general hospital care? A qualitative study', *BMC Geriatrics*, 12(57): 1471–2318.

Kempen, G.I., Yardley, L., van Haastregt, J.C., et al. (2008) 'The Short FES-I: a shortened version of the falls efficacy scale-international to assess fear of falling', *Age and Ageing*, 37(1): 44–50.

Kitwood, T. (1997) *Dementia Reconsidered: The Person Comes First*. Buckingham: Open University Press.

Knoops, K.T., de Groot, L.C., Kromhout, D., Perrin, A.E., Moreiras-Varela, O., Menotti, A. and van Staveren, W.A. (2004) 'Mediterranean diet, lifestyle factors, and 10-year mortality in elderly European men and women: the HALE project', *JAMA*, 292(12):1433–9.

Lamb, S.E., Jorstad-Stein, E.C., Hauer, K. and Becker, C. (2005) 'Development of a common outcome data set for fall injury prevention trials: the prevention of falls network Europe consensus', *Journal of the American Geriatrics Society*, 53: 1618–22.

LeBlanc, A., Schneider, V., Krebs, J., Evans, H., Jhingran, S. and Johnson, P. (1987) 'Spinal bone mineral after 5 weeks of bed rest', *Calcif Tissue Int*, 41: 259–61.

Levenson, R. (2007) *The Challenge of Dignity in Care: Upholding the Rights of the Individual*. London: Help the Aged.

Magee, H., Parsons, S. and Askham, J. (2008) *Measuring Dignity in Care for Older People: A Research Report for Help the Aged*. London: Help the Aged.

McCormack B. and McCance T. (2006) 'Development of a framework for person centred nursing', *Journal of Advanced Nursing*, 56 (5): 472–9.

McCormack, B. and McCance, T. (2010) *Person Centred Nursing: Theory and Practice*. Oxford: Wiley Blackwell.

McKeown, J., Clarke A. and Repper J. (2006) 'Life story work in health and social care: systematic literature review', *Journal of Advanced Nursing*, 55(2): 237–47.

Minkler, M. (1996) 'Critical perspectives on ageing: new challenges for gerontology', *Ageing and Society*, 16: 467–87.

Mitniski, A., Song, A. and Rockwood, K. (2004) 'The estimation of relative fitness and frailty in community-dwelling older adults', *Journal of Gerontology: Medical Sciences*, 59A(6):627–632.

Mitnitski, A., Song, X., Skoog, I., Broe, G.A., Cox, J., Grunfeld, E. and Rockwood, K. (2005) 'Relative fitness and frailty of elderly men and women in developed countries and their relationship with mortality', *J Am Geriatr Soc* 53: 2184–9.

Nandy, S., Parsons, S., Cryer, C., Underwood, M., Rashbrook, E., Carter, Y., Eldridge, S., Close, J., Skelton, D., Taylor, S. and Feder, G. (2004) 'On behalf of the falls prevention pilot steering group: development and preliminary examination of the predictive validity of the falls risk assessment tool (FRAT) for use in primary care', *Journal of Public Health*, 26 (2): 138–43.

National Institute for Clinical Excellence (2008) 'Mental well-being and older people', NICE Public Health Guidance 16. Available at: www.guidance.nice.org.uk/ph16 (last accessed 7 July 2014).

National Institute for Clinical Excellence (2013) *Falls: Assessment and Prevention of Falls in Older People, NICE Public Health Guidance CG161*. Available at: www.nice.org.uk/guidance/CG161 accessed on 07/07/14 (last accessed 7 July 2014).

Newbronner, L., Chamberlain, R., Borthwick, R., Baxter, M. and Glendinning, C. (2013) *A Road Less Rocky: Supporting Carers of People with Dementia*. London: Carers Trust.

NMC (2010a) *Standards for Pre-registration Nursing Education*. Available at: http://standards.nmc-uk.org (last accessed 19 November 2014).

NMC (2010b) *Standards for Competence for Registered Nurses*. Available at: www.nmc-uk.org/Documents/Standards/Standards%20for%20competence.pdf. (last accessed 19 November 2014).

Nordenfelt, L. and Edgar, A. (2005) 'The four notions of dignity', *Quality in Ageing*, 6(1): 17–21.

Office for National Statistics (2011) *Mid-2010 Population Estimates UK*. London: ONS.

Orrell, A., McKee, K., Dahlberg, L., Gilhooly, M. and Parker, S. (2013) 'Improving continence services for older people from the service-providers' perspective: a qualitative interview study', *BMJ Open*, 3 (7).

Pickard, S. and Glendinning, C. (2002) 'Caring for a relative with dementia: the perceptions of carers and CPNs', *Quality in Ageing*, 2: 3–11.

Podsiadlo, D.A. and Richardson, S. (1991) 'The timed up and go: a test of functional mobility for frail elder persons', *Journal of the American Geriatrics Society*, 39: 142–8.

Robertson, M.C., Campbell, A.J., Gardner, M.M. and Devlin, N. (2002) 'Meta-analysis of the four trials', *Journal of the American Geriatric Society*, 50: 905–11.

Rockwood, K. and Koller, K. (2013) 'Frailty in older adults: implications for end of life care', *Cleveland Clinic Journal of Medicine*, 80 (3): 168–74.

Rockwood, K., Fox, R., Stolee, P., Robertson, B. and Beattie, L. (1994) 'Frailty in elderly people: an evolving concept', *Can Med Assoc J*; 150 (4): 489–95.

Rockwood, K., Mitnitski, A., Song, X., Steen, B. and Skoog, I. (2006) 'Long-term risks of death and institutionalization of elderly people in relation to deficit accumulation at age 70', *J Am Geriatr Soc*: 1–5.

Rogers, S., Martin, G. and Rai, G. (2014) 'Medicines management support to older people: understanding the context of systems failure', *BMJ Open*, 4: 7.

Roper N., Logan W.W. and Tierney A.J. (2000) *The Roper-Logan-Tierney Model of Nursing: Based on Activities of Living*. Edinburgh: Elsevier Health Sciences.

Rossiter-Fornoff, J.E., Wolf, S.L., Wolfson, L.I., Buchner, D.M. and FICSIT Group (1995) 'A cross-sectional validation study of the FCSIT common database static balance measures', *Journal of Gerontology: Medical Sciences*, 50A: M291–7.

Røsvik, J.J., Kirkevold, M., Engedal, K., Brooker, D. and Kirkevold, Ø. (2011) 'A model for using the VIPS framework for person-centred care for persons with dementia in nursing homes: a qualitative evaluative study', *International Journal of Older People Nursing*, 6: 227–36.

Royal College of Physicians (2011) *Falling Standards, Broken Promises: Report of the National Audit of Bone Health in Older People in 2010*. London: RCP.

Royal College of Physicians (2012) *Hospitals on the Edge*. London: RCP.

Sherrington, C., Whitney, J.C., Lord, S.R., Herbert, R.D., Cumming, R.D. and Close, J.C. (2008) 'Effective exercise for the prevention of falls: a systematic review and meta-analysis', *Journal of the American Geriatric Society*, 56(12): 2234–43.

Siddiqi, N., Holt, R., Britton, A.M. and Holmes, J. (2007) 'Interventions for preventing delirium in hospitalised patients', *Cochrane Database of Systematic Reviews 2007*, Issue 2. Art. No.: CD005563. doi: 10.1002/14651858.CD005563.pub2.

Skelton, D.A., Dinan, S.M., Campbell, M.G. and Rutherford, O.M. (2005) 'Tailored Group Exercise (Falls Management Exercise - FaME) reduces falls in community-dwelling older frequent fallers (an RCT)', *Age and Ageing*, 34: 636–9.

Smith, M.E., Dunphy, L.M. and Mainous, R.O. (2011) 'Innovative nursing educational curriculum for the 21st century'. In National Research Council (ed.), *The Future of Nursing: Leading Change, Advancing Health*. Washington, DC: The National Academies Press.

Social Care Institute for Excellence (n.d.) *Dignity in Care*. Available at: www.scie.org.uk/publications/guides/guide15/selectedresearch/whatdignitymeans.asp (last accessed 13 March 2015).

Sorensen, L., Waldorff, F. and Waldemar, G. (2008) 'Early counselling and support for patients with mild Alzheimer's Disease and their caregivers: a qualitative study on outcomes', *Ageing and Mental Health*, 12 (4): 444–50.

Stanmore, E.K. (2011) 'Choice, appropriateness and adequacy of care for older people: utilising patients and professionals views to identify future service improvements', *The International Journal of Person-Centered Medicine*, 1(3): 522–6.

Stanmore, E.K. (2013) 'The importance of falls assessment in patients with rheumatoid arthritis', *Journal of Health Visiting*, 1(2): 5.

Stanmore, E.K., Oldham, J., Skelton, D.A. et al. (2013a) 'Fall incidence and outcomes of falls in a prospective study of adults with rheumatoid arthritis', *Arthritis Care Res*, 65(5): 737–44.

Stanmore, E.K., Oldham, J., Skelton, D.A., et al. (2013b) 'Risk factors for falls in adults with rheumatoid arthritis: a prospective study', *Arthritis Care & Research*, 65(8): 1251–8.

Steventon, A., Bardsley, M., Billings, J., Dixon, J., Doll, H., Beynon, M., Hirani, S., Cartwright, M., Rixon, L., Knapp, M., Henderson, C., Rogers, S., Hendy, J., Fitzpatrick, R. and Newman, S. (2013) 'Effect of telecare on use of health and social care services: findings from the Whole Systems Demonstrator cluster randomised trial', *Age and Ageing*.

Tadd, W., Hillman, A., Calnan, S., Calnan, M., Bayer, T. and Read, S. (2011) *Dignity in Practice: An Exploration of the Care of Older Adults in Acute NHS Trusts: Service Delivery and Organisation Programme*. Available at: www.sdo.nihr.ac.uk/files/project/SDO_FR_08-1819–218_V01.pdf (last accessed 25 July 2014).

The National Council on Ageing (2013) *Debunking the Myths of Older Adult Falls*. Available at: www.ncoa.org/ (last accessed on 19 August 2014).

The Social Care Institute for Excellence (2013) *Dignity*. Available at: www.scie.org.uk/publications/guides/guide15/index.asp (last accessed on 19 August 2014).

van Diest, M., Lamoth, C.J., Stegenga, J., Verkerke, G.J. and Postema, K. (2013) 'Exergaming for balance training of elderly: state of the art and future developments', *J Neuroeng Rehabil*, 10: 101.

Wilmoth, J,M. and Ferraro, K.F. (eds) (2013) *Gerontology Perspectives and Issues*. New York: Springer.

World Health Organization (2002) *Ageing: A Policy Framework*. Geneva: World Health Organization. Available at: http://whqlibdoc.who.int/hq/2002/WHO_NMH_NPH_02.8.pdf (last accessed 30 March 2012).

World Health Organization (2007) *WHO Global Report on Falls Prevention in Older Age*. Geneva: World Health Organization.

13   The Provision of Effective Palliative Care for Adults

JOHN COSTELLO

Most people in the UK die in hospital (National End of Life Care Intelligence Network, 2013), with around 58% of people dying in acute hospital settings (Gardiner et al., 2013). An essential part of adult nursing involves you having the competence and confidence to care for patients with a life-limiting illness, providing them with high quality palliative care. The challenges associated with this lie in your ability to not only give high quality care to the patient but also to offer psychosocial support to the family. In many respects palliative care constitutes the essence of what is referred to as holistic care in the real sense of enabling both the patient and the family to experience what is referred to as *a good death* (Costello, 2006).

This chapter introduces some of the key issues relating to palliative care for adult nursing, providing explanations about terms such as 'a good death' and how these can be applied in the context of adult nursing. End of life care should reflect contemporary developments in policy and practice, as well as considering the challenges of caring for patients who live with a life-limiting illness and are cared for in hospitals, community and hospice settings.

The main focus of the chapter will be placed in the acute hospital context as this is where most patients in the UK die. The essence of much end of life care for adults has been to transfer the gold standards of care often seen in hospices into the acute hospital care context. Strategies and contemporary developments that have formed part of contemporary palliative care (e.g. Integrated Care Pathways, the Gold Standard Framework and Preferred Priorities of Care (DH, 2004)) will be explained and discussed. I will explain and discuss the strategies and contemporary developments that have formed part of contemporary palliative care. In writing this chapter, I make the assumption that you are aware that end of life care (in the past referred to as terminal care) is an integral and important part of the palliative care approach. One of the central features of end of life care is the ability of an adult nurse to demonstrate effective communication skills with the patient, family and other multi-professional team colleagues. The development of a therapeutic relationship with the patient forms a significant part of the final section of the chapter and constitutes a key element of its take-home message. Before reading and working with this chapter, it is appropriate to point out that some of the content and interactive text could potentially cause some readers to become emotional as the case studies reflect authentic situations. The text may cause you to recall sad and painful experiences or you may feel empathy with what is being discussed. It is entirely natural that you may feel this way. As a way of helping you consider your feelings in relation to thinking about loss, try to reflect on your past loss experiences and consider undertaking Activity 13.1 (using loss lines). The completion of this should help you focus on the loss and its impact. It is not uncommon for nurses to feel emotional and upset when managing patients with a life-limiting illness, it is an indication that we feel for others. It is perhaps more worrying when we do not feel slightly emotional when working with patients and families at the end of life.

After reading this chapter you should be able to:

- Develop a clear understanding of the way in which palliative care for adults has been developed in the UK.
- Discuss the importance of the development of a therapeutic relationship in palliative care.
- Be able to describe and discuss what constitutes a good death for the patient, the family and for health practitioners.
- Discuss and describe effective end of life care for the patient and the family and how to initiate, implement and carry out this care effectively and sensitively.

Related NMC competencies

An overarching NMC requirement is that adult nurses must:

... recognise and respond to the challenges of adults, families and carers during terminal illness. They must be aware of how treatment goals and service user choices may change at different stages of progressive illness, loss and bereavement. (NMC, 2010: 7)

To achieve entry to the register as an adult nurse you should be able to:

- Promote and support the health, well-being, rights and dignity of people whose lives are affected by ill health, disability, ageing, death and dying.
- Plan, deliver and evaluate safe, competent, person-centred care in partnership with patients, paying special attention to changing health needs during different life stages, including progressive illness and death, loss and bereavement.
- Recognise and address ethical challenges relating to people's choices and decision making about their care and act within the law to help them and their families find acceptable solutions.
- Understand and apply current legislation, paying special attention to those with complex needs who are approaching the end of their life.

(Adapted from NMC, 2010a, 2010b.)

Background

The term 'palliative' in its Latin translation means *to cloak* and can cause confusion amongst health professionals and lay care givers. It is often used by medical staff when other active methods of intervention are ineffective, or when it is clear that the patient's condition is no longer susceptible to curative methods of treatment. The confusion regarding when and what constitutes palliative care is part of the problem that many nurses have in explaining to families what is happening to patients. Palliative care is focused on patients with a life-limiting illness (not necessarily cancer) when the chances of curative treatment are diminished.

Historically, palliative care emerged from the hospice movement during the 1960s when one of the first hospices (St Christopher's) was built in 1967 based on the pioneering work of Dame Cecily Saunders. Saunders trained as a nurse in 1948, became a medical social worker and finally a physician. Not only did she care for dying patients, she was also a prolific writer, publishing her work internationally. She is regarded as the founder of St Christopher's Hospice, the first research and teaching hospice linked with clinical care and focused on palliative medicine. Saunders was dismayed when, as a nurse, she cared for dying patients experiencing distress at the end of life. Her motivation to improve standards partly stemmed from the poor prescribing habits of medical staff who, at the time, were reluctant to prescribe morphine to patients in pain. Saunders wanted patients to receive what is referred to as tender loving care (TLC) and for both patients and family members to experience a good death (Saunders et al., 2003). Her famous quote follows: 'You matter because you are you, and you matter to the end of your life. We will do all we can not only to help you die peacefully, but also to live until you die', epitomises her concept of total pain, the notion that patients are more than a set of symptoms. Her philosophy was based on the provision of physical, psychological, social and spiritual care from the time of diagnosis until death.

Contemporary end of life policy and standards

Contemporary end of life care has received a lot of attention through the government's strategy to develop, maintain and improve end of life care, encapsulated in the End of Life Care Programme (DH, 2008) which sets out to improve end of life care through effective communication, education and the development of high quality evidence-based care. The evidence is summarised in the quality standards from NICE (2011) where quality standard QS13 *End of Life Care for Adults* indicates the best practice to adopt for patients at the end of life. This covers all settings and services providing end of life care to adults in the UK, including adults who die suddenly or after a very brief illness. The quality standard does not cover condition-specific management and care, clinical management of specific physical symptoms, or emergency planning and mass casualty incidents.

Principles of palliative care

Palliative care is focused on a number of key principles that are largely associated with quality of life. Becker (2009) discusses the importance of ensuring that the patient is considered to be the central feature of care management, with the needs of the family a close second.

Many of the key principles of palliative care are encapsulated in Figure 13.1. These principles suggest that like other nursing specialisms holistic care is required in order to ensure the philosophy described by Saunders earlier is adhered to. In order to do this, nurses providing palliative care need to consider the needs of the family/significant others as very important. For example, there may come a point in the patient's illness trajectory when they are not conscious or may be in a *Persistent Vegetative State* (PVS). In such circumstances, the nurse provides all the care to the patient but should also pay attention to the emotional needs of the family who may require as much emotional support as possible (Main, 2002). In circumstances whereby the patient does not have any meaningful social contact with those around them, it is important to enhance communication with family members. Sweeting and Gilhooley (1992) refer to patients unable to have any significant social contact with others as being 'socially dead'. This could include patients receiving artificial ventilation and or those with advanced dementia. It is in such cases that the nurse and the rest of the team need to focus closely on family needs. Working as a team and collaborating together is one of the ideals of palliative care, although as McIlfatrick (2013) points out embracing this ideal is easier said than done. Despite this, working together as a team (including social workers, physiotherapists and the spiritual care team) is vital to the provision of high standards of care. The latter is often more successful in hospice contexts than in hospitals where a curative ideology prevails (Costello, 2004).

- Neither hastens or postpones death
- Views death as a natural healthy process
- Emphasis on the importance of quality of life
- Embraces the notion of team working
- Control of symptoms is a priority
- Focuses on the patient and the family
- Considers spiritual and psychosocial needs

Figure 13.1   Principles of palliative care
Adapted from Becker, R. (2010) *Fundamental Aspects of Palliative Care Nursing*, 2nd edition.

ACTIVITY 13.1

We are all affected by loss, be it the death of a family pet or the death of a relative, grandparent, friend, or a patient that we felt emotionally close to. The impact of loss can influence our thoughts, feelings and ideas and how we approach palliative provision. It is useful to reflect on your own losses. This activity requires you to make a short list of three or four significant losses that have occurred in your life. 'Loss lines' asks you to draw a line for every loss that you have experienced in your life. The length of each horizontal line denotes its emotional internsity. Some lines may be shorter than others. The aim of the activity is to get you to reflect on loss and its impact on how you felt. It's also worth considering what sources of support were available and how you used these.

BIRTH

NOW

Loss lines is a useful exercise to do with family members who may be feeling confused or uncertain about what their feelings are. It can help put their thoughts and ideas into perspective. It is therefore helpful if you do the exercise yourself and consider what helped you manage the loss and how you feel as a result of it. Do you still feel that there are issues that you could and should have resolved, or do you as the proverb states feel stronger as a result of the experience on the basis of that which does not kill you makes you stronger?

BIRTH

Aged 5: My mum took me to school but did not explain that she would leave me there, I felt as if I had lost my relationship with my mother (very long line).

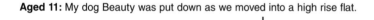

Aged 11: My dog Beauty was put down as we moved into a high rise flat.

Aged 15: My grandmother died but I was not emotionally close to her so I felt very little loss even though it was my first bereavement.

My mum died in 1981, I was very distressed, it was a bad death and I was very unprepared and felt unsupported (very long line).

My father died at home after a long illness, we cared for him until he died, it was a good death but sad.

NOW

Figure 13.2   Author's loss line

Diagnosing dying

A major challenge for palliative care practitioners is knowing when a patient is approaching death. The need for preparation and planning is important if the patient's death is to be well managed. Effective palliative care involves closely monitoring patients whose medical condition has become life threatening. Moreover, one of the major challenges facing many healthcare practitioners, and particularly nurses, has always been to identify when a patient has reached the point where active treatment is no longer an option (Broeckaert, 2008). Ellershaw and Wilkinson (2011: 21) point out that when it is suspected that a patient is dying because of a significant deterioration in their condition a number of considerations need to be made. In the early days of the Liverpool Care Pathway, ideas around when was a patient dying were based on key criteria. This consisted of a series of questions such as is the patient bed bound? What is the patient's level of consciousness, are they semi comatose? Are they able to swallow and take sips of water? Finally, can they take oral medication? Should the patient fulfil two of these criteria then it may be considered that they are likely to be in the advanced stages of dying or near to death. Elliot and Nicholson (2014) suggest that practitioners considering patients' proximity to death ask the 'surprise' question: 'Would you be surprised if the patient were to die in the next few months, weeks or days? If the answer is yes then the patient may be considered to entering the dying phase'.

Successful assessment of a patient's illness trajectory involves a thorough multidisciplinary team (MDT) assessment. Initially this is carried out when the patient is showing signs of deterioration. It is important to eliminate potentially reversible causes for the deterioration (such as an infection or opioid toxicity).

STOP AND THINK

Identify the role of each member of the multidisciplinary team in the assessment highlighted above. Which professionals might contribute to the assessment process and what might their individual roles involve?

The nurse would probably be the first person to recognise deterioration in the patient's condition. Assessment may involve the speech and language therapist assessing swallowing ability, or the physiotherapist assessing respiratory function. A patient who is very dehydrated, especially an older person who has stopped eating and drinking for whatever reason, may show signs consistent with an acute deterioration and be temporarily confused and unable or unwilling to drink. All reversible causes should be acted upon where possible to improve the patient's condition. Secondly, should the patient not respond positively to such steps, the next step is the clinical decision-making stage. This is where the MDT decide if the patient is to receive palliative care. Thirdly, and most importantly, it is at this stage that this decision involves the patient if appropriate, and/or the family, relatives and significant others. For many healthcare practitioners this can be the most difficult situation that requires tact, sensitivity, and a good relationship with the family.

Once a patient is considered to be no longer eligible for active treatment, it is important to communicate this effectively with them and/or their relatives, family or significant others. This can be one to the most challenging situations a healthcare practitioner can face.

Disclosing sensitive information

Whilst we touched upon the topic of disclosing sensitive information briefly in Chapter 2, it would be useful to revisit it again here in more detail. Often referred to as *breaking bad news*, this term has been used for many years to identify the point at which the diagnosis of a life-threatening illness is disclosed (Arnautska, 2010). However, since many patients and family members may have become aware of the condition, the disclosure will not be news but a confirmation. Moreover, in terms of the extent to which sensitive information can be disclosed, there are many other things that practitioners can tell a patient/family that are just as sensitive, such as the withdrawal/ withholding of treatment, or a decision not to resuscitate in the event of a cardiac/respiratory arrest, that can have a devastating impact on their well-being. It seems logical therefore to consider some guidance based on published work around breaking bad news. Numerous authors have identified ways of disclosing sensitive information. These include Buckman (1992), Baile et al. (2000) and Fallowfield (2005). Notable amongst these is the Spikes Model (Baile et al., 2000) which offers a clear and concise series of steps to follow that are both understandable and sensitive.

Step 1: S – SETTING UP the Interview

Step 2: P – Assessing the Patient's PERCEPTION

Step 3: I – Obtaining the Patient's INVITATION

Step 4: K – Giving KNOWLEDGE and Information to the Patient

Step 5: E – Addressing the Patient's EMOTIONS with Empathic Responses

Step 6: S – STRATEGY and SUMMARY

However, taking an eclectic approach by utilising the key components of a number of models, various principles emerge that can be seen as guidance for best practice. These principles are summarised below.

─────────── Principles of breaking bad news ───────────

Preparation of the setting, including the availability of documents such as medical notes. This can include giving the patient the opportunity to invite a friend.

Warning shot: This is an important principle that helps prepare the patient psychologically: *'I am afraid the news is rather bad, I am sorry but the results are not good'.*

Pause: Allow the patient time to consider the news.

Provide a clear/concise account: *'I am afraid you have cancer, or ... The results indicate cancer'.*

Clarify: *'The cancer is malignant',* meaning it is possible that it will spread.

Elicit the patient's concerns: *'You may be feeling shocked by this result'.*

Express treatment aspirations: *'We can and will, provide treatment and care'.*

Nurses will rarely disclose a diagnosis to a patient but many will deal with the aftermath of the encounter with the doctor, something Costello (2004) calls the emotional rescue. Evidence suggests that despite many years of education and training to improve communication about a life-threatening illness many healthcare practitioners get it wrong (Smith et al., 2012). The role of the nurse in relation to receiving bad news is to provide comfort, sometimes in the form of reassurance arising not from platitudes that *things will be all right* but from clear reassurance and knowledge based on sound evidence. Moreover, nurses are in a position to provide information about the diagnosis and the likely reactions people make when they are given bad news.

ACTIVITY 13.2

In the following situation consider what you, as a nurse, could do to help a patient in relation to trying to provide comfort and improve their well-being without being patronising.

Brenda was in bed and had just had a wash. Whilst undertaking his usual ward round, Brenda's consultant decided to give her the result of her recent bronchoscopy. As the consultant was reading Brenda's medical notes, he gestured to the staff nurse to close the curtains. Then, without looking up from the notes, he initially told Brenda in a very matter of fact manner that the result of the bronchoscopy showed that she had a large mass in her windpipe that was causing the problem with breathing, but (then looked up and said) 'We have no way of removing a cancer this large as it has progressed rather rapidly'.

Brenda went pale and sagged in the bed in a type of shock. 'What does that mean?' she said. The consultant replied that in his opinion she had a few weeks or months left and she should consider being admitted to a hospice for further care. The consultant pointed out that he appreciated that it was a difficult time but suggested she discuss things with the nurse and the hospital social worker. He then went on to continue with his rounds, leaving you alone with Brenda.

This sad and insensitive situation was obviously badly managed but could and should have been carried out in a more sensitive way. What could have been done to improve the situation in light of your reading and understanding of the SPIKES Model.

Responding to a patient's emotions is one of the most difficult challenges of breaking bad news as their emotional response may vary from silence to disbelief, crying, denial, or anger. When told bad news, a patient's emotional reaction can be expressed in many ways such as anger, shock, isolation and grief. The role of the nurse is to try to accurately identify the patient's reaction and make an empathic response. An empathic response consists of observing the patient's emotions, identifying their emotions (be they sad, angry or very distressed), and by expressing this in an understanding way (e.g. 'You sound very angry'). It is important to make an empathic response such as 'I can understand your anger' or 'You have every right to feel angry'. It is also important to connect the feeling with the response, e.g. 'I can see you are angry and this is justified'. Throughout the period after the bad news is broken the patient should be allowed time to express their feelings. Use open questions if you are unsure of what emotions are being expressed.

Breaking bad news: where things go wrong

Sadly breaking bad news is very difficult to get right as what may work for one patient will not always work every time, hence having a set of principles like the SPIKES Model is useful to enable a consistent approach to be made based on sound evidence. In relation to the previous case scenario it is easy to pick out what went wrong here. However it is more difficult to work out why the consultant chose to disclose the bad news then and there.

For example, why did he not chose a more private place, with the patient's family there to provide support? Why did he not provide a sense of hope and discuss the possibility of palliative radiotherapy to arrest the growth and enable the patient to have some hope?

One of the reasons why medical staff develop this type of approach is due to the context in which care takes place. In an acute hospital context many doctors (but by no means all!) will chose to impart news during the ward round. This is because it symbolises the major mode of communication between consultant and patient (Willard and Luker, 2006; Costello, 2004). It is the accepted norm for imparting information about, and to, the patient. Not only does the doctor consider this to be the norm, patients and relatives also regard the ward round as the place where they are updated on what is going on. In some cases relatives will plan a visit before or just after the ward round in anticipation of being updated on the latest news.

Policy context: Advanced Care Planning

Advance Care Planning (ACP) is a key part of end of life care and an integral part of the NHS End of Life Care Strategy (DH, 2008). Improving the pre-planning of care is one of the ways that nurses can ensure reliable patient-focused care. Effective palliative care includes open discussion and advanced care planning in order to enable the patient to experience a good death. This involves the use of a number of relatively recent innovations, such as Integrated Care Pathways (ICPs), the Gold Standard Framework (GSF) and the use of the Preferred Priorities of Care (PPC) document (DH, 2004). However, such organisation can be very difficult to initiate if, for example, the patient is not aware they are dying (Skilbeck and Payne, 2003). In these situations, the notion of ACP becomes problematic. Once it is established that curative treatment is no longer an option and this has been discussed with the patient and/or family, it is recommended that ACP can become a feature of the patient's end of life care (Ellershaw et al., 2010). However, when a patient dies suddenly or when their death is unexpected, ACP is not possible. The following three innovations are important aspects of ACP in end of life care and provide a broad structure of how effective care can be organised.

Advanced Care Planning 1: Integrated care pathways

Up until 2013, one of the most significant elements of Advanced Care Planning was the Liverpool Care Pathway (LCP) (Ellershaw and Wilkinson, 2003). For many years, the LCP was considered the epitome of good care at the end of life. It provided a documentary framework that helped to guide and facilitate practitioners to ensure completeness of care. It did this by devising procedures to enable patients with a life-limiting illness near the time of death to be provided with the highest standard of care resources allowed. Unfortunately, due to a series of media portrayals pointing out that both the pathway and the practitioners using it were not doing what was required, its use was discontinued in the UK towards the end of 2013. In an independent review of the LCP, the Department of Health (2013) made the comment that: ' .... what we have heard at relatives' and carers' events ... is that there have been repeated instances of patients dying on the LCP being treated with less than the respect that they deserve'. The academic response to the withdrawal of the LCP questioned the lack of research underpinning the pathway (Seymour and Horne, 2013), together with a lack of communication and multidisciplinary collaboration by clinical practitioners (Seymour and Horne, 2013).

Much of the media publicity focused around the latest changes to the document (version 12) and centred on hydration. The LCP guidance advocated clinicians not over-hydrating patients towards the end of life but correcting dehydration wherever possible. However, in clinical practice many hospital wards adopted an approach based on non-hydration. As a result, a small number of patient were portrayed in the media as being left to die without adequate food and hydration. Subsequently the LCP came under sustained criticism, with some authors citing that it was a back door to euthanasia (Granger, 2012). Following a number of highly publicised cases where family members were not made aware that the patient was dying (*Newsweek*, May 2013), use of the LCP was discontinued. On reflection, it may be argued that the pathway was an excellent tool for monitoring the patient's progress, although issues such as the diagnosis of dying remained problematic, and the communication of the purpose of the pathway between health professionals, the patient and the family was not all that it could have been.

Advanced Care Planning 2: The Gold Standards Framework

Approximately 20% of patients are cared for at the end of life in a community setting. The Gold Standards Framework (GSF) is a community-based model of best practice originally designed by Kerri Thomas (Thomas and Noble, 2007), a GP concerned about the need to develop and co-ordinate care for those at the end of their life in the community. The GSF has been adopted by almost a third of GP practices in the UK and the model consists of seven components (known as the 7Cs: *Communication, Co-ordination, Control (of symptoms), Continuity, Continued learning, Carer support* and *Care in the dying phase.* Each is interlinked to ensure that community resources and support for those at the end of life who choose to be cared for at home can be optimised by community care staff using available resources. It begins with communication and is summarised below.

———————— Components of the Gold Standards Framework ————————

1. Communication

A supportive care register is compiled to record, plan and monitor patient care. This is used as a tool for discussion at healthcare team meetings which are held regularly to improve the flow of information.

2. Co-ordination

A nominated co-ordinator (e.g. a district nurse, practice manager or GP) is appointed to maintain a register of concerns and problems. The co-ordinator also organises team meetings for discussion, planning, case analysis and education.

3. Control of symptoms

Patient symptoms are assessed, discussed and treated. Anticipatory prescribing is practised.

4. Continuity

Palliative care patient details are passed on to local palliative care specialists, with a transfer of information to the local out-of-hours service. Patients and carers are given information about the contacts needed for out-of-hours advice.

5. Continued learning

Meetings are organised to discuss patients' care and to share ideas and problems. Significant event analysis takes place to consider good examples of care and possible improvements for future work.

6. Carer support

Carers are supported, listened to, encouraged, and educated to play as full a role in the patient's care as they wish. A link with social services is made to ensure that practical support is available. Healthcare professionals plan support for the carer when bereavement occurs.

7. Care in the dying phase

The period when the patient is approaching the terminal phase (i.e. death is likely in the next two weeks) is recognised and this information communicated to family and carers. Medicines for the control of all terminal symptoms are made available in the home.

Adapted with permission from Amass, J. (2006) *Pharmacological Journal*, 276: 353.

Advanced Care Planning 3: Preferred Priorities of Care (PPC) document

Palliative care practice upholds the right of the individual to express their autonomy and places high regard for the wishes of the patient and the family to be taken into account. The Preferred Priority of Care document originated in the Lancashire and South Cumbria Cancer Network in June 2004 and was endorsed by the NHS End of Life care programme (DH, 2008). The End of Life care programme endorsed the view that patient choice was important and encapsulated this in the End of Life Care Strategy (DH, 2008). The PPC is a patient-held document designed to facilitate individual choice at the end of life care. Documenting and responding to individual preferences and wishes can enable both the person and their carers to express their desires, beliefs and wishes to be cared for in the place of their choice. The PPC document is part of the wider assessment made of a patient at the end of life. Moreover, it is part of a process of care and assessment designed to empower patients at the end of life and to enable and encourage nurses to ensure that the patient's wishes are included in advanced care planning. The document encourages patients to state their individual preferences. Moreover, its importance lies more in the fact that it demonstrates that the practitioner and patient had had a discussion about the wishes of the patient, and it represents that the patient has been involved in the decision-making process when it becomes clear that they are nearing the end of their life. Once documented, it is necessary (with the individual's permission) that these wishes are shared with key care facilitators such as community nurses. The PPC document provides an opportunity to discuss concerns that may not otherwise be addressed. As such, it is a very useful tool to enable nurses to initiate and record the patient's wishes. The explicit recording of individual wishes can form the basis of care planning in multidisciplinary teams and other services, therefore reducing unplanned admissions and avoiding inappropriate and/or unwanted interventions. The PPC document is used more widely in the community as a means of enabling patients to exercise choice over where they receive care at the end of life (Reynolds and Croft, 2011).

Legal and ethical issues

The PPC document provides patients with the freedom to express their preferences but it does not constitute a legal document binding nurses to carry out all of the patient's wishes. For example, it is not the appropriate place to record decisions concerning a refusal of treatment. Furthermore, should the person lose the capacity to make a decision about issues, the previously completed PPC acts as an advanced statement. This means that information included within the PPC can be used as part of an assessment of a person's best interests when making decisions about their care. However, from a legal and ethical perspective, the PPC document is not the place to state the patient's refusal to have, for example, a naso-gastric tube, or to comment on Do Not Actively Resuscitate (DNAR) orders. The latter are medical directives and form part of the overall treatment medically determined by competent medical practitioners. This does not mean that the patient is excluded from such discussions. They are however separate issues.

Evidence suggests that the PPC is having a significant impact and enabling individuals to receive care in their preferred place at the end of life.

The quality of care: enabling patients to experience a good death in hospital

The concept of the so-called 'good death' is ambiguous and the attributes varied and numerous. Good death concepts have received a lot of attention since the hospice movement and the development of palliative care focused on the quality of care for dying patients (Conway, 2007). What constitutes a good death includes various attributes that have been described by numerous authors, such as open and honest communication about end of life care (McNamara, 2004), effective pain and other symptom control (Tadman and Roberts, 2007), and enabling the patient and family to be involved in the decision making about end of life care (Morrison and Garland, 2004; Smith et al., 2012). Further attributes of the good death include upholding the patient's dignity and self-respect (Stringer, 2007) and a focus on spiritual well-being (Mootoo, 2005; Murray, 2010; Milligan, 2011).

The literature has drawn attention to the differing perceptions of a good death with some authors asking *for whom is the death good?* (Gazelle, 2003; Schwartz et al., 2003). Specifically, what the patient may regard as a good death in terms of a quick and sudden departure from life may leave the family and hospital staff shocked, unprepared and grief stricken. The literature relating to the good death concept has grown rapidly in the last decade, with writers highlighting the difficulties of being able to achieve a good death for all (Ellershaw et al., 2010), and the importance of context in shaping the experience of a good death (Costello, 2004; Paddy, 2011). What in fact many describe as a good death is often a term meaning the process of dying and not the actual death event itself (Costello, 2006).

One of the key features of enabling patients and families to experience a good death is recognising advanced disease and the inevitability of death (Gadoud and Johnson, 2011). The sooner advanced care planning can take place – in an ideal situation from the time of diagnosis – the more likely it will be that steps can be taken to ensure the patient's wishes become an integral part of end of life care and treatment. Evidence suggests that it is often too late to include the patient in care planning once the illness becomes more advanced (Skilbeck and Payne, 2003). Dying well should also involve the patient and the family.

Others have focused on the influence of context in shaping the experience of good death, with hospitals being the most challenging areas for good deaths to occur (Costello, 2006). The time spent once the life-limiting illness has been diagnosed (also known as *the dying trajectory*) may help to prepare both the patient and family for death. If the wishes of the patient and family in relation to dying are considered and implemented, despite the sadness that this involves, death may be seen as appropriate or good. In some cases, the death of some patients who have suffered and experienced pain and other adverse symptoms may be seen as *a blessing and a relief* to families.

Enabling patients to experience good death often means finding out what their wishes are and what they consider to be in their best interests. This could mean discharging them to die at home or alternatively a place of their choice, utilising the Preferred Priorities of Care documentation (DH, 2004) if home is not appropriate due to a lack of care facilities or the vulnerability of family care. Patient and family perceptions of a good death experience can also involve a range of scenarios, for example not attempting to resuscitate, providing the patient with adequate symptom relief, and considering and responding to requests for assisted dying.

As a way of clarifying how nurses and others can help patients experience a good death, the following case study of an authentic patient experience illustrates difficulties associated with experiencing a good death in an acute hospital context.

Mary was a 58-year-old lady admitted to the surgical ward with a suspected 'acute' abdomen, resulting from a prolonged period at home where her symptoms became out of control. Her husband John was her primary care giver and they received help from friends, neighbours and their daughter who lived 60 miles away. Mary did not want to be in hospital and was hoping to be cared for at home. On admission, she was found to be in pain, distressed and tearful. After being settled into the ward and medically examined, it was confirmed that Mary was dehydrated, constipated, and had been experiencing nausea and vomiting for two weeks. As a

Case Scenario

(Continued)

(Continued)

consequence of her symptoms she was not eating well, she had lost weight, and her heels, sacrum and hips were red from prolonged periods in bed. She also had a urinary tract infection. Psychologically she was depressed and felt frustrated at having to be admitted to hospital when she wanted to be at home. On further examination it was found that she had an acute abdomen and a hard mass suggestive of an obstruction or tumour. Ultrasound investigations indicated a need for an explorative laparotomy which was performed as an emergency procedure. Unfortunately this revealed an abdominal tumour and widespread metastases.

STOP AND THINK

Consider the following questions in relation to the care of Mary and the emotional support of her husband John:

- How do you think Mary's husband John felt about her admission to hospital?
- What were Mary's immediate needs when she was first admitted?
- How would you try to assess her psychological state?
- How could you inform them about the need for emergency surgery?

The above case study highlights a reasonably typical situation of a patient being cared for at home by a relative under the medical treatment of the GP. Mary's husband John is likely to feel both a sense of relief that his wife is receiving professional care and also perhaps guilty that he was not able to provide the care himself. Mary's immediate care needs involved the management of her symptoms (specifically pain, nausea and vomiting) and to prevent further problems. Clearly Mary required palliative care. The nurse could assess her psychological state by getting to know her, accompanying her through the investigations and tests, explaining what was going on, involving her husband in care, and making sure that, as far as possible, a good therapeutic relationship was developed. Clearly, Mary and John needed a lot of support as the long-term prognosis was poor. Nurses and other members of the multidisciplinary team can help patients like Mary experience a good death by actively listening to her and enabling Mary, John and their important others to express their needs, wishes and fears.

If in doubt about what to do about Mary's situation, the medical staff could refer her to the hospital's Palliative Care Support Team for advice on further treatment. All hospitals in the UK have such teams. Patients like Mary need to have each symptom (physical, psychosocial and spiritual) responded to appropriately. Once Mary's physical symptoms are well managed, a discussion with Mary and her family needs to take place about future care. This would involve Mary, her husband and other members of the multidisciplinary team. It is important to stress that in order to provide and maintain quality of life, emergency surgery is needed to help alleviate her distressing symptoms. Mary needs to have the news broken sensitively with her husband and possibly other family members present. Explanations and information about her care and treatment need to be provided in a careful and sensitive way. Her future care plan depends very much on what her personal wishes are for palliation. A stay in a hospice may be in her best interests. Alternatively, Mary may wish to stay in hospital and possibly be transferred to a ward that is more appropriate to her needs. Moreover, she needs to have her psychosocial needs assessed and responded to in a professional and sensitive way. At this stage she and her husband need a compassionate approach based on her need for comfort, symptom management and an acknowledgement that Mary and John were experiencing a crisis. Her situation requires the highest quality of communication.

The importance of communication

Developing effective communication with patients and families about the diagnosis and prognosis of a life-limiting illness is an essential part of quality care (Wilkinson, 2002; Davies et al., 2003; Skilbeck and Payne, 2003; Fallowfield, 2005; Kurtz et al., 2005; Seymour and Horne, 2013). Hospitals in particular have been criticised for not providing effective communication to patients and examples of poor communication such as 'blocking behaviour', where nurses avoid discussing perceived sensitive areas of care or answer questions such as 'What is wrong with me?' or 'Do I have cancer?' by changing the subject and blocking attempts at communication. Indeed, a failure to develop more open communication with patients has resulted in the UK health ombudsman receiving complaints from the public about poor end of life communication (DH, 2008). A study by Rogers et al. (2000) over a decade ago highlighted issues of poor communication that are still evident today (Gardiner et al., 2013) and that have influenced the development of advanced communication courses throughout the UK. These courses use up-to-date, humanistic communication methods to prepare healthcare staff, emphasising the need for hospital staff to develop compassion and the need for nurses and doctors to demonstrate empathy and develop what O'Connell (2008) and others call 'therapeutic relationships with patients'.

The role of the nurse providing palliative care

In the past, nursing and nurses working in acute hospital settings were criticised for being too impersonal in their approach to patients in hospital by failing to discover the patient needs (Peplau, 1996). The contemporary development of therapeutic relationships with patients represents a response to the objectification of patients in hospital (May, 1992). In particular, palliative care is the area of nursing using a relatively new vocabulary that focuses on holistic and personal care. Palliative care nurses advocate the use of therapeutic relationships as they represent the essence of holistic care. Central to such care is the nurse's ability to develop emotional intelligence, the ability to elicit and consider the patient's feelings and how they influence the dynamic of the relationship (Goleman, 2000). Emotional intelligence (EI) in this situation is the ability of the nurse to recognise their own emotions, and using self-awareness understand what they are telling you and how they affect others around them. In relation to nursing patients at the end of their life and supporting their families, EI can be utilised to help nurses consider the situation and distress of the family, how they may be feeling, and how the nurses can help them.

As highlighted previously in Chapter 2, a therapeutic relationship between patient and healthcare practitioner involves the practitioner focusing their attention on the needs of the patient at the expense of the needs and demands of the organisation. A key element of interpersonal relations between healthcare practitioners and patients in contemporary times has been the development of a more meaningful level of emotional engagement between nurses and patients, especially at the end of life. Informed by the work of Peplau (1996), therapeutic relationships focus on the need for nurses to develop more patient-centred nursing. In palliative care this is seen as especially poignant and resonates with others writing about nursing care for vulnerable patients (Dexter and Walsh, 2001; O'Connell, 2008). As the social group with the most patient contact, nurses who form therapeutic relationships can become what Peplau (1996) and others call 'a professional friend'.

ACTIVITY 13.3

Drawing upon your knowedge and understanding from reading this and previous chapters, consider what attributes are required to fulfil the important role of being what Peplau calls *a professional friend*. Make a list of the things you consider to be important in order to develop a therapeutic relationship.

You will already be aware that the development of therapeutic relationships involves the promotion of trust and understanding between the patient and the nurse. Central to the development of such relationships is mutual respect for the patient and their situation. Considering the patient's situation and expressing empathy are very important, although difficult to achieve in some cases. A therapeutic relationship is often focused on enabling the patient's needs to be met in their current situation (O'Connell, 2008). By finding out what the patient's needs are (e.g. for dignity, privacy and respect) nurses can tangibly help to improve their situation.

In practical terms, developing and maintaining a therapeutic relationship with a patient requires the nurse to consciously spend time actively listening to that patient, developing trust and respect for each other, and for the nurse to elicit the patient's needs and concerns about care and treatment. The development of empathy is a very difficult thing to do as often there may be many barriers to understanding a patient's situation, such as age, gender, culture, beliefs, religion and a lack of understanding of the attitude and relationship between the patient and others. Many nurses find this hard to understand and have empathy for patients who attempt suicide, take drugs and self harm (McAllister et al., 2002).

The development of empathy is central to the provision of effective palliative care. Nyatanga (2013) points out that empathy for others is an ability to identify the emotional experience of others. In doing so we need to try see things from the other person's view point or to stand in their shoes and see the world as they see it. Sharing the suffering and grief of others and considering what it may be like to have a limited time left to live are a very challenging prospect for any individual, but are especially difficult if you are young. Noddings (2002) states that care providers must step out of their frame of reference and into the patient's situation and world view. Whilst very noble and idealistic, this is by no means an easy task.

However, one way of helping to develop empathy is through education and training. The Sage and Thyme model of communication (Connolly et al., 2010) was designed to assist healthcare professionals to learn to recognise and respond effectively to psychological distress, avoiding causing psychological harm, communicating honestly and compassionately, and knowing when they have reached the boundary of their competence. 'SAGE & THYME' is a mnemonic which guides healthcare professional/ care workers into and out of a conversation with someone who is distressed or concerned. It provides a structure to psychological support by encouraging the health worker to hold back with advice and prompting the concerned person to consider their own solutions (Connolly et al., 2010).

In the recommendations to improve the safety and well-being of patients, the Berwick Report (DH, 2013a) pointed out the need for nurses to treat patients with respect and enable respect to develop from the basis of compassion for and an understanding of vulnerable patients. It may be argued therefore that nurses have a professional duty to develop therapeutic relationships with patients and their families, not only at the end of life but also at the beginning of their illness trajectory. Moreover, at the end of life, there is only one chance to get it right and therefore it is essential that nurses provide high quality competent care, from committed practitioners who demonstrate a desire to ensure that all deaths are good experiences, and that this becomes the professional aim of all practitioners. From reading Chapter 2, you may remember that the development of a therapeutic relationship between a patient and a nurse is encapsulated in what Cummings (2012) called the 6Cs: commitment, courage, compassion, communication, competence and a caring attitude. O'Connell argues that the development of therapeutic nurse-patient relationships in certain contexts can expose nurses to emotional pain. However, by reflecting on their situation through for example clinical supervision, nurses have an opportunity to learn about the emotional intelligence required to develop and maintain this important relationship. The vital characteristics of therapeutic relationships involve the development of trust and understanding, a key element of the 6Cs. This requires the nurse to consciously spend time actively listening to the patient, developing trust and respect for each other, and for the nurse to elicit the patient's needs and concerns about care and treatment. By undergoing additional preparation to develop their skills further, for example learning to apply models of communication (Connolly et al., 2010), nurses can learn to recognise and respond effectively to psychological distress, avoiding causing psychological harm, communicating honestly and compassionately and knowing when they have reached the boundary of their competence. However, whilst subsequent evaluative studies (Connolly et al., 2014) have demonstrated increased knowledge and self-efficacy amongst participants, the impact upon patients and carers of such approaches is a little less clear.

Developing competence in palliative care

Becoming an effective palliative care practitioner may require some nurses to make a number of changes. Some might argue that in order to provide effective care at the end of life you need to have had personal experience of loss. Whilst this may help some people it is not a prerequisite for becoming a competent practitoner. An important element of any specialism is the need for education and additional preparation. Specialist nurses often receive regular educational and training updates (for example Macmillan Nurses). As professional nurses we are required to be able to respond autonomously and confidently to planned and uncertain situations, managing ourselves and others effectively. It is important to be aware of medical directives such as DNAR orders and their implications for patients and families. In many trusts palliative care link nurses are a good source of help, guidance and support. To ensure that you are able to maintain your professional accountability, it is necessary to be aware of and work through local governance and policies, ensuring that you know the link nurse for palliative care in your area. At the same time try to make contact with the Specialist Palliative Care team for your placement area. Part of their role is to support others caring for patients with a life-limiting illness. As student nurses it is also important you are able to maximise the potential of clinical placements and utilise the expertise of specialist nurse. All nurses are required to create and maximise opportunities to improve services. One of the attributes of many nurses in palliative care is their educative role in helping others developing the skills to become competent practitioners.

ACTIVITY 13.4

Make a list of things you can do to develop competence in palliative care nursing.

No doubt you will have identified a number of things that you can do to help you achieve and maintain your competence in this area of nursing. Your list may include the following:

- Maximising opportunities for improving services by improving your knowledge and experience, such as volunteering to work in a hospice, through selective spoke placements.
- Shadowing those who have a specialist role in palliative care.
- Keeping up to date can be achieved by reading journals, books and short research reports.
- Attending seminars and study days.
- Enrolling on a palliative care course at your School of Nursing.
- Attending additional education and training in the form of study days, short courses and conferences. These are helpful to ensure that your practice is not only based on up-to-date evidence but will also help you to develop the confidence required to provide effective palliative care.

Chapter summary

This chapter has focused on the importance of palliative care for ensuring experiences at the end of life are positive and fulfilling for the patient and the family as well as the healthcare professional. Nurses are often the group who have the most intimate contact with and spend a lot of time with patients and families. It is worth reconsidering the famous quote from Saunders at the beginning of this chapter: 'You matter because you are you, and you matter to the end of your life. We will do all we can not only to help you die peacefully, but also to live until you die'.

We have explored the importance of enabling all those involved in end of life care to experience a good death. In particular, advanced care planning, effective symptom control from the time of diagnosis, respect for patient autonomy and engaging in frank discussions are important and made easier when a nurse is able to develop a therapeutic relationship with the patient and family. The 6Cs of nursing (Cummings, 2012), often discussed and publicised, particularly in the wake of the Francis Report: Mid Staffordshire NHS Foundation Trust Public Inquiry (Francis, 2010), are central features of effective palliative care.

We only have one chance to get it right for patients with a life-limiting illness and we can do this by enabling the patient and the family to play an active part in the planning and implementation of care, by respecting their wishes and putting their needs at the forefront of care planning.

Suggested further reading

Albarran, A. J. W. and Hills, M. (2012) 'Managing end of life care'. In I. Bullock, J. Macleod-Clark and J. Rycroft-Malone (eds), *Adult Nursing Practice*. Oxford: Oxford University Press. pp. 302–327.

Baldwin, M.A. and Woodhouse, J. (2011) *Key Concepts in Palliative Care*. London: Sage.

Department of Health, Social Services and Public Safety (DHSSPS) (2010) *Living Matters, Dying Matters: A Palliative and End of Life Care Strategy for Adults in Northern Ireland*. Belfast: DHSSPS.

NHS Wales (2013) *Together for Health: Delivering End of Life Care*. Cardiff: Welsh Assembly Government.

Payne S., Seymour J. and Ingelton C. (2008) *Palliative Care Nursing*, 2nd edition. McGraw-Hill Open University Press.

The Scottish Government (2008) *Living and Dying Well: A National Action Plan for Palliative and End of Life Care in Scotland*. Edinburgh: The Scottish Government.

Wiienberg-Lyles, E., Goldsmith J., Ferrell, B. and Ragan, S.L. (2013) *Communication in Palliative Nursing*. Oxford: Oxford University Press.

References

Amass, J. (2006) 'The Gold Standard Framework', *Pharmacological Journal*, 276: 353.

Arnautska E. (2010) 'Breaking bad news', *Trakia Journal of Sciences*, 8 (Suppl. 2): 491–492.

Baile, W., Buckman, B., Renato, L., Globera, G., Bealea, E.A. and Kudelkab, A.P. (2000) 'SPIKES: A six-step protocol for delivering bad news: application to the patient with cancer', *Clin J Oncol Nurs*, 14 (4).

Becker, R. (2009) 'Palliative Care 1: Principles of palliative care nursing and end of life care', *Nursing Times*, 105: 13.

Becker, R. (2010) *Fundamental Aspects of Palliative Care Nursing*, 2nd edition. London: Quay Books.

Broeckaert, B. (2008) 'Treatment decisions at the end of life: a conceptual framework'. In S. Payne, J. Seymour and C. Ingleton (eds), *Palliative Care Nursing*. McGraw-Hill/Open University Press. pp. 402–422.

Buckman, R. (1992) *Breaking Bad News: A Guide for Healthcare Professionals*. Baltimore: Johns Hopkins University Press. p. 15.

Connolly, M., Perryman, J., McKenna, Y., Orford, J., Thomson, L., Shuttleworth, J. and Cocksedge, S. (2010) 'SAGE and THYME: a model for training health and social care professionals in patient-focussed support', *Patient Education and Counselling*, 79: 87–93.

Connolly, M., Thomas, J.M., Orford, J., Schofield, N., Whiteside, S., Morris, J. and Heaven, C. (2014) 'The impact of the SAGE & THYME foundation level workshop on factors influencing communication skills in healthcare professionals', *Journal of Continuing Education in the Health Professions*; 34 (1): 37–46.

Conway, S. (2007) 'The changing face of death: implications for public health', *Critical Public Health*, 3: 195–202 .

Costello, J. (2004) *Nursing the Dying Patient: Caring in Different Contexts*. London: Palgrave.

Costello, J. (2006) '"Dying well": nurses' experiences of good and bad deaths in hospital', *Journal of Advanced Nursing*, 54 (5): 1–8.

Cummings, J. (2012) '"I want to achieve pride in the profession": The 6 Cs of nursing', *Nursing Times*. Available at: www.nursingtimes.net/nursing-practice/leadership/jane-cummings-i-want-to-achieve-pride-in-the-profession/5048241.article# (last accessed 7 October 2013).

Davies, J., Kristjanson, L.J. and Blight, J. (2003) 'Communication with families of patients in an acute hospital with advanced cancer: problems and strategies identified by nurses', *Cancer Nursing*, 26: 337–45.

Department of Health (2004) *Preferred Place of Care*. London: DH. (Revised December 2007 by the National PPC Review Team.)

Department of Health (2008) *Promoting High Quality Care for Adults at the End of Their Lives*. London: DH.

Department of Health (2013) *More Care, Less Pathway: A Report on the Liverpool Care Pathway*. London: DH.

Department of Health (2013a) *The Berwick Report into Patient Safety*. London: DH.

Dexter, G. and Walsh, M. (2001) *Psychiatric Nursing: A Patient Centred Approach*. Bath: Nelson Thornes.

Ellershaw, J. and Wilkinson, S. (2003) *Care of the Dying: A Pathway to Excellence*. Oxford: Oxford University Press.

Ellershaw, J.E., Dewar, S. and Murphy, D. (2010) 'Achieving a good death for all', *British Medical Journal*, 341:c4861.

Elliot, M. and Nicholson, C. (2014) 'A qualitative study exploring use of the surprise question in the care of older people: perceptions of general practitioners and challenges for practice', *BMJ Support Palliative Care*, doi:10.1136/bmjspcare-2014-000679.

Fallowfield, L. (2005) 'Learning how to communicate in cancer settings', *Support Cancer Care*, 13: 349–50.

Francis, R. (2010) *Mid Staffordshire NHS Foundation Trust Inquiry*. London: HMSO.

Gadoud, A. and Johnson, M. (2011) 'Recognising advancing disease', *British Journal of Hospital Medicine*, 78 (2): 432–36.

Gardiner, C., Gott, M., Ingleton, C., Seymour, C. and Cobb, M. (2013) 'Extent of palliative care need in the acute hospital setting: a survey of two acute hospitals in the UK', *Palliative Medicine*, 27 (1): 76–83.

Gazelle, G. (2003) 'A good death: not just an abstract concept', *Journal of Clinical Oncology*, 21 (9): 95–6.

Goleman, D. (2000) *Working with Emotional Intelligence*. New York: Bantram.

Granger, K .(2012) 'The Liverpool Care Pathway for the Dying Patient improves the end of life', *Guardian*, 13 November.

Kurtz, S., Silverman, J. and Draper, J. (2005) *Teaching and Learning Communications Skills in Medicine*. Oxford: Radcliffe.

Main, J. (2002) 'Management of relatives of patients who are dying', *Journal of Clinical Nursing*, 11 (6): 794–801.

May, C. (1992) 'Individual care? Power and subjectivity in therapeutic relationships', *Sociology*, 26 (4): 589–602.

McAllister, M., Creedy, D., Moyle, W. and Farrugia, C (2002) 'Nurses' attitudes towards clients who self-harm', *Journal of Advanced Nursing*, 40 (5): 578–86.

McIlfatrick, S. (2013) 'Interprofessional collaboration in palliative care: rhetoric or reality?', *International Journal of Palliative Nursing* (Editorial), 19 (9): 419.

McNamara, B. (2004) 'Good enough death: autonomy and choice in Australian palliative care', *Social Science & Medicine*, 58 (5): 929–938.

Milligan, S. (2011) 'Addressing the spiritual needs of people near the end of life', *Nursing Standard*, 26 (4): 12–15.

Mootoo, J.S. (2005) 'A guide to cultural and spiritual awareness', *Nursing Standard*, 19: 17.

Morrison, J. and Garland, E. (2004) 'Developing palliative care services in partnership', *Cancer Nursing Practice*, 3 (31): 22–25.

Murray, R.P. (2010) 'Spiritual care, beliefs and practices of special care and oncology RNs at patients end of life', *Journal of Hospice and Palliative Nursing*,12(1): 12–14.

National End of Life Care Intelligence Network (2013) *End of Life Care Profile*. Available at: www.endoflifecare-intelligence.org.uk/home (last accessed 8 October 2013).

Newsweek (May 2013) BBC Television programme, 'Death in Hospital'.

NICE (2011) *End of Life Care for Adults (QS13)*. Available at: http://guidance.nice.org.uk/QS13 (last accessed 20 January 2015).

Noddings, N. (2002) *Starting at Home: Caring and Social Policy*. Berkeley, CA: University of California Press.

Nursing and Midwifery Council (2010) *Standards for Competency for Registered Nurses*. London: NMC.

Nyatnaga, B. (2013) 'Editorial: Empathy in palliative care: is it possible to understand another person', *International Journal of Palliative Nursing*, 19 (10): 471.

O'Connell, E. (2008)'Therapeutic relationships: a reflection on practice', *Critical Care Nursing*, 13(3): 138–43.

Paddy, M. (2011) 'Influence of location on a good death', *Nursing Standard*, 26 (1): 12–13.

Peplau, H. (1996) *Interpersonal Relations in Nursing*. New York: Springer.

Reynolds, J. and Croft, S. (2011) 'Applying the preferred priorities for care document in practice', *Nursing Standard*, 25: 36.

Rogers, A., Karlsen, S. and Addington-Hall, J. (2000) '"All the services were excellent. It is when the human element comes in that things go wrong": dissatisfaction with hospital care at the end of life', *Journal of Advanced Nursing*, 31 (4): 768–74.

Saunders, Y., Ross, J.R. and Riley, J. (2003) 'Planning for a good death: responding to unexpected events', *British Medical Journal*, 327 (7408): 204–206.

Schwartz, C.E., Mazor, K., Rogers, J., Ma.,Y. and Reed, G. (2003) 'Validation of a new measure of concept of good death', *Journal of Palliative Medicine*, 6 (4): 575–84.

Seymour, J. and Horne, G. (2013) 'The withdrawal of the Liverpool Care Pathway in England: implications for clinical practice and policy', *International Journal of Palliative Nursing*, 19 (8): 369–71.

Skilbeck, J. and Payne, S. (2003) 'Emotional support and the role of clinical nurse specialist in palliative care', *Journal of Advanced Nursing*, 43: 521–30.

Smith, S., Pugh, E. and, McEvoy, M. (2012) 'Involving families in end of life care', *Nursing Management*, 19 (4): 72–7.

Stringer, S. (2007) 'Quality of death: humanisation v medicalisation', *Cancer Nursing Practice*, 6 (3): 12–19.

Sweeting, H. and Gilhooly, M. (1992) '"Doctor, am I dead?": a review of social death in modern societies', *Omega: Journal of Death and Dying*, 24 (4): 251–69.

Tadman, M. and Roberts, D. (2007) *Oxford Handbook of Cancer Nursing*. Oxford: Oxford University Press.

Thomas, K. and Noble, B. (2007)' Improving the delivery of palliative care in general practice: an evaluation of the first phase of the Gold Standards Framework', *Palliative Medicine*, 21: 49-52.

Wilkinson, S. (2002) 'The essence of cancer care: the impact of training on nurses' ability to communicate effectively', *Journal of Advanced Nursing*, 40 (6): 731–38.

Willard, C. and Luker, K.A. (2006) 'Challenges to end of life care in the acute hospital setting.', *Palliative Medicine*, 20 (6): 611–615.

Glossary

Accountability   Taking personal responsibility for your actions and being able to clearly explain your rationale for taking particular courses of action.

Active listening   A way of listening and responding that focuses entirely on the speaker. This can involve asking open questions, observing both your own and their body language and demonstrating empathy and understanding of their situation

Advocacy   Championing a particular concept, such as public health. This can also mean defending and promoting an individual's rights, speaking out on behalf of someone who is not able to fully act on their own behalf.

Anti-discriminatory   Ensuring that all individuals are treated fairly and equally.

Aphasia   Partial or total loss of the ability to articulate ideas or comprehend spoken or written language, resulting from damage to the brain from injury or disease.

Bio-psychosocial   Taking into account the biological, psychological and social aspects of an issue. For example making a bio-psychosocial assessment of a patient.

Clinical decision making   Using a balance of experience, awareness, knowledge, information and appropriate assessment tools in order to make a decision about patient care options.

Clinical judgement   The process by which nurses are able to make logical, rational decisions about patient care.

Compassion   Empathising with a patient and/or their family. To show compassion is to show genuine regard for their bio-psychosocial needs.

Competence   Having the knowledge, skills and experience to deliver safe and effective nursing care.

Complex care interventions   Activities that contain a number of components with the potential to produce a range of different outcomes.

Continuous professional development   The means by which professionals continuously develop and expand their knowledge and skills.

Cultural competence   Having the attitude, knowledge, and skills necessary to provide care for diverse populations, irrespective of their ethnicity or cultural background.

Delirium   A state of mental confusion.

Dignity   To treat someone with dignity is to treat them with respect in a way that values them as an individual.

Disclosure   Providing or revealing information.

Dysphasia   A partial or complete impairment of the ability to communicate verbally resulting from brain injury.

Empathy   The capacity to understand what another person is experiencing from their perspective rather than your own.

Empirical evidence   Evidence derived from experience rather than research.

Epidemiology   The study of patterns and causes of health related conditions, including disease, in a defined population.

Ethics   Moral principles that inform or govern behaviour.

Evidence-based practice   The informed and careful use of current best evidence in making decisions about the care of an individual.

Gerontology   The study of the social, psychological, cognitive and biological aspects of aging.

Health promotion   The process of enabling people to increase control over, and to improve, their health. It moves beyond a focus on individual behaviour towards a wide range of social and environmental interventions.

Hypothesis   An idea or statement which you can test through research or experimentation.

Inequalities in health   Differences in the health status of people or in the distribution of health determinants between different social classes, ages and ethnic groups.

Informed consent   Giving permission and agreeing to something in the knowledge of all the related facts.

Interpersonal   The interaction or relationship between individuals.

Interprofessional   When different professional groups such as nurses and counsellors work and/or learn together and communicate effectively towards a mutual goal.

Jargon   Complex terms which a lay person cannot understand.

Justice   Defining if something is fair or proportionate.

Locus of control   Refers to the extent to which individuals believe that they have control over events affecting them.

Mental health   A state of psychological and emotional well-being.

Mentor A registered nurse who, following successful completion of an NMC approved mentor preparation programme, facilitates practice learning and assesses the competence of a student nurse.

Moral engagement A cognitive process in which an individual makes a reasoned judgement about harmful behaviours and resists engaging with such behaviours.

Motivational interviewing A collaborative conversation which aims to strengthen a person's own motivation and commitment to change.

Multi-agency working Different services, agencies and/or professionals working together to provide seamless healthcare that fully meets the needs of an individual.

Occupational therapy A client-centred health profession which aims to promote health and well-being through occupation.

Orthopaedics A medical speciality that focuses on injuries and diseases affecting the musculoskeletal system.

Palliative care End of life care; care provided for a person who is terminally ill, through the relief of suffering by early identification and treatment of symptoms.

Paralanguage The way something is said, such as the pitch and tone, the softness or loudness of words, all of which can give an implication on what the speaker really means

Patient empowerment Sharing information and knowledge to enable individuals to make informed decisions about their care.

Pharmacology Relating to medicines, drugs and remedies.

Postpartum After birth

Preceptorship A period of supervised practical training and support provided to new NMC registrants.

Professional portfolio A place where you keep multiple examples of your skills and achievements.

Proprioception The ability to sense stimuli arising within the body regarding position, motion, and equilibrium.

Quality If a product or service is of good quality then it meets or exceeds its objectives.

Randomised controlled trial A type of scientific experiment in which people are randomly allocated (by chance alone) to receive one of several interventions.

Reasonable adjustments Making changes based on a person's needs or the situation.

Reciprocity A positive act being returned via another positive deed between two individuals.

Reflective practice   Constantly reviewing your actions and thinking what could be improved in future.

Research   Studying and investigating a subject to learn more about it.

Root cause analysis   A problem solving method or approach that can help to identify the root causes of a fault or problem.

Safeguarding   Protecting a person from harm.

Self-awareness   Understanding yourself as a person and how your own views and experience impact on your decisions.

Service users   Patients or clients.

Social cognitive theory   A psychological model of behaviour that suggests people learn by watching others.

Socioeconomic   The social and economic conditions which may affect a situation or a person.

Stereotype   An entrenched view of a particular group.

Stigma   Perceived shame.

Supervision   Monitoring the activities of another person or group.

Team work   Working as a group towards mutual goals.

Therapeutics   Treatment and care of a patient for the purpose of both preventing and combating disease or alleviating pain or injury.

Values   A person's values relate to their moral code or ethics.

Vulnerable   An individual in need of special care, support or protection because of age, disability, or risk of abuse or neglect.

Well-being   Holistic interpretation of a person's mental, emotional and physical health.

Whistleblowing   Reporting a wrongdoing within an organisation or making a disclosure in the public interest.

Index

Note: Page numbers in italics indicate tables and figures.

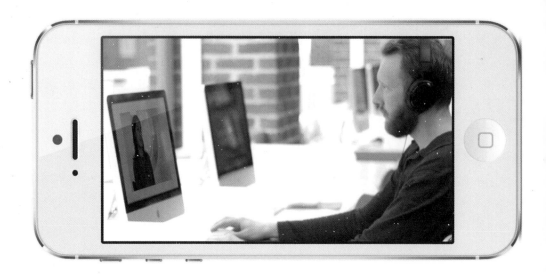
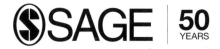